HEALTH & WELLNESS SERIES

DIABETES MEALS FOR GOOD HEALTH COOKBOOK

FOURTH EDITION

Low-Carb Recipes & Swaps for Every Meal

KAREN GRAHAM, RD, CDE
Registered Dietitian &
Certified Diabetes Educator

MANSUR SHOMALI, MD, CM
Endocrinologist & Diabetes Expert

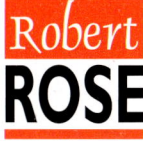

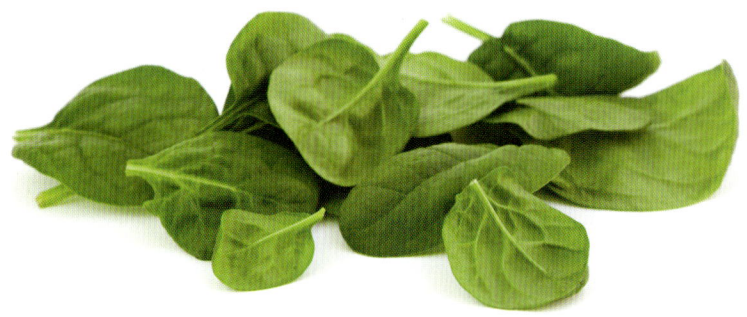

DIABETES MEALS FOR GOOD HEALTH COOKBOOK, FOURTH EDITION
Text copyright © 2023, 2020, 2012, 2008 Karen Graham, RD, CDE
Photographs and illustrations copyright © 2023, 2020, 2012, 2008 Durand & Graham, Ltd. (except as listed on page 288)
Cover and text design copyright © 2023, 2020, 2012, 2008 Robert Rose Inc.

Some of the content of this book was previously published as *Meals for Good Health* (Paper Birch Publishing, 1998–2007). No part of this publication may be reproduced, stored in a retrieval system or transmitted, in any form or by any means, without the prior written consent of the publisher or a license from the Canadian Copyright Licensing Agency (Access Copyright). For an Access Copyright license, visit www.accesscopyright.ca or call toll-free: 1-800-893-5777.

For complete cataloguing information, see page 288.

DISCLAIMER
The suggestions and information contained in this publication are based on a thorough assessment of the latest research and information. Reasonable steps have been taken to ensure the accuracy of the information presented. However, we cannot ensure the safety or efficacy of any product or service described in this publication. Individuals are advised to consult a physician or other appropriate health care professional before undertaking any diet, exercise, activity or treatment program or taking any herb or medication referred to in this publication. Professionals must use and apply their own professional judgment, experience and training and should not rely solely on the information contained in this publication before prescribing any diet, exercise, treatment or medication. While we thank the professional expertise of the reviewers of this publication, neither they nor the authors or publisher assumes any responsibility or liability for personal or other injury, loss or damage that may result from the suggestions or information in this publication.

The recipes in this book have been carefully tested by our kitchen and our tasters. To the best of our knowledge, they are safe and nutritious for ordinary use and users. For those people with food or other allergies, or who have special food requirements or health issues, please read the suggested contents of each recipe carefully and determine whether or not they may create a problem for you. All recipes are used at the risk of the consumer. For those with special needs, allergies, requirements or health problems, in the event of any doubt, please contact your medical adviser prior to the use of any recipe.

This book is not intended as a substitute for professional medical care. Only your doctor can diagnose and treat a medical problem.

Use of brand names is for educational purposes only and does not imply endorsement.

Editor: Janice Madill, Easy English
Robert Rose Proof Editor: Anne Louise Mahoney
Food Photographer (except as noted on page 288):
  Brian Gould, Brian Gould Photography Inc.
Food Stylists: Judy Fowler and Katie Fowler
Production & Design Updates: PageWave Graphics Inc.
Cover Design: PageWave Graphics Inc.
Nutrient Analysis: Karen Graham calculated the total and net carbs and any recipe and nutrient revisions in the 3rd and 4th edition. Canadian Nutrient File and USDA FoodData Central were primary sources of nutrient information. Nutrient calculations by Food Intelligence (Barb Selley and Cathie Martin) using ESHA Genesis software from earlier editions were used and adapted as needed.
Recipes: All recipes are developed by Karen Graham, often inspired by family and friends. The recipe on page 92 is by Sally McKenney and adapted with permission.
4th Edition Reviewers: Full book reviews by Jennifer Scarsi, RD, CDCES; Davis Knight, Chef and Diabetes Advocate; Margaret Graham; and Rick Durand. Early reviewer of usage of carb swaps: Jenna Walsh, RD, CDE; and of Dinner 28, Sue Mah, MHSc, RD. Gillian Watts developed the first draft of the index.

We acknowledge the support of the Government of Canada.

Canadä

Published by Robert Rose Inc.
120 Eglinton Avenue East, Suite 800, Toronto, Ontario, Canada M4P 1E2
Tel: (416) 322-6552 Fax: (416) 322-6936
www.robertrose.ca

Printed and bound in China

1 2 3 4 5 6 7 8 9 ESP 28 27 26 25 24 23

Contents

Seven Smart Features of This Book 5

This Book's for You! 13

What Affects Your Blood Sugar 21

Low-Carb Baking and Cooking 25

Meals, Recipes and Snacks 31

- Breakfast Meals 33
- Lunch Meals 65
- Dinner Meals 97
- Snacks 259

Read Food Labels for Carbs 268

Low-Carb Swap Charts 273

Index 283

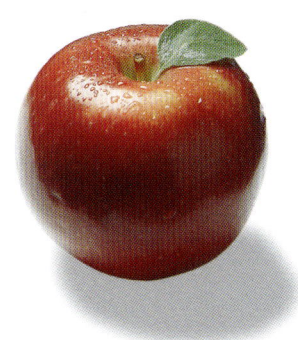

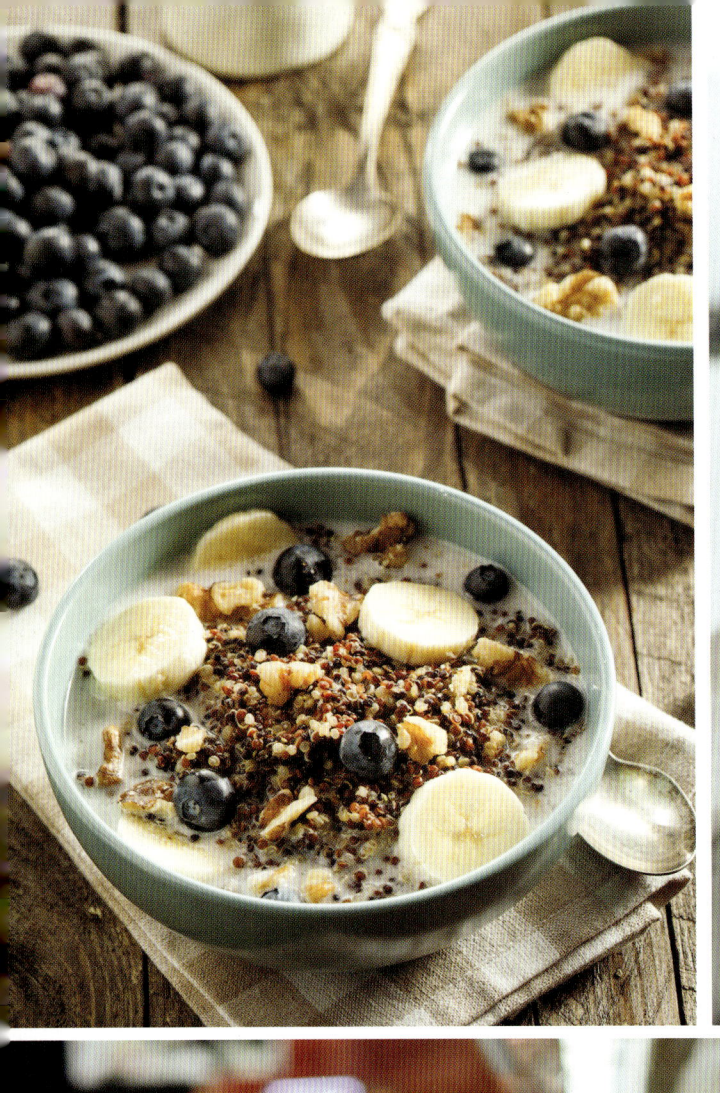
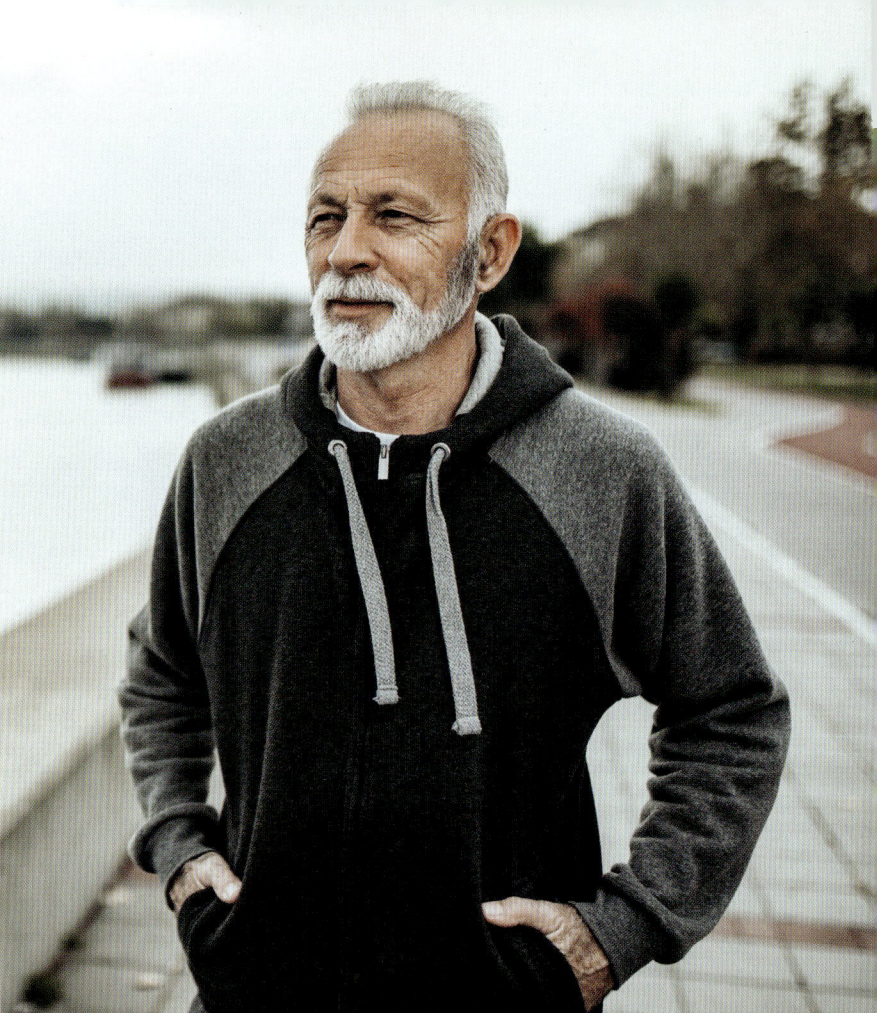
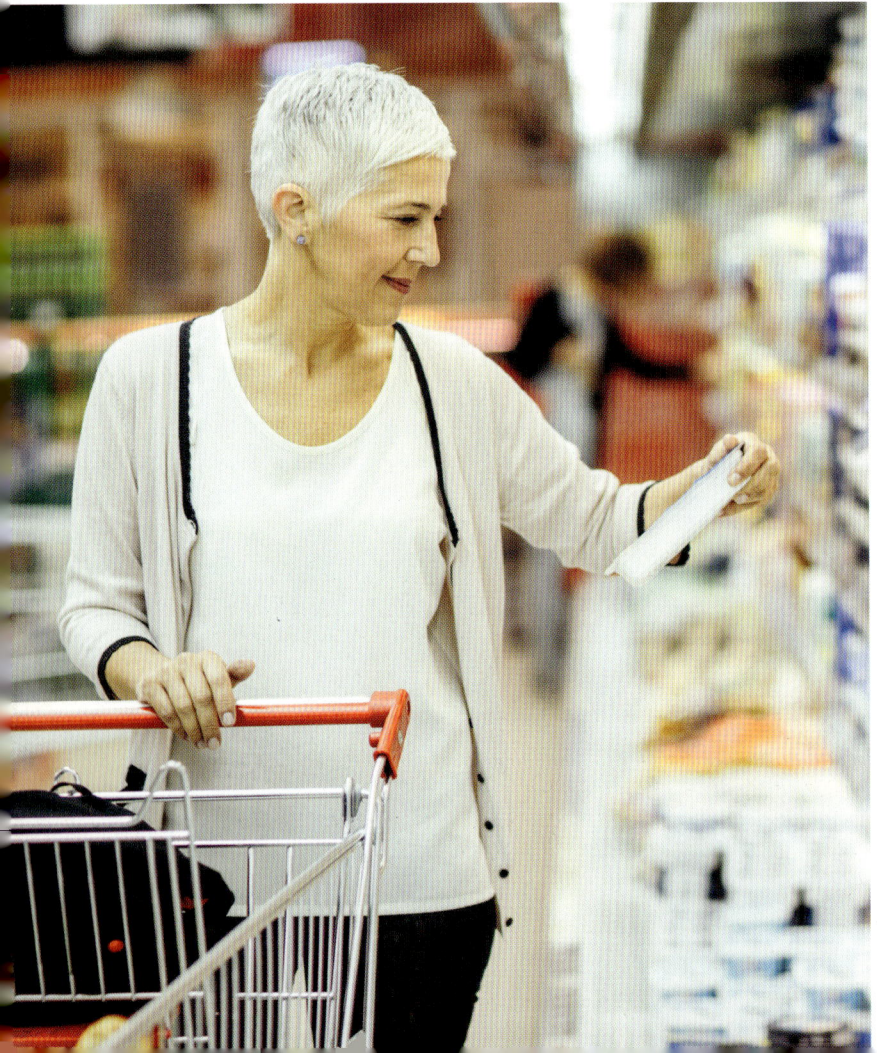
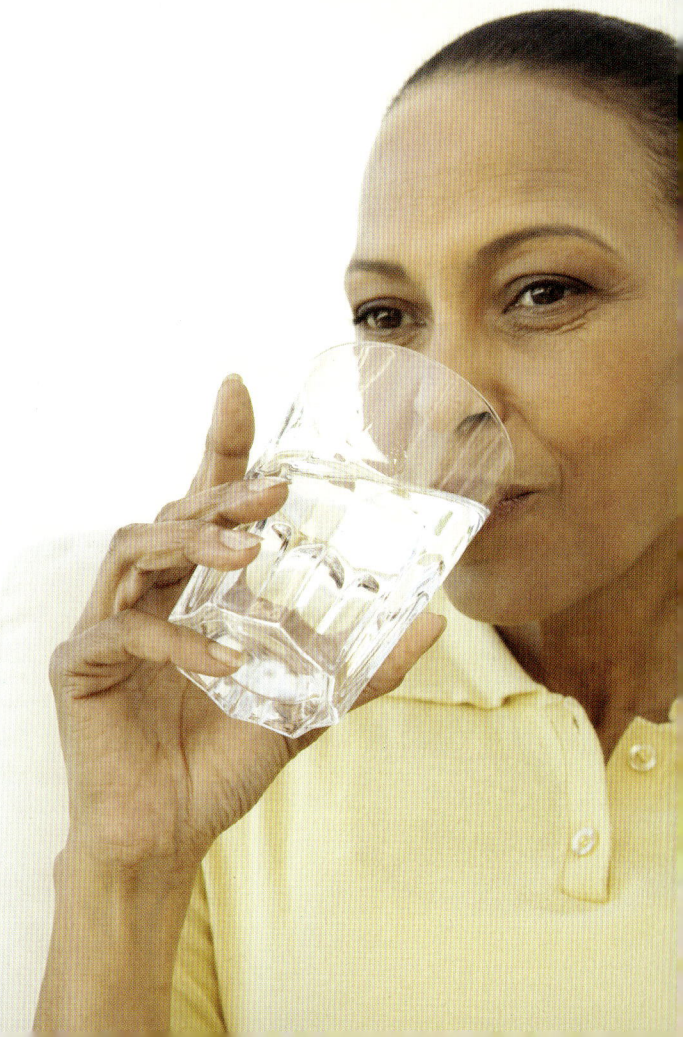

Seven Smart Features of This Book

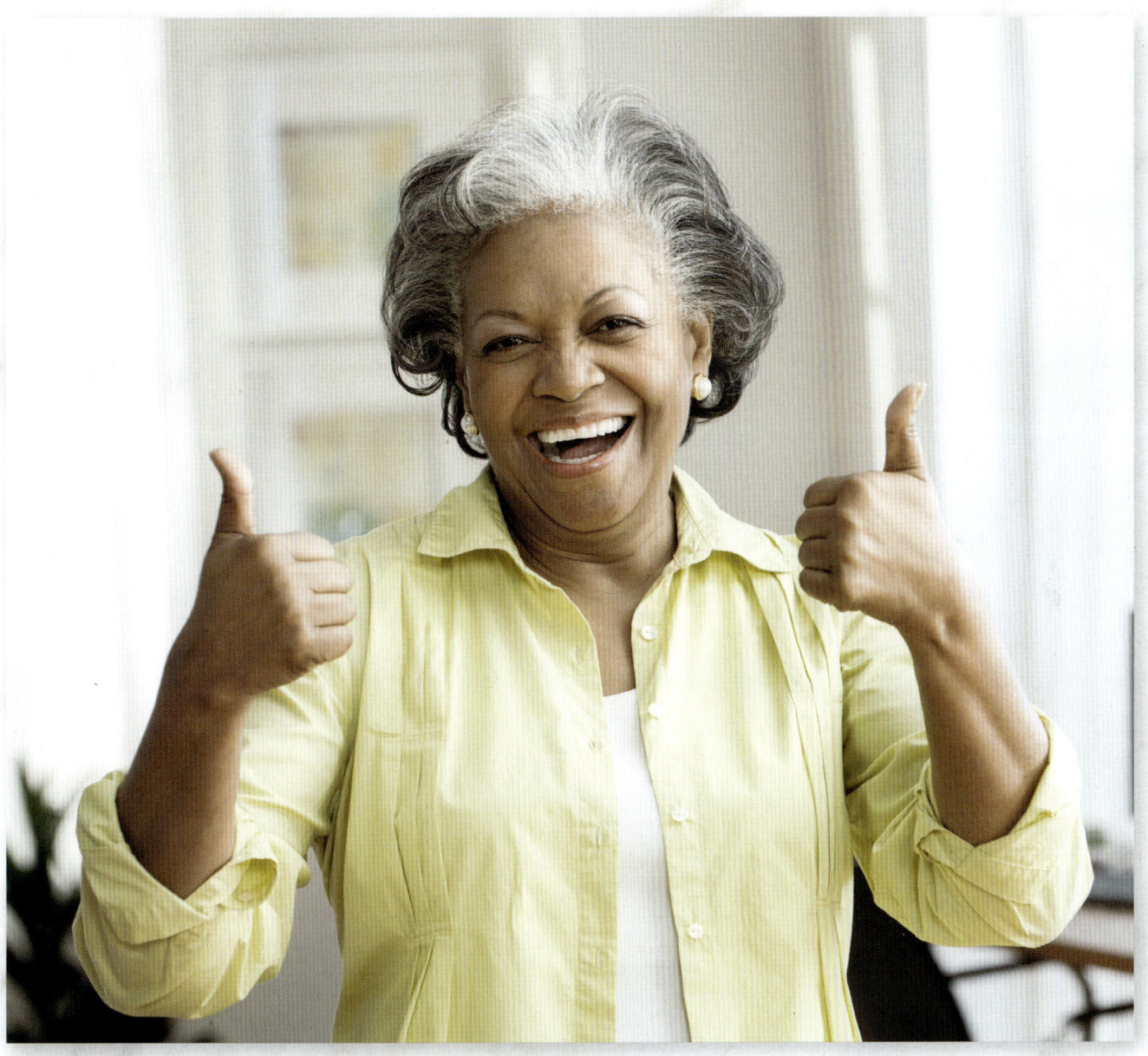

So many reasons to use this book.

SEVEN SMART FEATURES OF THIS BOOK

1 Sensible Lifelong Guidance

Our commitment: To provide you with meals for good health that will make you feel well and happy.

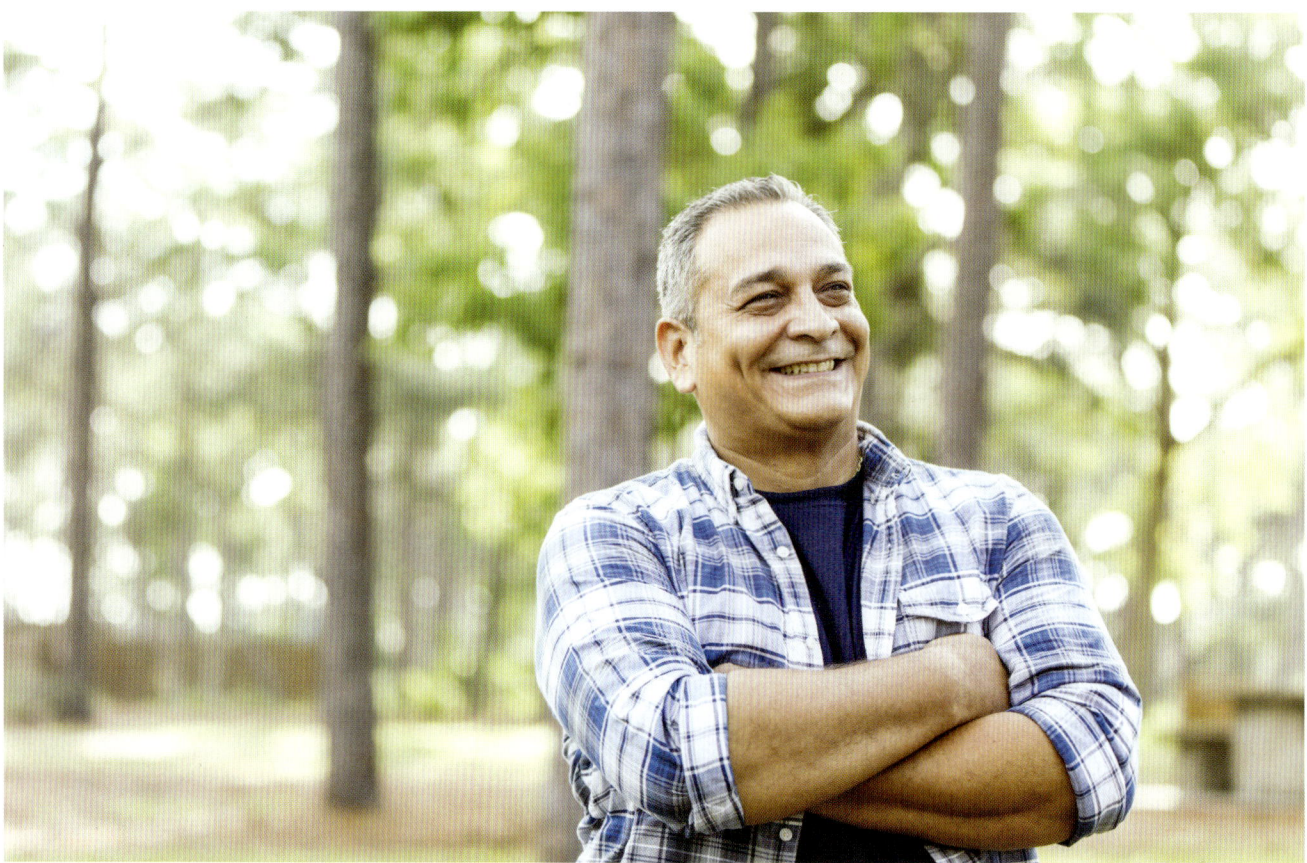

We understand that personal food choices are formed in the family kitchen, within our culture, from our income, and even where we live. In this book, we do not group foods into good or bad; rather, we encourage you to eat a variety of foods in the healthiest portions.

This cookbook promotes healthy, balanced eating of everyday foods. We include five or more fruits and vegetables every day.

We are excited about this new edition, which introduces lower-carb options for the recipes and all the meals. They have been meticulously tested for great taste and are easy to prepare. Enjoy!

Over 100 low-carb, low-calorie recipes, including desserts, keeping you satisfied at every meal.

SEVEN SMART FEATURES OF THIS BOOK

2 Diabetes Healthy Plate Method

Variations of the Plate Method are recommended by diabetes associations around the world.

When you fill half your plate with vegetables and the remainder with starch and protein, you will get a balance of essential nutrients, carbohydrates, fiber, proteins and healthy fats.

The 70 meals in this book include breakfast, lunch and dinner and follow this plate method. The breakfast meals often have fruit instead of vegetables, and fruit is a common dessert choice for many lunches and dinners.

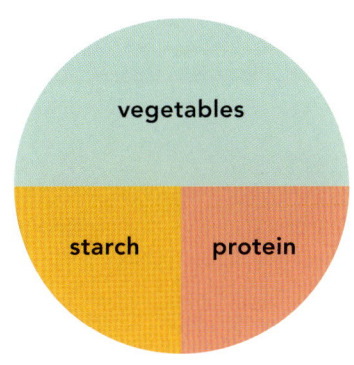

This is not just a cookbook!

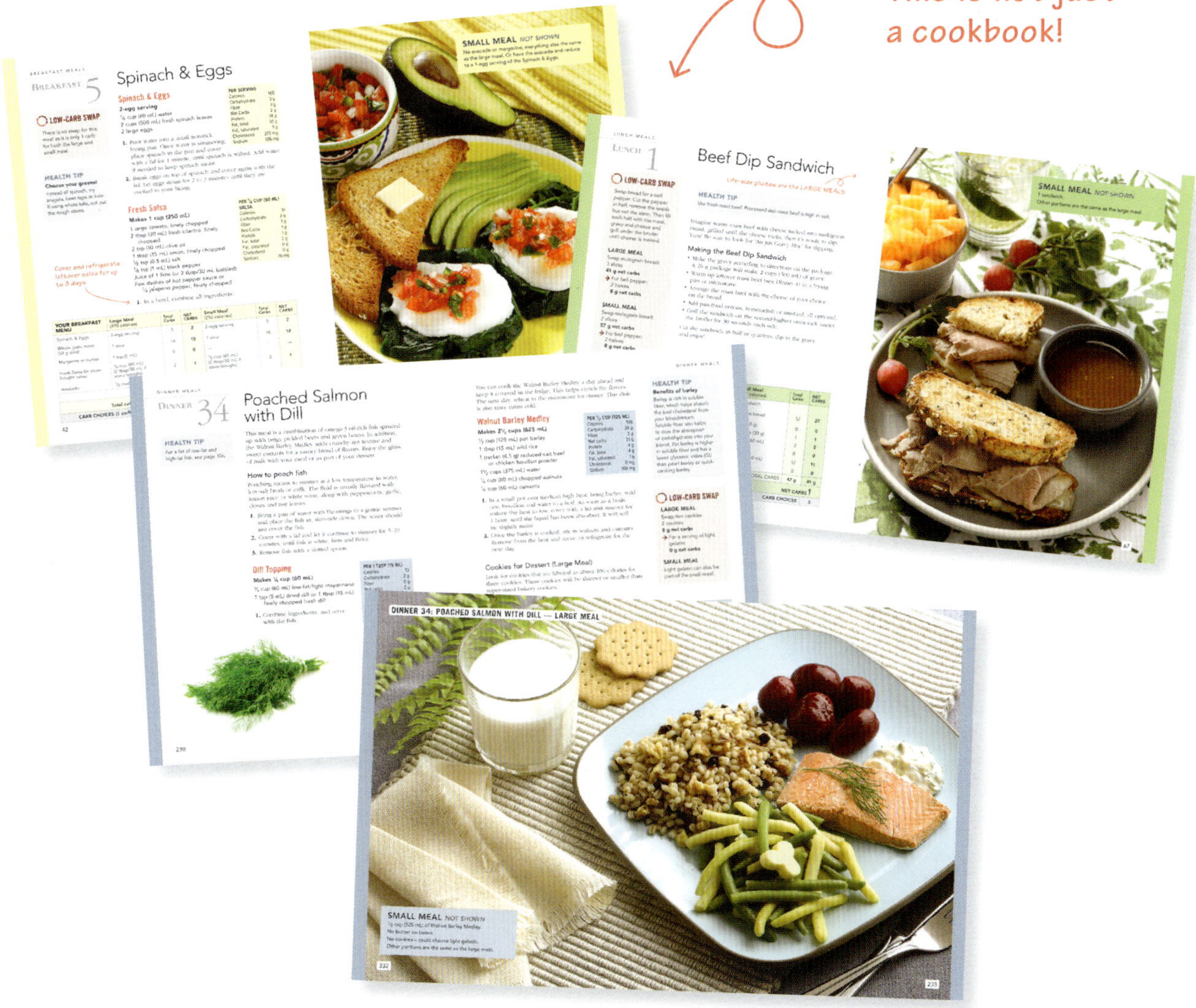

7

SEVEN SMART FEATURES OF THIS BOOK

3 Life-Size Photos of Exact Portions

The user-friendly feature of the life-size photographs means you can compare the large meal portions to the portions on your plate.

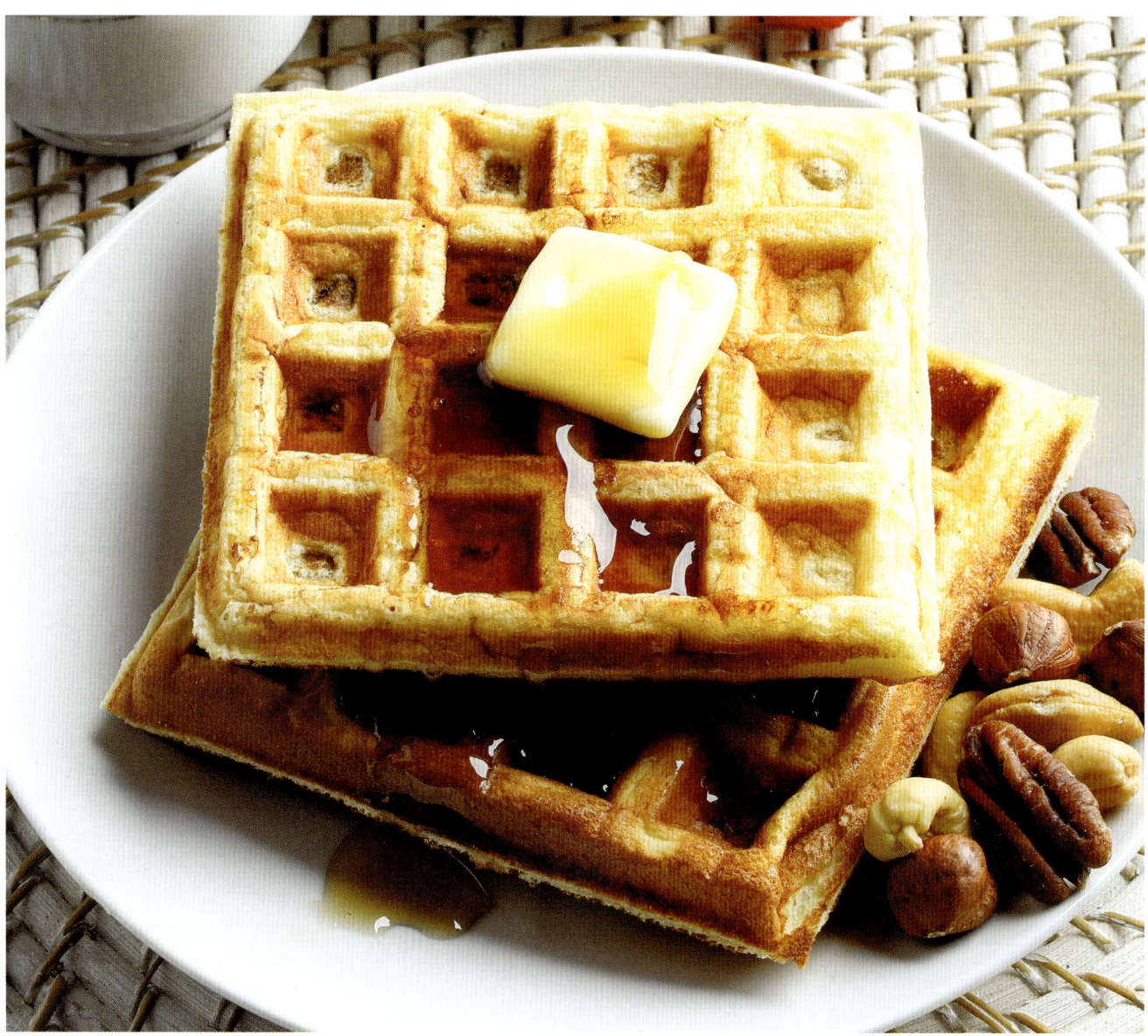

Correct portions are the answer to healthy eating.

SEVEN SMART FEATURES OF THIS BOOK

④ Large and Small Meals & Snacks

Every meal has two options:

1) the **Large Meal** shown in life-size photos, a special highlight of the cookbook, and

2) the **Small Meal** portions shown in a side box. The Small Meals have 25% fewer calories.

Snacks are listed in four calorie groups, each with a choice of carb amounts.

Snacks can be included as wholesome food options and still keep you within your daily food plan.

Whichever meal or snack size you choose, you don't have to diet or count calories. This book shows correct portions which can help you maintain your weight or lose weight safely.

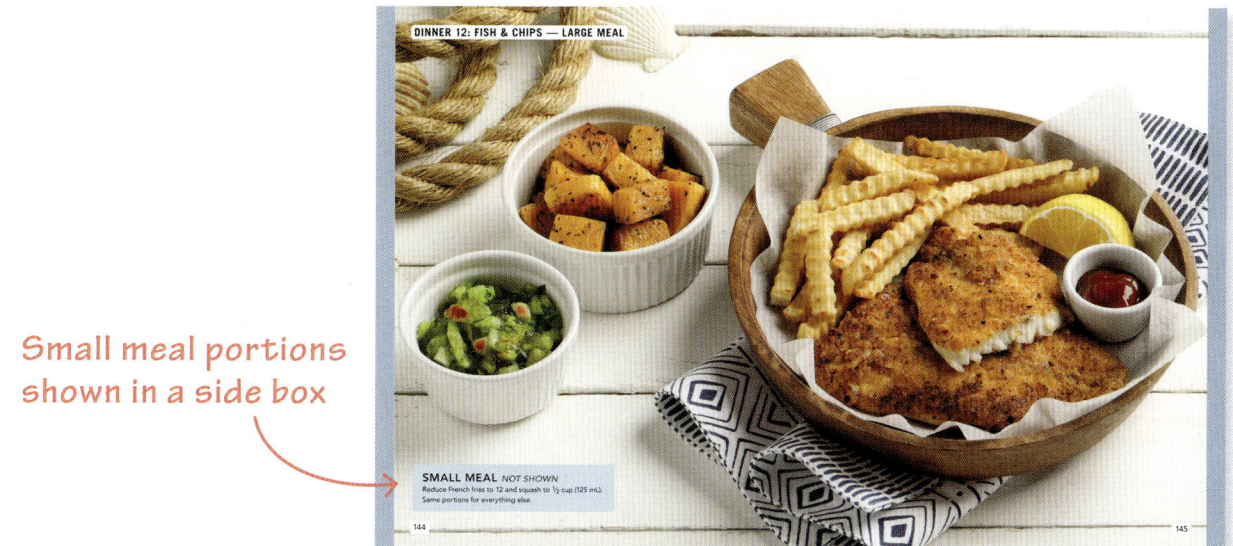

Small meal portions shown in a side box

Here are some examples of how you can select large or small meals and snacks to meet your calorie goals (search online "calorie calculator"). These examples show a range from 2,200 to 1,200 calories.

See page 30 for calories of each meal and snack.

CALORIES

- **2,200:** Large breakfast, lunch and dinner, with three large snacks
- **1,870:** Large breakfast, lunch and dinner, with one small and two medium snacks
- **1,620:** Large breakfast, lunch and dinner, with no snacks
- **1,550:** Small breakfast, lunch and dinner, with one small, one medium and one large snack
- **1,300:** Small breakfast, lunch and dinner, with two small snacks
- **1,200:** Small breakfast, lunch and dinner, with no snacks

5 Carb Choices

Carb Choices are a simplified number used to do easy carb counting.

ONE CARB CHOICE = 15 NET CARBS

Here are some examples of one Carb Choice:

- 1 slice of bread
- 1 small bun
- ⅓ cup (75 mL) cooked rice
- ½ cup (125 mL) corn or potato
- 1 small apple
- ½ large banana
- 1 cup (250 mL) strawberries
- 1 cup (250 mL) peas or carrots
- 1 cup (250 mL) milk or plain yogurt
- 1 tbsp (15 mL) regular sugar

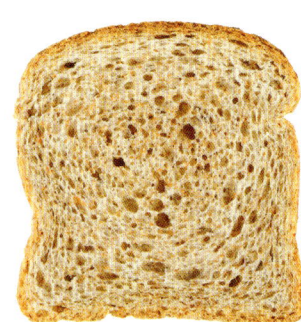

A Carb Choice is also known as a Diabetes Exchange, Diabetes Food Group or Carb Serving.

Large Meal Carb Choices		Small Meal Carb Choices	
Breakfasts	1 to 3	Breakfasts	1 to 2
Lunches	3 to 4	Lunches	2 to 3
Dinners	4 to 5	Dinners	3 to 4

Sample Menu: Lunch 13 – Avocado Salad & Bruschetta. This meal has:
- **Large Meal:** 3 Carb Choices
- **Small Meal:** 2 Carb Choices

YOUR LUNCH MENU	Large Meal (520 calories)	Total Carbs	NET CARBS	Small Meal (400 calories)	Total Carbs	NET CARBS
Avocado Salad	1 serving	22	14	1 serving	22	14
Light salad dressing	1½ tbsp (22 mL)	4	4	1 tbsp (15 mL)	3	3
Bruschetta	6 baguette slices	29	27	3 baguette slices	14	13
	TOTAL CARBS	55 g	45 g	TOTAL CARBS	39 g	30 g
	Total carbs minus fiber = NET CARBS				NET CARBS	
	CARB CHOICES (1 carb choice = 15 g net carbs)		3	CARB CHOICES		2

SEVEN SMART FEATURES OF THIS BOOK

 Total Carbs and Net Carbs

If you're counting total carbs or net carbs to manage your blood sugar or to adjust insulin units at mealtimes, then please read on.

All the total carbs and net carbs are listed for every single menu item and all meal totals!

What are Total Carbs?

Total Carbs = starches, sugar, fiber and sugar alcohols

Why use Total Carbs?

Some people adjust their insulin dose using Total Carbs because it is easier to count Total Carbs, especially as food labeling of Net Carbs can be complicated to interpret.

 Keep in mind that not all the Total Carbs will be absorbed and affect blood sugar.

What are Net Carbs?

Net Carbs = Total Carbs minus fiber and minus most sugar alcohols

Net Carbs are the carbs that are absorbed and directly affect blood sugar.

- Fiber, such as bran, is not digested.
- Sugar alcohols, such as sorbitol, maltitol and erythritol, are only partly absorbed.

Why use Net Carbs?

The Net Carbs in this book accurately subtracts fiber and sugar alcohols, so you'll see the direct effect of food on your blood sugar.

Sample Menu: Lunch 13 – Avocado Salad & Bruschetta. This meal has:
Large Meal Option: Total Carbs = 55 g   Net Carbs = 45 g
Small Meal Option: Total Carbs = 39 g   Net Carbs = 30 g

YOUR LUNCH MENU	Large Meal (520 calories)	Total Carbs	NET CARBS	Small Meal (400 calories)	Total Carbs	NET CARBS
Avocado Salad	1 serving	22	14	1 serving	22	14
Light salad dressing	1½ tbsp (22 mL)	4	4	1 tbsp (15 mL)	3	3
Bruschetta	6 baguette slices	29	27	3 baguette slices	14	13
	TOTAL CARBS	55 g	45 g	TOTAL CARBS	39 g	30 g
Total carbs minus fiber = NET CARBS						NET CARBS
CARB CHOICES (1 carb choice = 15 g net carbs)			3	CARB CHOICES		2

NOTE: The guidance on carb counting is changing as we learn more, including the effects of protein and fat on blood sugar levels (see page 23).

SEVEN SMART FEATURES OF THIS BOOK

7 Low-Carb Swaps

The essential feature of low-carb swaps gives you meal-by-meal options to better manage your blood sugar.

An example of an easy low-carb swap:

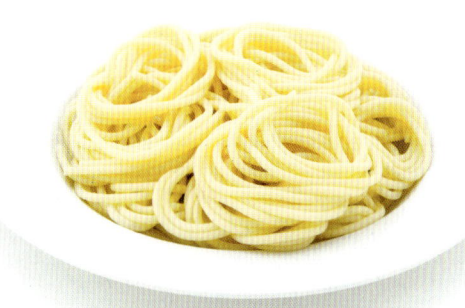

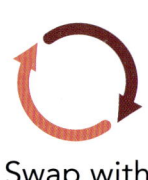
Swap with

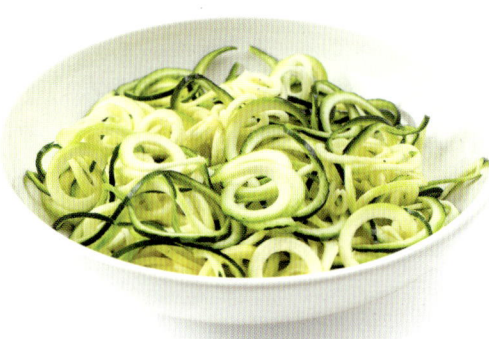

Regular pasta

Zucchini noodles

What are low-carb swaps?

Low-carb swaps have fewer carbs. They are often higher in fiber, protein or fat.

Reasons to choose a low-carb swap:

- Your blood sugar is running high one day
- Your blood sugar is always high at a certain meal, and medication or exercise hasn't helped to bring it down
- You want to take less insulin before a meal

Example of a Low-Carb Swap Chart

You'll find these charts in the Low-Carb Baking and Cooking chapter and the Low-Carb Swap Charts chapter.

PASTA SWAPS ½ cup (125 mL) cooked	CALORIES	TOTAL CARBS	FIBER	NET CARBS	PROTEIN
Konjac spaghetti, see page 275	15	4	3	1	0
Zucchini noodles	10	2	0	2	0
Edamame spaghetti	81	9	6	3	11
Spaghetti squash	21	5	1	4	0
Spelt spaghetti	84	16	3	13	3
Whole-grain spaghetti	**88**	**19**	**2**	**17**	**3**
Regular spaghetti	90	20	1	19	3

This Book's for You!

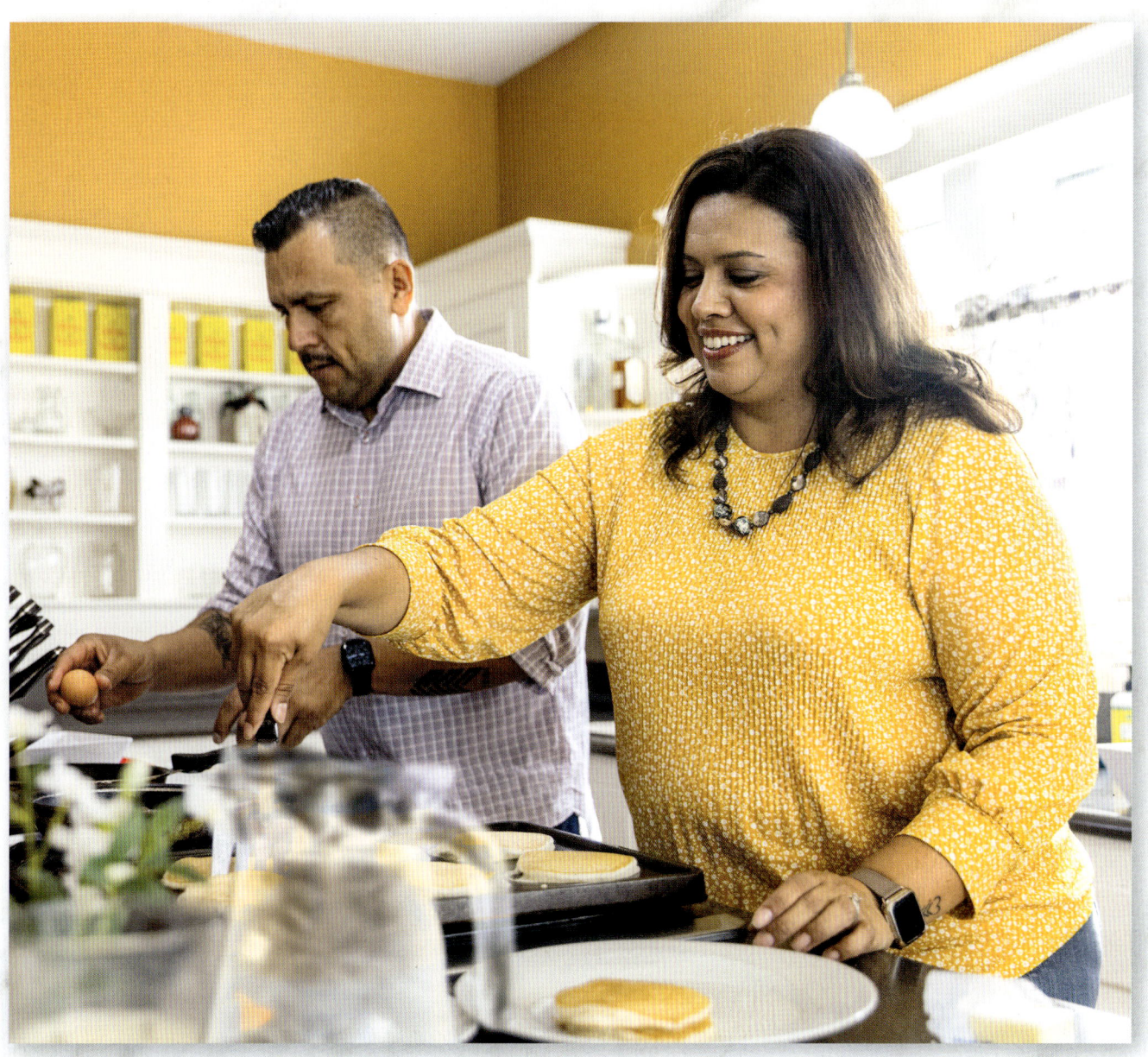

Making Protein-Power Pancakes (page 38).

THIS BOOK'S FOR YOU!

To Delay or Prevent Diabetes

"We have a history of diabetes and high blood pressure in my family. I'm worried I'll get diabetes and that someday my son will too."

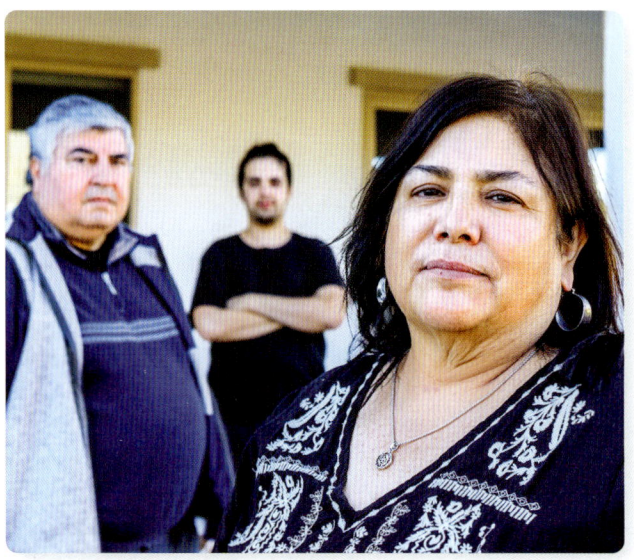

Start now. Look at the life-size photos that show you the correct portions, and use the Plate Method (see pages 7–8).

This cookbook has healthy meals to help you make easy changes to your diet to help delay or prevent the onset of diabetes.

There is a varied selection of meals, and in no time at all you will discover your favorites.

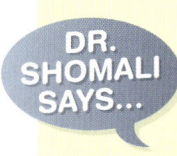 There are proven, achievable lifestyle changes that can delay or prevent type 2 diabetes, even if you are at high risk. It is essential to maintain a healthy weight and exercise regularly. What is so beneficial about these meals is that they all have fewer calories and carbs, and less saturated fat and salt. This helps with prevention of both diabetes and high blood pressure.

For Prediabetes

"My doctor said I have prediabetes. She said my blood sugar is higher than normal and that I could get diabetes if I don't do something about it. I love to eat and don't want to give up all my favorite foods."

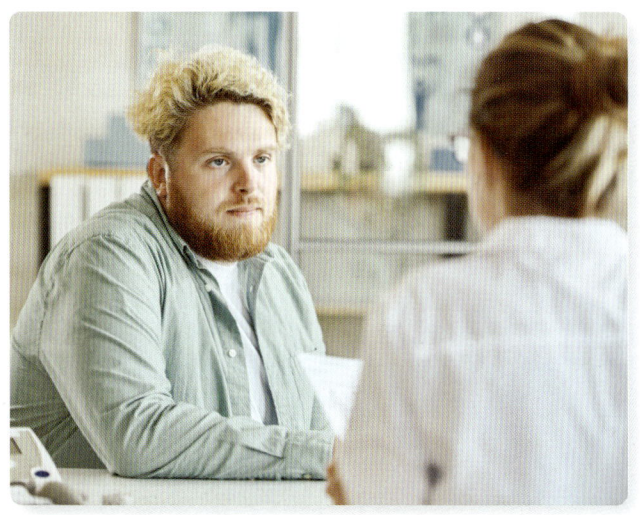

The meals in this cookbook are favorite foods. You will learn how easy it is to cook them yourself. Home cooking means less take-out food and helps save money too.

Start with the Large Meal portions and Medium and Large Snacks (see page 9). They are wholesome and filling.

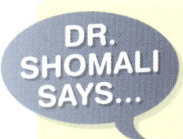 In diabetes prevention studies, three things had a significant impact on preventing prediabetes from becoming diabetes: eating healthy foods, regular physical activity and modest weight loss.

Youth with Type 2 Diabetes

"It's hard because my friends don't have diabetes. Now I'm not allowed to drink pop or eat potato chips."

There are no bad foods, only a variety of foods in the right portions.

You can choose potato chips occasionally; they are in the Snacks section on page 266. Also see low-carb Potato Chips Swaps on page 282.

Most soda pop has sugar-free options. Choose them, because one can of regular pop has 9 teaspoons of sugar you don't need. See the low-carb Sugary Drinks chart on page 279.

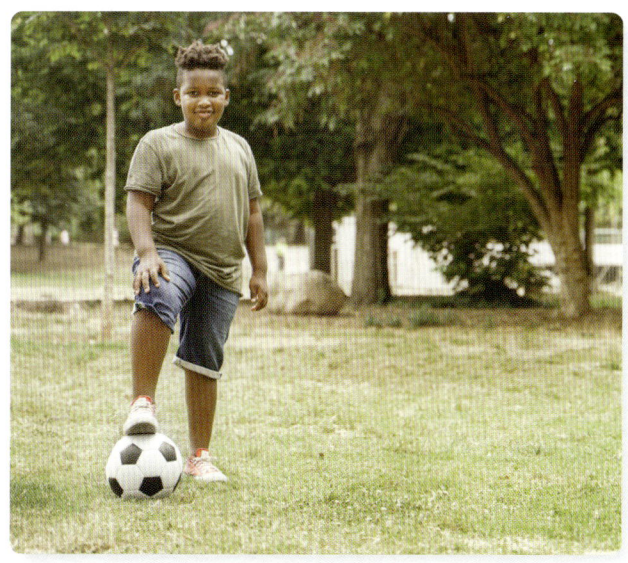

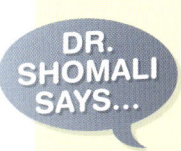 I advise all parents to get active with their children around the home and outside the home. Parents are the best role models for children to learn healthy ways to eat and exercise. As children grow, they need extra calcium and vitamin D for healthy bone growth. Milk or milk alternatives (cheese and yogurt) have those important minerals.

Gestational Diabetes

"I felt overwhelmed when my doctor told me I had gestational diabetes. I want to do what is best for my baby."

When you are pregnant, it is especially important to keep your blood sugar in the target range and gain the recommended amount of weight.

The book's low-carb meals have vitamins, minerals, proteins and healthy fats.

Choosing these meals will help you manage your blood sugar and increase your chances for a healthier pregnancy and a healthier baby.

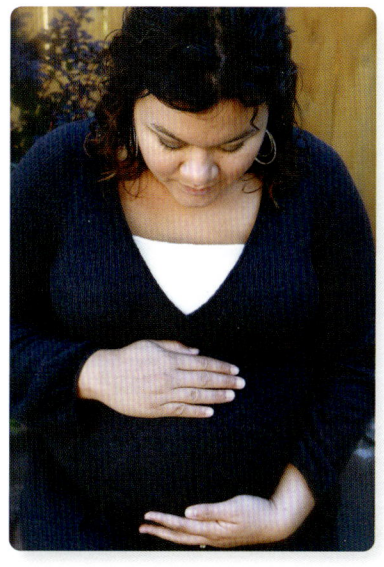

Continue to see your doctor or health care provider on a regular basis.

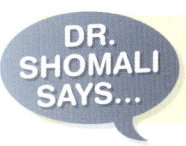 Add high-protein snacks (see pages 266–267) to keep up your calories as your baby grows.

THIS BOOK'S FOR YOU!

Adults with Type 2 Diabetes

"I'm not that active anymore, so I choose the Small Meals. I have a sweet tooth and I like the options for desserts with the dinners."

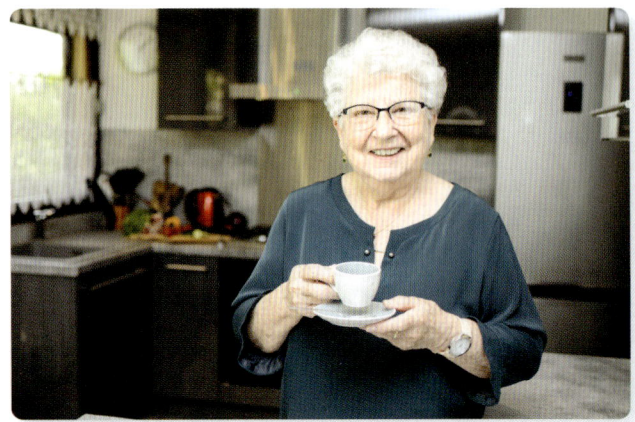

For many seniors, the Small Meals and Small Snacks have the right calories and carbohydrates (see page 30).

Good health is not just about eating less: it's also about moving more. Walking every day helps manage blood sugar levels.

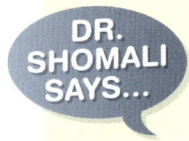

When you reduce your portions and carbs, you may need fewer diabetes medications. Always check in with your health care team if you are experiencing an increase in low blood sugars. For more information on medications and low blood sugars, please see the *Complete Diabetes Guide*, described on page 20.

"Breakfast is our favorite meal; we take our time and make our plans for the day. Together we follow the Carb Choices. It makes meal planning so easy for us. Depending on our appetite at breakfast, we'll have the small or large meal which gives us up to 3 Carb Choices."

At a glance, Carb Choices show how many carbs are in each meal (see page 10).

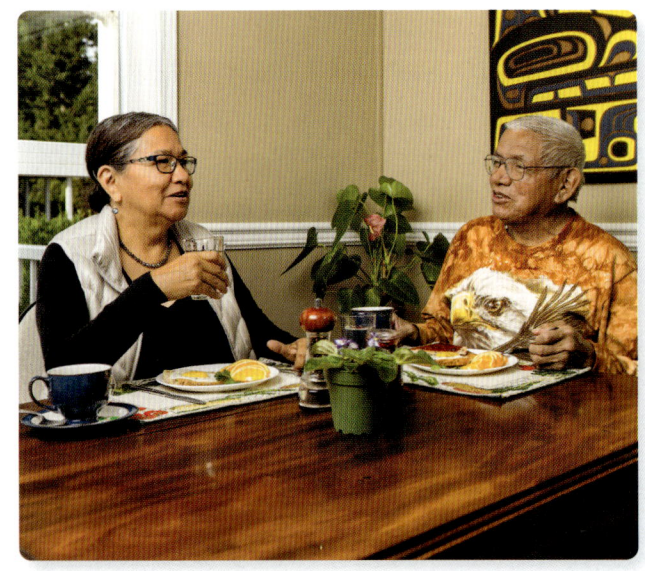

One Carb Choice = 15 g net carbs

A carb choice is also known as a diabetes exchange or a diabetes food group.

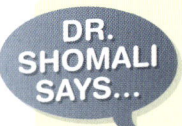

People who eat breakfast find it easier to lose weight and keep it off. Research also shows that people who eat breakfast are more likely to establish a healthy eating pattern and get the nutrients they need each day for best health.

"I look at the portions in the large meal photos, and say, 'Okay, this is how much I can eat.' It's all laid out for me! I've been dieting for years, but with these meals I don't go hungry. A terrific bonus is that my kids eat these meals too."

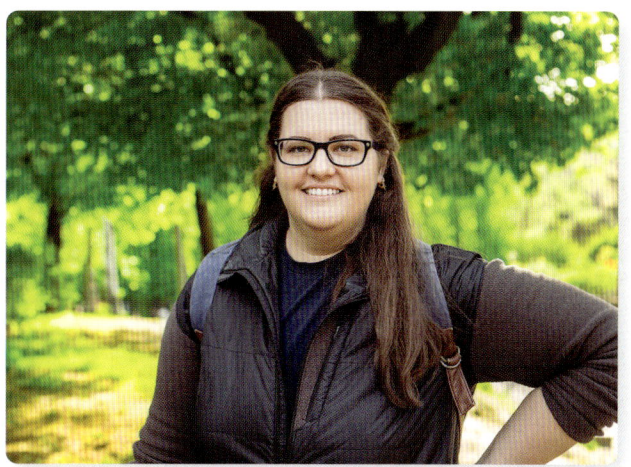

Every meal has been carefully calculated to have the same calories. For example, all large breakfasts have the same calories.

See page 30 for breakfast, lunch and dinner calorie and carb counts.

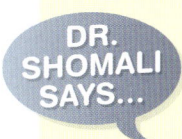

DR. SHOMALI SAYS… Most of my patients with type 2 diabetes have learned to manage their medications and insulin but struggle with staying on a consistent eating pattern. This cookbook can help. Follow these well-laid-out healthy meal plans for optimal nutrition to help you reach your blood sugar targets and goal weight and to feel well.

And yes, these meal plans support families to cook and eat together.

Note: This book does not include recommendations for infants and toddlers.

"I have type 2 diabetes and take insulin and wear a CGM. Having diabetes is a lot of work, and sometimes I just don't know what to cook for dinner. That's why I love this cookbook: it has so many quick and easy recipes. For each meal plan, I look at the carb counts and adjust my portions based on my blood sugar."

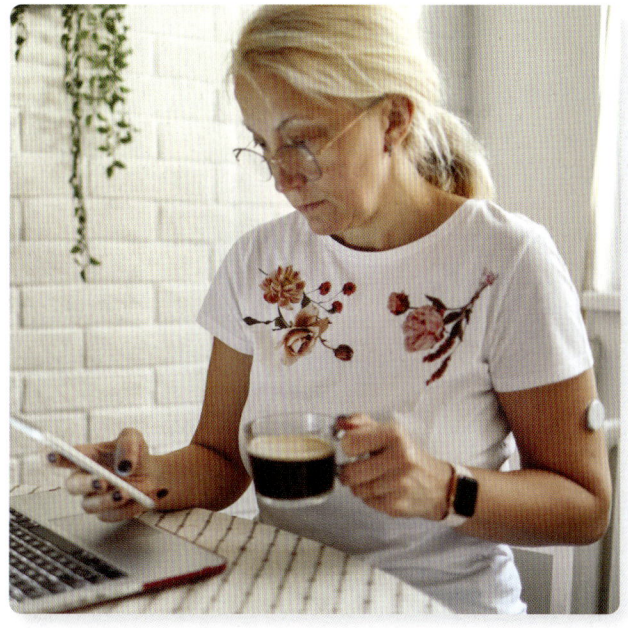

A continuous glucose monitor (CGM) gives you frequent blood sugar readings on your phone. It is based on glucose levels in the fluid that is just under your skin.

Total carbs and net carbs are listed for all the recipes, meals and snacks in this cookbook (see page 11).

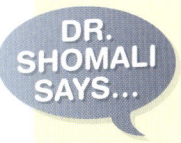

DR. SHOMALI SAYS… A CGM is helpful if you inject mealtime insulin. It helps you understand how insulin, food, exercise and other factors (see pages 21 to 24) affect your blood sugar, and if you need to adjust your insulin. A CGM will alert you each time your blood sugar drops too low.

THIS BOOK'S FOR YOU!

To Transition Off Keto

"I've got type 2 diabetes. I've been on the keto diet for four months and have lost 20 lbs. My blood sugar and A1C have improved. Now I want to live a normal life, but I'm afraid I'll gain back the weight."

If you want to gradually transition off a very-low-carb diet such as keto or Atkins and still maintain your weight loss, the balanced low-carb meals in this book will help you.

Choose the meal and snack sizes that match your current calorie intake: see page 30. At first, choose the low-carb swaps (see page 12), and gradually you can choose fewer carb swaps and switch to the large or small meals.

Gently, your body will get used to a variety of foods again.

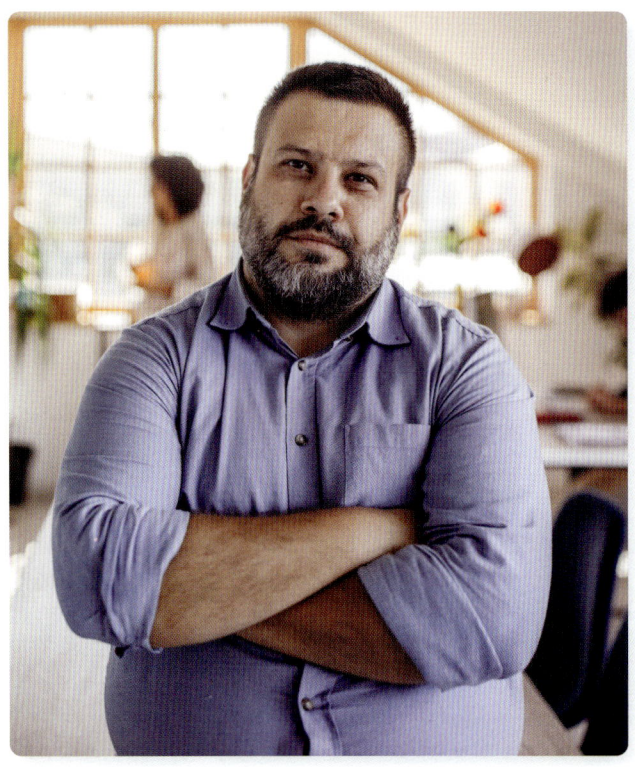

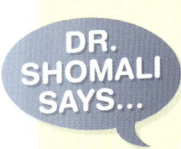

DR. SHOMALI SAYS... To minimize weight regain, I recommend that you reintroduce carbohydrates gradually. Increase your carbs by no more than 10 to 15 grams per week over the first month. This gradual reintroduction will help prevent your body from making a surge of insulin that would then make you hungry. Less hunger equals less weight regain. During your transition off the keto diet, keep physically active. See your doctor and dietitian for follow-up support, including lab tests.

To Transition Off Diabetes Remission Diets

Under supervision by a doctor and dietitian team, these remission diets are adapted for fast weight loss over 3 to 5 months. These are very-low-calorie diets, 800 to 900 calories a day, typically consisting of liquid shakes or soups. Once weight loss is achieved, a small whole-food meal is introduced into daily eating. Gradually, over another several months, the liquid diet is replaced with complete whole-food meals. The Small Meal plans in this cookbook support a 1200-calorie range per day. All necessary nutrition by calories and carbohydrates has been calculated for each meal plan in this book; this means less work for you. This cookbook will move you forward into a life of healthy eating. Talk with your dietitian.

Adults with Type 1 Diabetes

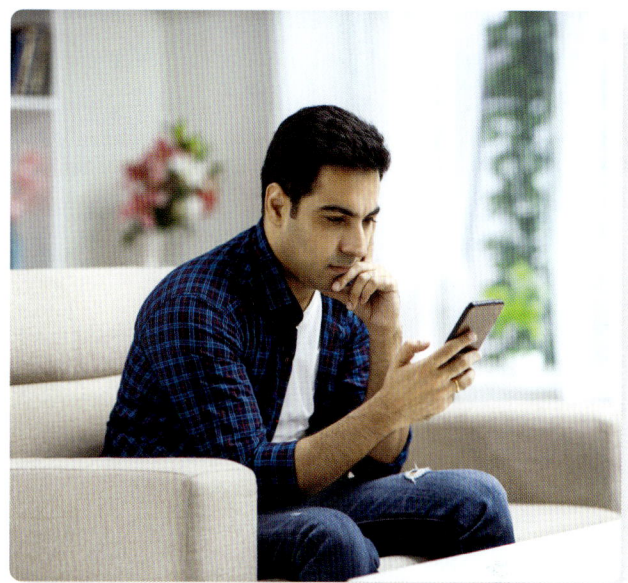

"I've had type 1 diabetes since I was 15 years old. I wear an insulin pump and a CGM. I mostly do pattern management. I love this book's set of go-to recipes that have a consistent effect on my blood sugar."

If you use an insulin-to-carbohydrate ratio, you can use the carb data (see page 11) to calculate your insulin dose.

If you do pattern management, you can track your blood sugar before and after a meal or snack. If your blood sugar goes too high or too low, then next time you'll know to adjust that meal or the insulin dose.

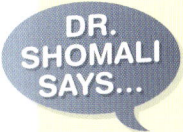 **DR. SHOMALI SAYS...** What makes this book so valuable is that the total carbs and net carbs are listed not just for the recipes but for every food item in the meals. So you can easily figure out your insulin dose even if you adjust what you eat.

Youth with Type 1 Diabetes

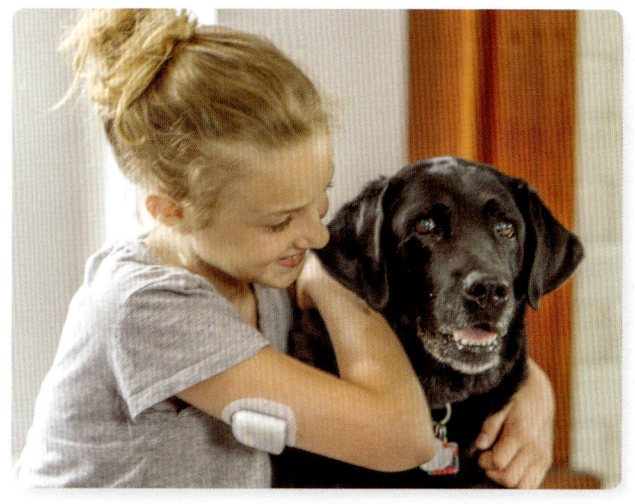

"I'm 12 and I've had diabetes for two years. I like to help my mom make meals out of this cookbook; my favorite is Sausages & Cornbread. If there is a food that I want to eat that's not in the meal, we add the net carbs for that food to the total. Then I know how much insulin I need to take."

Every food in the book has a carb count. It's so easy to add or omit a food item from any meal and still quickly work out the carbs. You can use a marker to write in the book as needed.

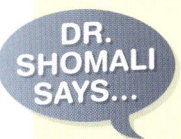 **DR. SHOMALI SAYS...** For those with a flexible insulin dosing plan, their insulin dose can be adjusted to match their carbs in this cookbook. Keep in mind that the nutritional and calorie needs of children with type 1 diabetes change as they grow; follow the individualized diet advice from your diabetes team.

THIS BOOK'S FOR YOU!

For Diabetes Educators

"I love this book because I use it with people who want to lose weight, those who want to count their carbs, and those who want to mix Large and Small Meals to meet their calorie needs."

Show your clients the life-size photos so they can see the right portions to eat for each meal. Clients can easily learn how to put a healthy meal together and not be overwhelmed.

The Snacks section is always popular; here again, the calories and carbohydrates are counted. People don't have to guess portions.

All Carb Choices are listed for every meal. This makes it handy for educators to explain the importance of carbs for everyone with diabetes.

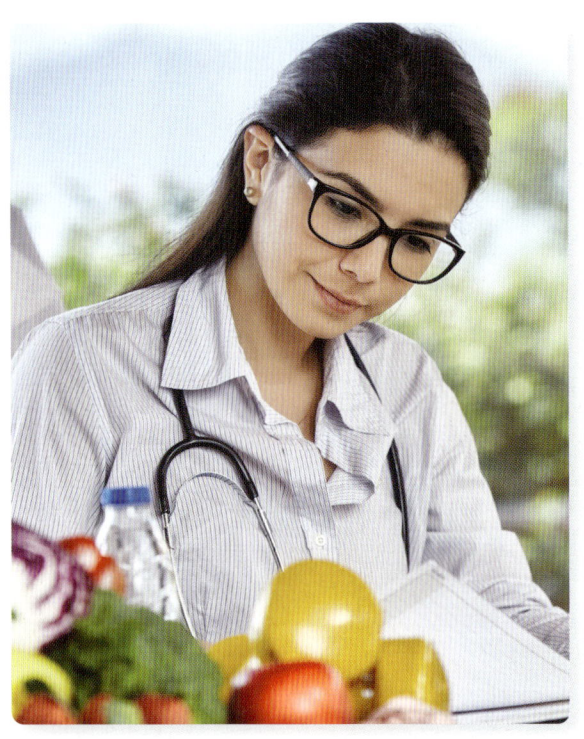

DR. SHOMALI SAYS... The Health and Wellness Series includes this book, the *Complete Diabetes Guide* and *Diabetes Essentials*. Together, these three books provide you with excellent resources to teach and educate your clients about diabetes.

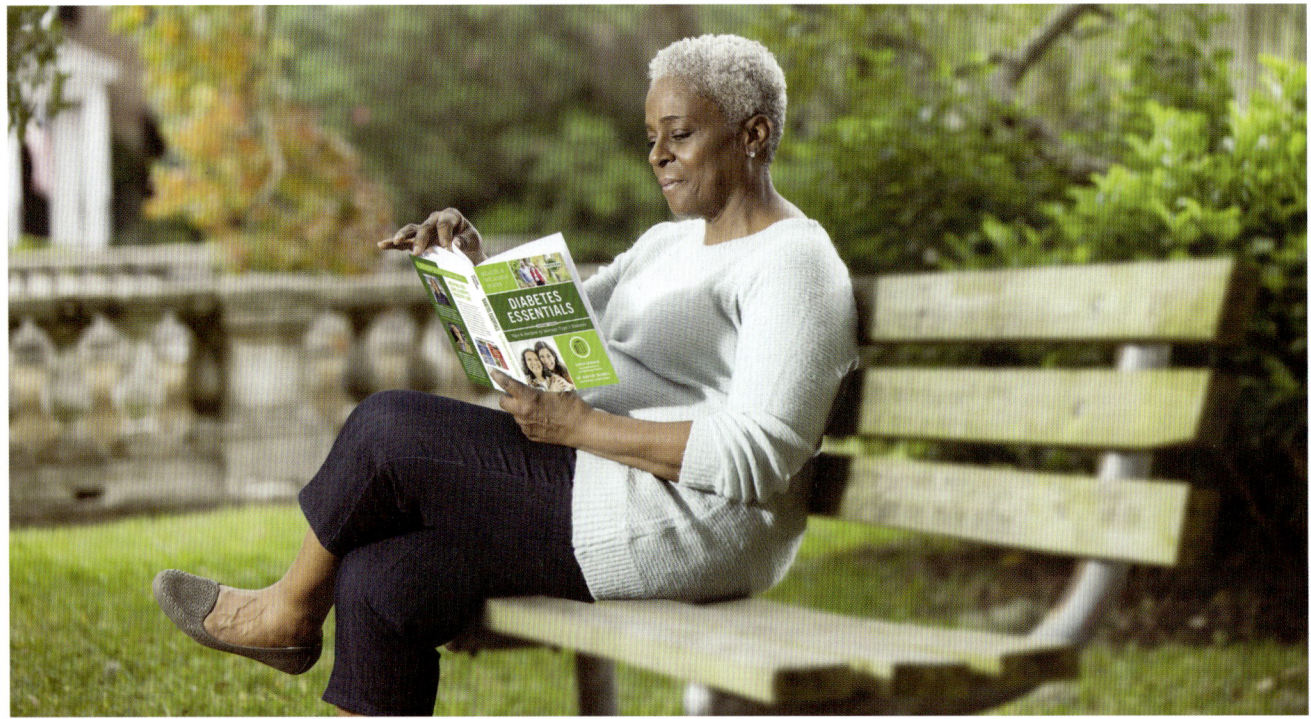

What Affects Your Blood Sugar

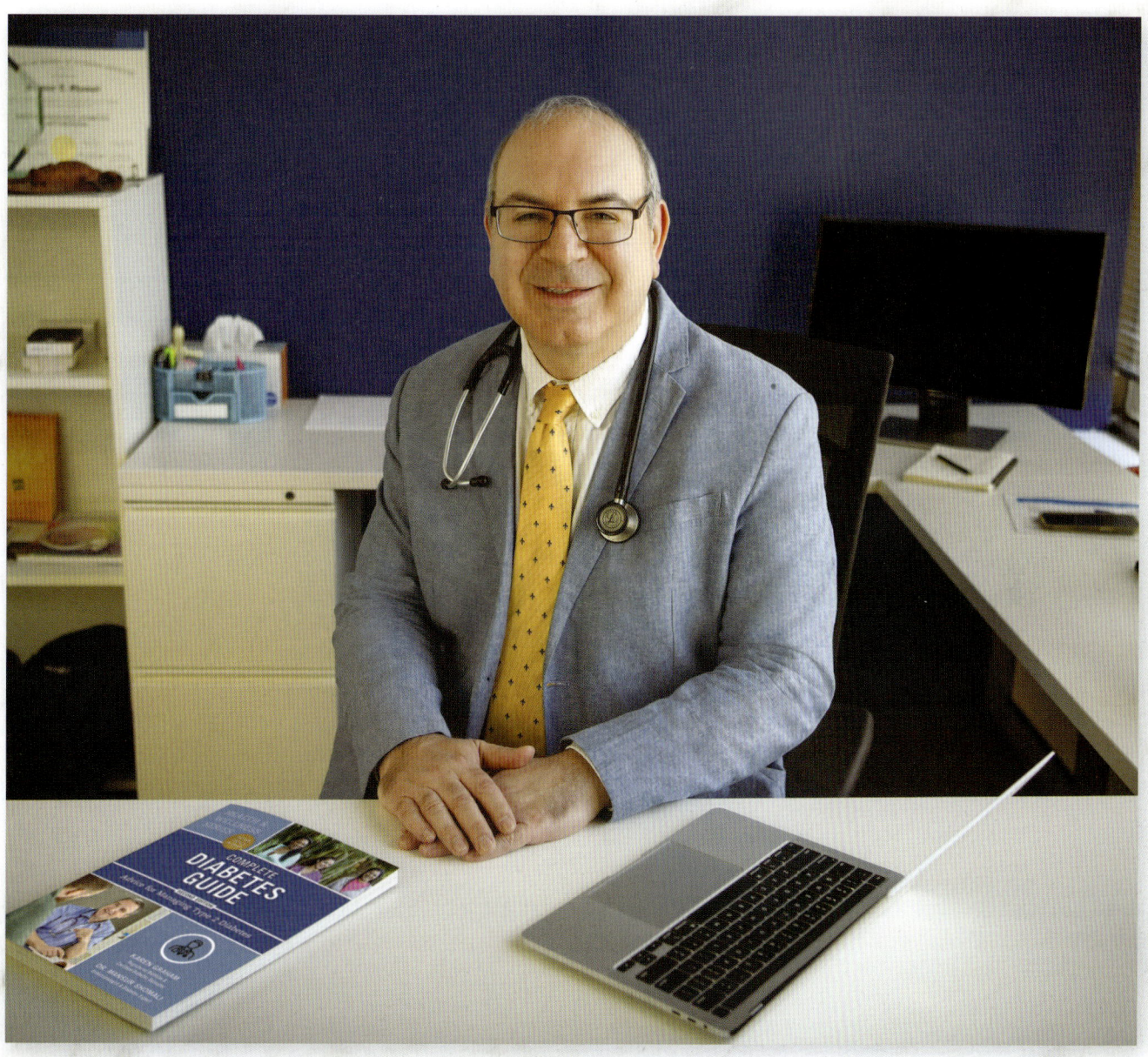

Dr. Shomali provides research-based diabetes facts and information.

WHAT AFFECTS YOUR BLOOD SUGAR

For more information on ALL the topics on pages 22–24, please see the other two books in our Health & Wellness Series: *Complete Diabetes Guide* **and** *Diabetes Essentials.*

Carbohydrates have the greatest effect on blood sugar levels. Yet, it's not as simple as "eat fewer carbs and your blood sugar will go down." Our bodies are complex; we each digest food differently and respond to insulin differently. This is why your blood sugar can vary, even after meals that have similar amounts of food and carbohydrates. This section will highlight other factors that can affect your blood sugar.

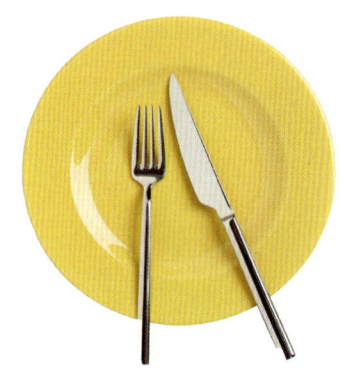

Morning Blood Sugar Rise

Your blood sugar rises naturally in the morning. This is because there is a release of sugar from your liver in response to the hormones that help wake you up. To moderate this morning blood sugar rise, the Breakfast Meals have fewer carbohydrates than the Lunches and Dinners.

Eating protein with your breakfast makes it easier to manage blood sugar later in the day.

Diabetes Medications

A common type 2 diabetes medication is metformin, yet there are many new diabetes medications and types of insulin. Some medications tend to lower your blood sugar before you eat, while others help after you eat. Some require that you eat consistently throughout the day to avoid low blood sugar; others allow for flexibility with eating. Some help insulin work better, and still others help to protect your heart and blood vessels.

Several diabetes and heart medications usually work better together than just one. With any changes in your routines, it is important to consult with your diabetes care team to monitor and adjust medications as needed.

Taking your medication or insulin at the prescribed time is important for good blood sugar. If you forget a dose of insulin or pills, then your blood sugar will spike.

Infections

Any infection, such as inflamed gums, an open sore or a bladder infection, will increase your blood sugar, and it will remain high until the infection is gone.

Get the appropriate medical attention.

Smoking

Smoking or using other nicotine products reduces how well insulin works, which leads to an increase in blood sugar.

Timing

Eating, walking, resting and taking your medications all affect your blood sugar, and these activities may happen at different times each day.

So, an important part of diabetes management is to organize the timing of your daily activities to be as consistent as possible. Then, if there is an unexpected high or low in your blood sugar, you will probably know what you did differently in your daily routine.

Sleep and Stress

We know how important sleep is to reduce stress and to help us be alert during the hours we are awake. If we don't sleep well or we are feeling stressed during the day, the body produces stress hormones such as adrenalin. Stress hormones increase blood sugar.

Gut Bacteria

Healthy probiotic bacteria that live in your large intestine (gut) help to slow down the digestion of certain nutrients and can reduce a blood sugar rise after a meal.

Probiotic bacteria occur naturally in food, from yogurt to sauerkraut. High-fiber foods help these bacteria to grow and sustain a healthy gut.

Protein and Fat

When you eat protein and fat, this helps slow down digestion. The slower the digestion time, the slower the rise in your blood sugars.

The meals in this cookbook have lean protein and healthy fats and carbohydrates. Because of this healthy balance, these meals have a lower glycemic index (or GI), and so food is digested more slowly.

Water

When your blood sugar is high, drinking water helps dilute the amount of sugar in your blood.

Water also helps reduce stored fat and helps keep your bowel movements regular. Importantly, water reduces your risk of getting a urinary tract infection.

Try to drink six to eight 8 oz (250 mL) glasses of water a day.

If you have a sleepless night, you could have high blood sugar levels in the morning before you even have any food.

The meals in this cookbook include probiotic foods and are high in fiber.

Blood sugar is an essential source of energy. With a zero-carb meal, your body converts some of the protein or fat into blood sugar.

If the weather is hot, or you are exercising, or your blood sugar is high, you may need to drink more water.

Alcohol

For your best health, this book limits alcohol to an "Occasional" item in the meals or snacks.

Learn how alcohol affects you by testing your blood sugar before and after you drink. Some people experience a high blood sugar after drinking alcohol, while others have a low blood sugar.

Beer, sweet wines and mixed alcoholic drinks contain sugar, which may raise your blood sugar. Mixed drinks include coolers.

Drinking regularly can cause weight gain, which then can cause an overall increase in your blood sugar over time.

For those taking insulin or certain types of diabetes medications, alcohol can cause a low blood sugar reaction, often many hours later. This low blood sugar can happen even if the alcohol is mixed with juice or sugary drinks.

Beer lovers: check out page 282 for beer swaps that have little or no alcohol or few or no carbs.

Drink alcohol with food to help avoid low blood sugar.

Weight Loss or Weight Gain

Losing weight or gaining weight both affect your blood sugar levels.

When you eat less and make other important changes to your lifestyle, and if you start to lose some weight, you may need less insulin or diabetes medication. Your doctor will adjust your medications to reduce your risk for low blood sugar reactions.

With weight gain, blood sugar levels tend to increase. It is important to see your doctor or dietitian to talk about what has changed for you and how best to manage your weight gain and diabetes.

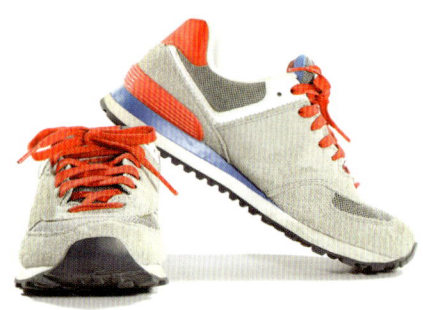

Exercise

Taking a brisk walk after a meal, even for 10 minutes, helps insulin work better and can reduce a post-meal blood sugar high. The great news is that aerobic exercise like walking, bicycling and swimming can help improve your blood sugar for several hours.

While regular exercise is essential for healthy blood sugar levels, the effects on your blood sugar may vary. For example, intense exercise such as weight lifting or moving heavy furniture can, in the short term, cause an increase in your blood sugar.

Test your blood sugar before and after exercise to understand the effect of exercise on your body.

Low-Carb Baking and Cooking

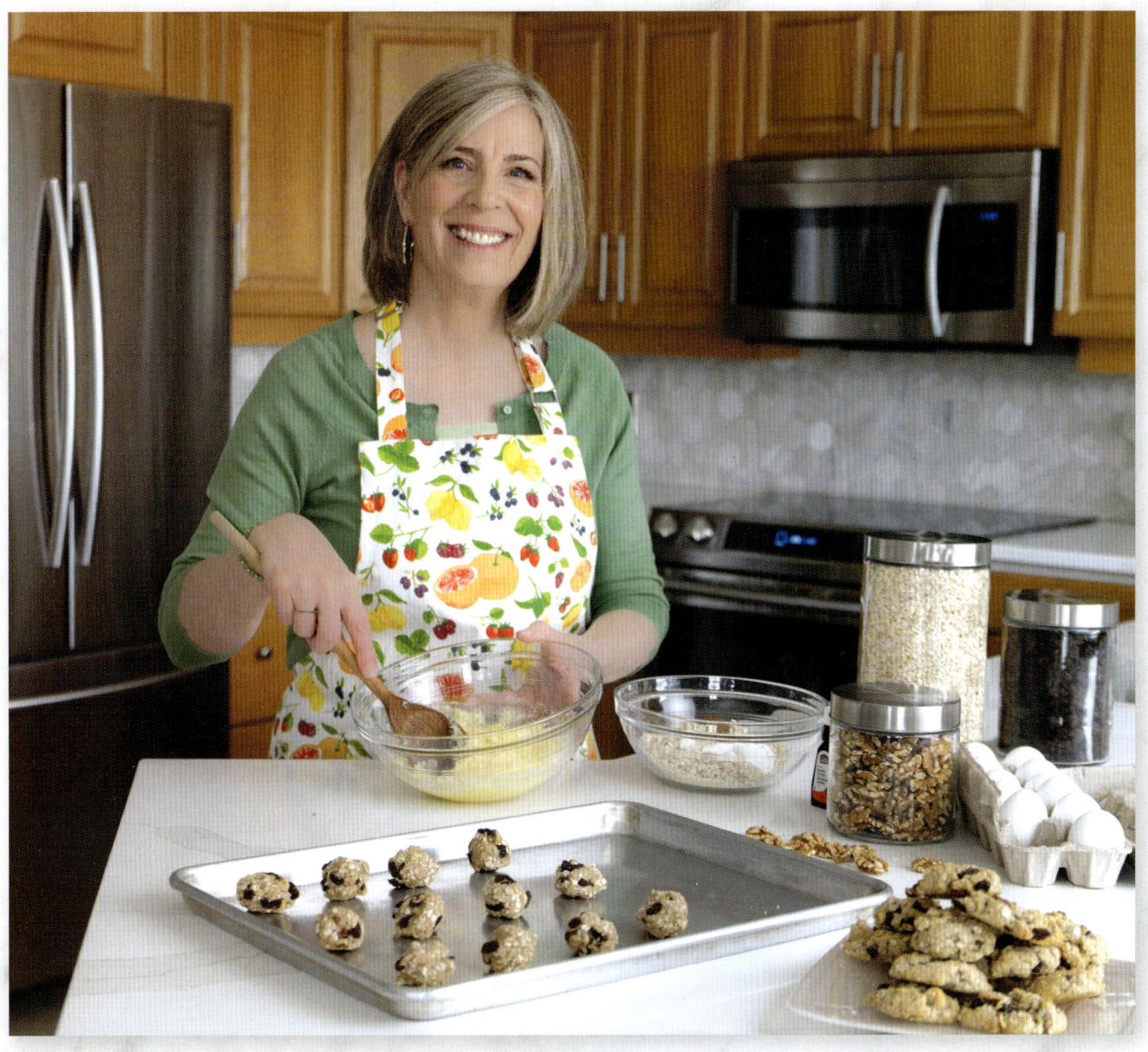

Karen Graham, author and creator of the recipes in this book, prepares the Oatmeal Cookies (page 131).

Do I Need to Buy Different Products to Cook the Low-Carb Way?

You will need to buy some different products so you can make healthy low-carb meals for yourself, but most often you'll be cooking with regular products.

Low-carb products to start with:
- almond flour or finely ground blanched almond flour
- ground flaxseed
- almond beverage, unsweetened
- soy beverage, unsweetened
- reduced-sugar pancake syrup
- zero-calorie sweeteners

Low-carb products may cost more than regular products. Consider this an investment in your health.

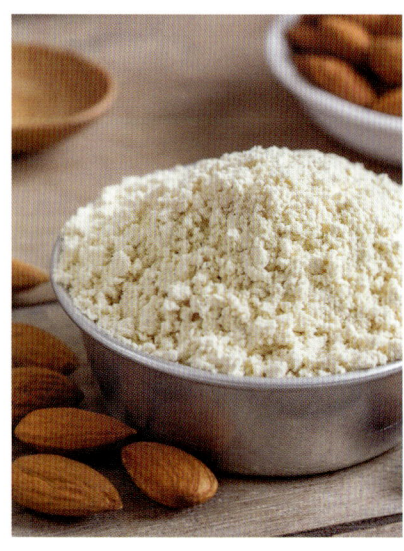

Almond flour

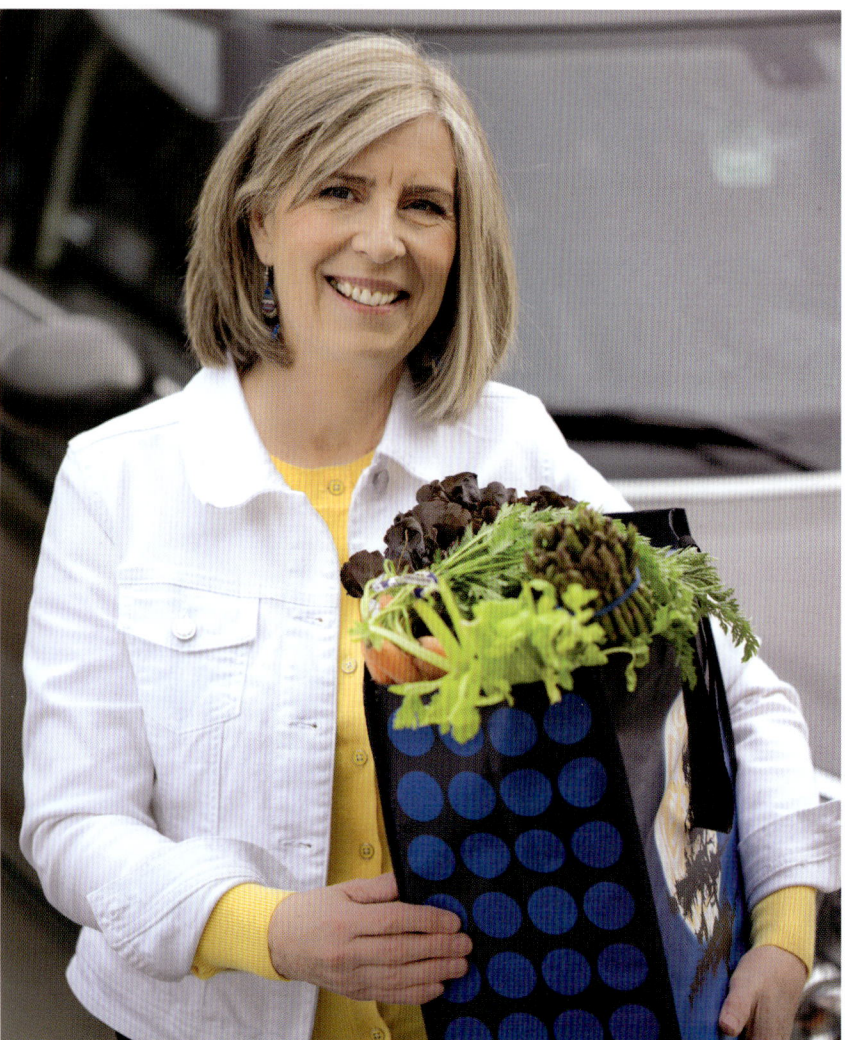

Look for low-carb products in the grocery store aisles under Health Food or Natural Products. Many low-carb products are now sold in health food stores, in bulk stores and online too.

Low-Carb Flours

Almond flour

This is my favorite alternative flour to reduce carbs in cooking or baking. Typically, I'll replace half of the all-purpose flour in my recipes with almond flour. I also like to use ground flaxseed or oats as alternatives.

COOKING TIP: Wheat flour contains gluten, which is essential to help baked products rise. This is why I keep some wheat flour in baked products for the best shape and texture.

Flour Swaps

¼ cup/60 mL portion

In all the Swap Charts, carbohydrates, protein and fat are in grams (g).

	CALORIES	TOTAL CARBS	FIBER	NET CARBS	PROTEIN	FAT	NOTES
Ground flaxseed*	138	8	7	1	5	11	Lowest in carbs, high in healthy fat
Almond flour*	170	5	3	2	6	15	Low in carbs, high in protein and healthy fat
Coconut flour*	120	18	12	6	5	3	In cooking, does not replace regular flour cup-for-cup. Typically, more eggs or liquid need to be added.
Wheat germ	104	15	4	11	7	3	
Oats, large flaked*	83	15	2	13	3	2	
Whole wheat flour	100	22	2	20	4	1	
All-purpose flour	110	22	1	21	4	1	**Excellent baking qualities**

*gluten-free: check labels for impurities

Other flours:

Spelt and rice flour are higher in net carbs than all-purpose flour, so I don't generally use these.

Nutrients vary between brands, and companies may change their ingredients over time. Always check the label.

Low-Carb Alternatives to Milk

Unsweetened almond beverage or soy beverage

These are my top lower-carb picks for plant-based beverages, commonly just called almond milk or soy milk. Both are readily available in cartons or fresh (refrigerated). As I do with flour, I often replace half of the cow's milk in my recipes with unsweetened almond or soy beverage.

A few other common milk alternatives are listed in the Milk Swaps chart below. Note that rice beverage is not listed, as it is higher in carbs than milk.

What to look for on the plant-based beverage label:

- Unflavored or Original usually means no added sugar.
- Flavored varieties can have more carbs than cow's milk.
- Fortified or Enriched will mean added calcium and vitamin D.

COOKING TIP: Cow's milk has proteins and casein which help baked products brown nicely and taste good. In baking and cooking, you can use half cow's milk and half almond beverage. You will have fewer carbs and little difference in flavor.

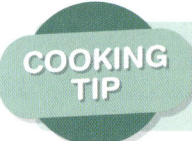
COOKING TIP: Soy beverage helps pudding to thicken better than almond beverage.

Milk Swaps
1 cup/250 mL portion

	CALORIES	TOTAL CARBS	FIBER	NET CARBS	PROTEIN	FAT	NOTES
Almond beverage, unsweetened	30	1	1	0	1	3	Zero net carbs and low in calories; poor source of protein
Coconut milk, unsweetened	45	1	0	1	1	5	
Cashew beverage, unsweetened	45	3	0	3	1	4	
Soy beverage, unsweetened	100	7	2	5	7	4	Similar protein and fat to 2% cow's milk, but with fewer carbs
Oat beverage, unsweetened	70	8	1	7	1	3	Thicker texture than almond milk
1% cow's milk	110	12	0	12	9	3	**Natural lactose helps absorb calcium**

Low-Carb Alternatives to Sugar

Most of my recipes have less sugar than a standard recipe, and some use zero-calorie sweeteners to help reduce the carbs. Examples of zero-calorie sweetener brands that measure cup-for-cup like sugar are Sugar Twin Stevia, Splenda, Truvia and Swerve. See the table below.

COOKING TIPS

In baked products, sugar gives texture and moistness and helps with rising and browning. That's why I often use some sugar along with zero-calorie sweeteners.

To give a nice sweetness to desserts instead of sugar, try no-sugar-added pancake syrup (often sweetened with sucralose). You may need to slightly reduce other liquids.

Sugars
Honey, brown sugar and maple syrup are NOT a low-carb swap for white sugar. They are all natural sugars that have similar carbs.

Sugar has 4 grams of carbs per teaspoon/ 5 mL (12 grams per tbsp/15 mL).

Zero-calorie sweeteners
Zero-calorie sweeteners have 0 grams of carbs per teaspoon/5 mL.

Sugar Swaps
1 tablespoon/15 mL equivalent

ZERO-CALORIE AND LOW-CALORIE SWEETENERS	CALORIES	TOTAL CARBS	FIBER	NET CARBS	NOTES / KEY INGREDIENTS
NutraSweet	12	0	0	0	Dextrose, maltodextrin, aspartame
Pure Via Stevia, granulated	0	0	0	0	Dextrose, steviol glycosides Measures cup-for-cup like sugar
Sugar Twin Stevia	0	0	0	0	Stevia Measures cup-for-cup like sugar
Swerve, granular	0	4	4	0	Erythritol Measures cup-for-cup like sugar
Truvia, granulated	0	4	4	0	Erythritol, chicory root, stevia Measures cup-for-cup like sugar
NutraSweet Natural	4	1	0	1	Erythritol, stevia
Equal, granular	6	2	0	2	Maltodextrin, aspartame, acesulfame potassium
Splenda, granulated	6	2	0	2	Maltodextrin, sucralose Measures cup-for-cup like sugar
Pancake syrup, no-sugar-added (ED Smith brand)	10	3	1	2	Sweetened with sucralose
Sugar, white	**48**	**12**	**0**	**12**	
Pancake syrup, regular	**47**	**12**	**0**	**12**	

LOW-CARB BAKING AND COOKING

Calories and Carbs of Meals and Snacks

The meals in this book are color-coded as follows:

15 Breakfast Meals
Large meals have 370 calories
Net carbs 16–45 grams: 1–3 Carb Choices
Small meals have 250 calories
Net carbs 12–32 grams: 1–2 Carb Choices

15 Lunch Meals
Large meals have 520 calories
Net carbs 41–66 grams: 3–4 Carb Choices
Small meals have 400 calories
Net carbs 28–50 grams: 2–3 Carb Choices

40 Dinner Meals
Large meals have 730 calories
Net carbs 57–75 grams: 4–5 Carb Choices
Small meals have 550 calories
Net carbs 41–55 grams: 3–4 Carb Choices

4 Snack Groups
- Freebie snacks: 20 calories and 0–5 g net carbs
- Small snacks: 50 calories and 0–15 g net carbs
- Medium snacks: 100 calories and 0–20 g net carbs
- Large snacks: 200 calories and 0–30 g net carbs

Low-Carb Swaps will further reduce carbohydrates.

Sample Daily Meal Plan

	Calories
Large breakfast	370
Small snack	50
Small lunch	400
Large snack	200
Large dinner	730
Medium snack	100
Total calories	**1,850**

Calories for the small meals:
- Breakfast has 250 calories
- Lunch has 400 calories
- Dinner has 550 calories

1,200 calories

Calories for the large meals:
- Breakfast has 370 calories
- Lunch has 520 calories
- Dinner has 730 calories

1,620 calories

Calories for the snacks:
- Freebies:
  20 calories or less
- Small:
  50 calories
- Medium:
  100 calories
- Large:
  200 calories

NOTE: There is a range in calories for the meals and snacks: plus or minus up to 10 percent.

Meals, Recipes and Snacks

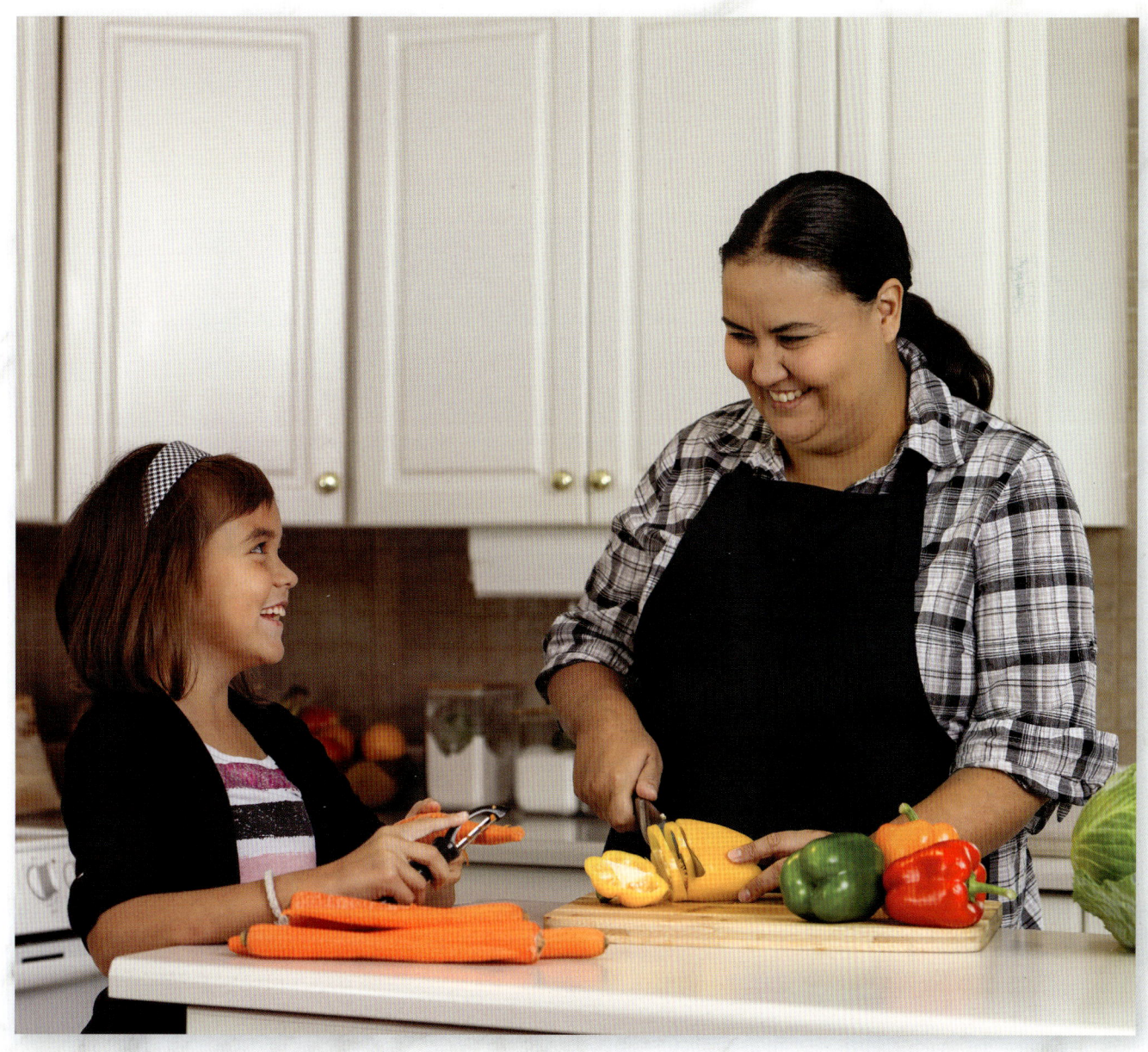

Cooking is more than food; it's family time.

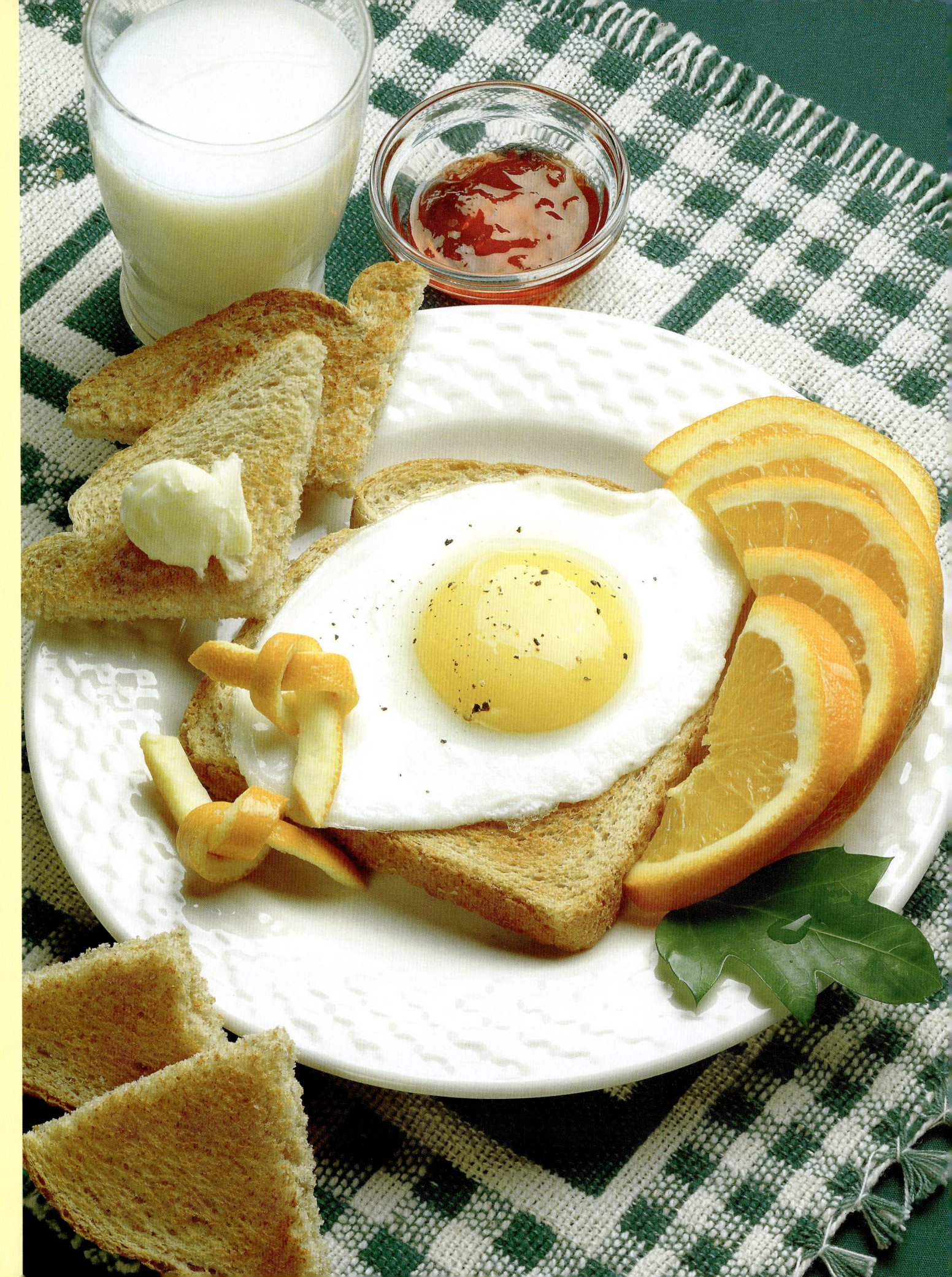

Breakfast Meals

- Each large breakfast has **370 calories** and 1–3 Carb Choices
  Total carbs: 52 g or less | Net carbs: 45 g or less
- Each small breakfast has **250 calories** and 1–2 Carb Choices
  Total carbs: 38 g or less | Net carbs: 32 g or less

1. Cold or Hot Cereal 34
2. Egg & Toast 36
3. Pancakes & Bacon 38
4. Toast & Peanut Butter 40
5. Spinach & Eggs 42
6. Muffin & Cheese 44
7. Raisin Toast & Fruit 46
8. Tuna Scramble 48
9. Homemade Waffles 50
10. Smoothie & Protein Bar 52
11. Fiesta Breakfast 54
12. Fast-Food Breakfast 56
13. Granola Combo 58
14. Prairie Quiche 60
15. Irish Currant Cake 62

ALL MEAL PHOTOS ARE LIFE-SIZE

BREAKFAST MEALS

BREAKFAST 1

Cold or Hot Cereal

Choose cereal brands with more fiber and less added sugar. The nuts with this meal add protein, which slows down the absorption of carbohydrates into your bloodstream. Fruit adds essential vitamins.

Life-size photos are the LARGE MEALS

🔴 LOW-CARB SWAP RECIPE: Chia Pudding

LARGE MEAL

Swap All-Bran Flakes with milk:
1 cup (250 mL) cereal and
¾ cup (175 mL) milk
30 g net carbs

→ For Chia Pudding made with almond beverage:
1 serving (1 cup/250 mL)
16 g net carbs

SMALL MEAL

Swap All-Bran Flakes with milk:
⅔ cup (150 mL) cereal and
½ cup (125 mL) milk
20 g net carbs

→ For Chia Pudding made with almond beverage:
1 serving (1 cup/250 mL)
16 g net carbs

See Cereal Swaps, page 277, or Milk Swaps, page 28.

Makes 1 serving (1 cup/250 mL)

Chia seeds are an excellent low-carb alternative to grain cereals. Ground chia, compared to whole chia, makes the most smooth textured pudding. Let the pudding set overnight so it's ready for breakfast the next morning. Before eating, add nuts and fruit as listed in the menu below. 2 tbsp (30 mL) of dried fruit has the same carbs as the half banana.

¼ cup (60 mL) chia (chia seeds), whole or ground

1 cup (250 mL) almond beverage, unsweetened

2 tsp (10 mL) sugar or regular syrup*

1. In a wide-mouthed glass jar (Mason jar), add chia seeds, almond beverage and sugar, and mix together with a spoon. Put the lid on, and leave on the counter for 10 minutes – set the timer!
2. After 10 minutes, give the jar a good shake, until there are no lumps in the pudding.
3. Refrigerate overnight to set.

* Note: Light syrup is not used, as it prevents the pudding from setting properly.

1 SERVING	
Calories	299
Total carbs	33 g
Net carbs	16 g

YOUR BREAKFAST MENU	Large Meal (370 calories)	Total Carbs	NET CARBS	Small Meal (250 calories)	Total Carbs	NET CARBS
Cereal – All-Bran Flakes	1 cup (250 mL)	25	21	⅔ cup (150 mL)	17	14
Skim or 1% milk	¾ cup (175 mL)	9	9	½ cup (125 mL)	6	6
Banana	½ medium	12	11	½ medium	12	11
Sliced almonds or other nuts	¼ cup (60 mL)	5	2	¼ cup (60 mL)	3	1
	TOTAL CARBS	**51 g**	**43 g**	TOTAL CARBS	**38 g**	**32 g**
	Total carbs minus fiber = NET CARBS ↑			NET CARBS ↑		
	CARB CHOICES (1 carb choice = 15 g net carbs)		3	CARB CHOICES		2

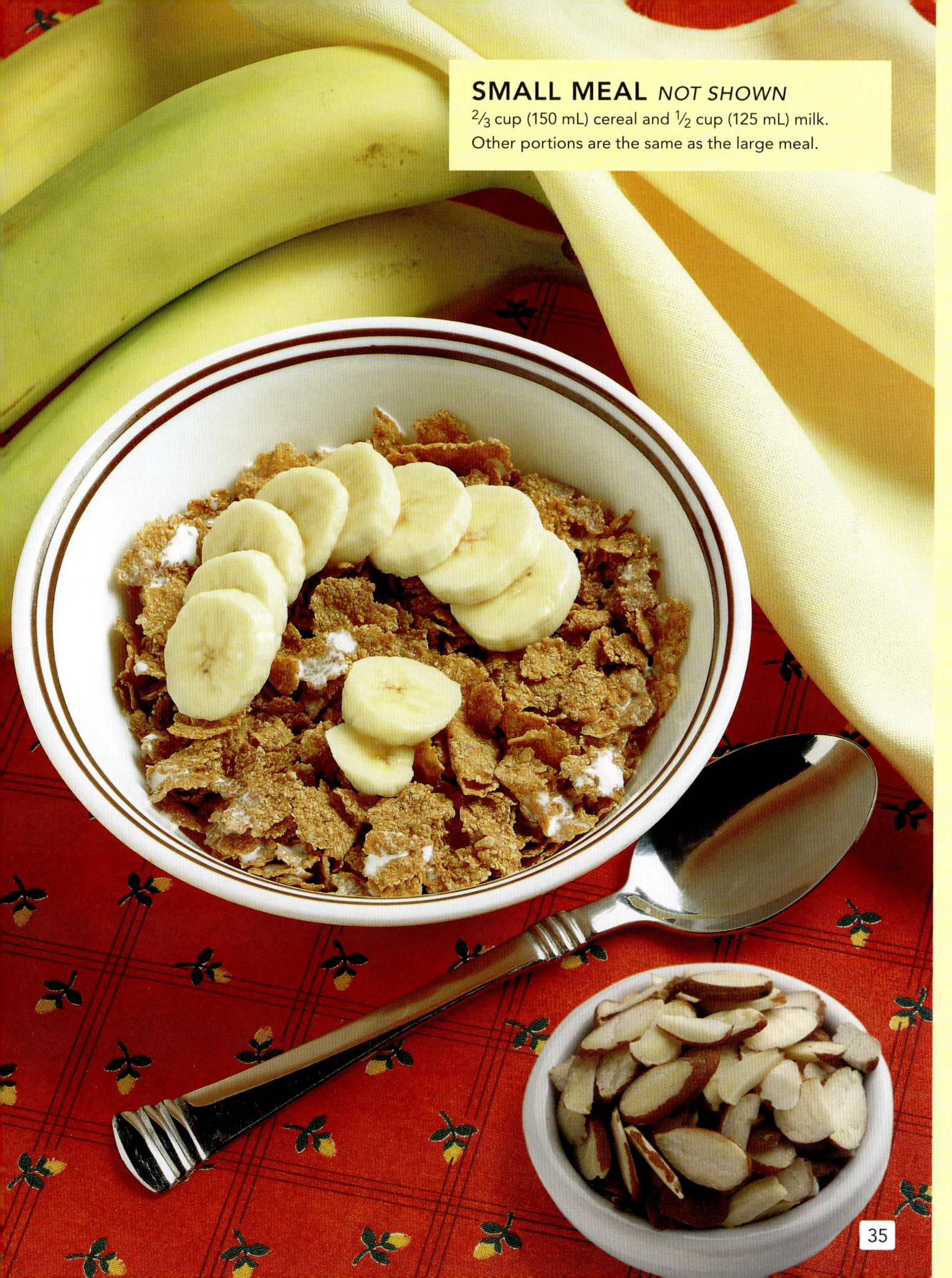

SMALL MEAL *NOT SHOWN*
2/3 cup (150 mL) cereal and 1/2 cup (125 mL) milk. Other portions are the same as the large meal.

BREAKFAST MEALS

BREAKFAST 2

Egg & Toast

Every morning, we need nutritious food to feed our brain. The brain consumes about a quarter of the calories that we need in a day, so we know breakfast is the best start for brain function.

Soft boil or poach the egg in a nonstick pan, which requires no fat in the cooking. If you prefer to fry the egg in fat, then have the toast unbuttered.

Large eggs and small eggs have similar-sized yolks and a similar amount of cholesterol. The difference is that large eggs have more egg white – so buy the large eggs.

When it comes to choosing your bread, check the label for a slice of bread that has less than 70 calories and 16 grams of carbohydrate per slice. Good choices are whole-grain, whole wheat and rye bread.

⭕ LOW-CARB SWAP

LARGE MEAL

Swap the second piece of toast with margarine and jam:
18 g net carbs

→ For half a medium avocado:
2 g net carbs

See Bread Swaps, page 274.

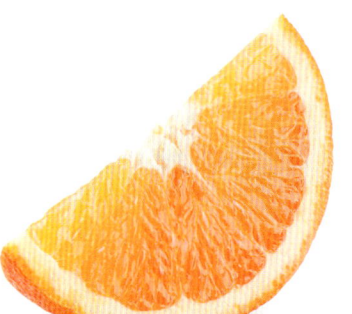

HEALTH TIP

Limit Juice

Because juice is liquid, it's very easy to drink too much. Juice raises your blood sugar very quickly.

Most days, eat fruit rather than drink fruit.

Fresh whole fruit has fiber, and juice has virtually none. So, whole fruit is more nutritious and more filling.

YOUR BREAKFAST MENU	Large Meal (370 calories)	Total Carbs	NET CARBS	Small Meal (250 calories)	Total Carbs	NET CARBS
Egg (cooked without fat)	1 large egg	0	0	1 large egg	0	0
Whole-grain or whole wheat toast	2 slices	32	27	1 slice	16	13
Margarine/butter	1 tsp (5 mL)	0	0	1 tsp (5 mL)	0	0
Jam or jelly	1 tsp (5 mL)	5	5	—	—	—
Skim or 1% milk	½ cup (125 mL)	6	6	½ cup (125 mL)	6	6
Orange slices	½ medium orange	8	7	½ medium orange	8	7
	TOTAL CARBS	**51 g**	**45 g**	TOTAL CARBS	**30 g**	**26 g**
	Total carbs minus fiber = NET CARBS ↑			NET CARBS ↑		
	CARB CHOICES (1 carb choice = 15 g net carbs)		3	CARB CHOICES		2

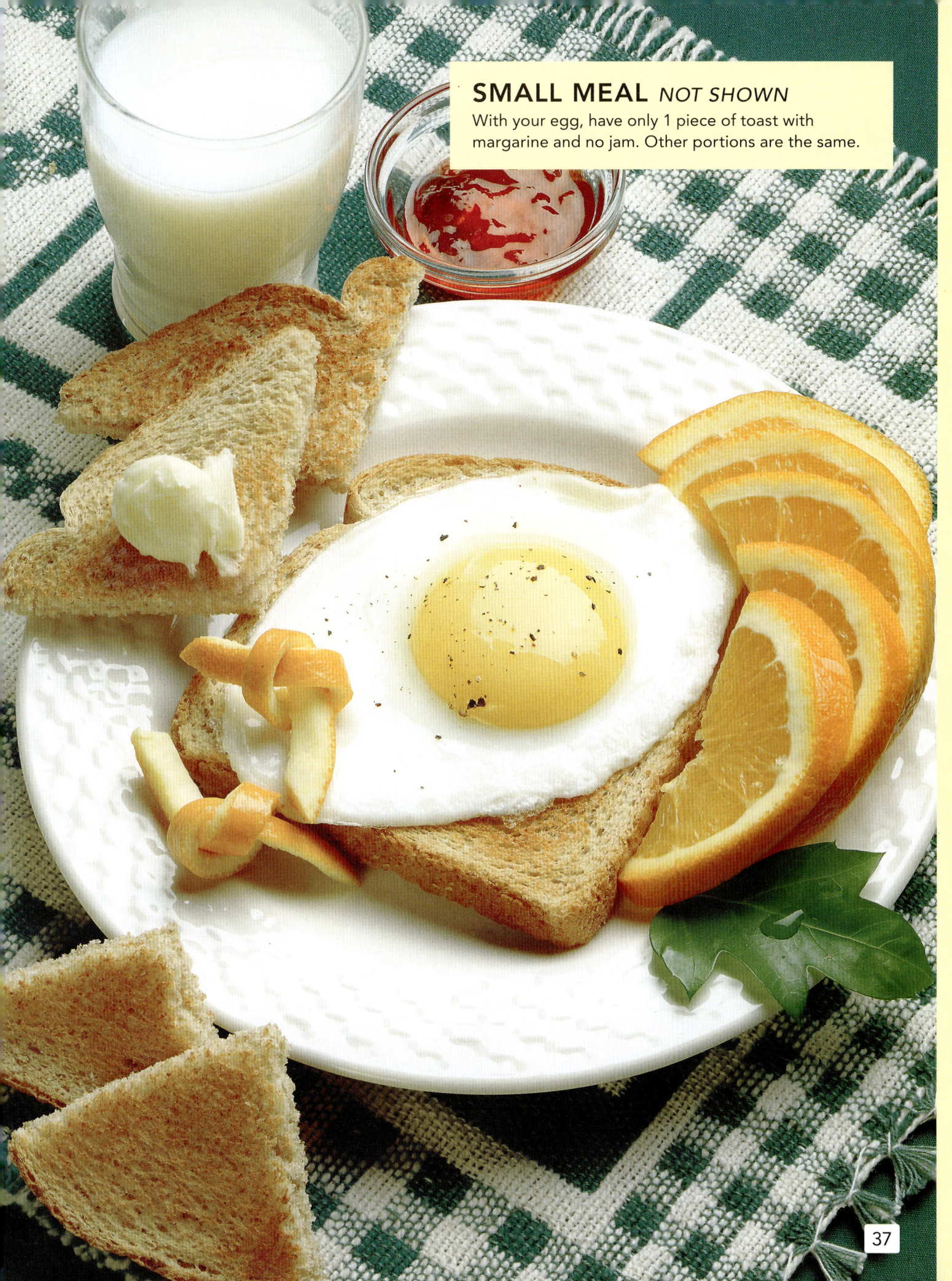

SMALL MEAL *NOT SHOWN*
With your egg, have only 1 piece of toast with margarine and no jam. Other portions are the same.

BREAKFAST MEALS

BREAKFAST 3

🔴 LOW-CARB SWAP

Swap 1 Protein-Power Pancake:

8 g net carbs

→ For 1 Protein-Power Pancake made with ½ cup (125 mL) almond flour and ½ cup (125 mL) regular flour in the recipe:

5 g net carbs

See Flour Swaps, page 27.

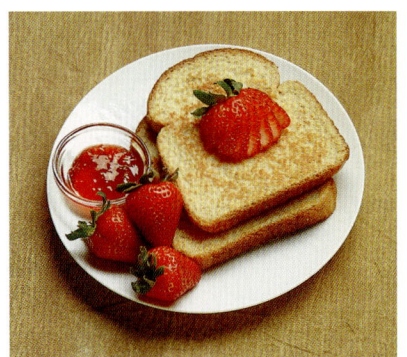

Pancakes & Bacon

Protein-Power Pancakes

Makes fourteen 4-inch (10 cm) pancakes

1 cup (250 mL) flour
½ tsp (2 mL) salt
1 tsp (5 mL) baking powder
1 tbsp (15 mL) sugar
3 large eggs
2 tbsp (30 mL) oil, margarine or butter, melted
1¼ cups (300 mL) skim milk
½ tsp (2 mL) vanilla

PER PANCAKE	
Calories	76
Carbohydrate	8 g
Fiber	0 g
Net Carbs	8 g
Protein	3 g
Fat, total	3 g
Fat, saturated	1 g
Cholesterol	40 g
Sodium	110 mg

1. In a large bowl, mix together flour, salt, baking powder and sugar.
2. In a medium bowl, beat eggs with a fork. Add the fat, milk and vanilla to egg, and mix well.
3. Add egg mixture to the flour mixture. Stir until smooth. It helps to stir with a wire whisk. If it is too thick, add a little more milk.
4. In a greased nonstick pan or griddle, cook on medium heat. Use just under ¼ cup (60 mL) of batter for each pancake. Once the pancakes have small bubbles, turn them over.

French toast instead of pancakes

Also boost the protein of your French toast. Use three large eggs and ¼ cup (60 mL) of milk for three slices of bread. Have two slices of French toast for the large meal and one slice for the small meal.

YOUR BREAKFAST MENU	Large Meal (370 calories)	Total Carbs	NET CARBS	Small Meal (250 calories)	Total Carbs	NET CARBS
Protein-Power Pancakes	3 pancakes	25	24	2 pancakes	17	16
Light syrup (40% less sugar), see page 29	3 tbsp (45 mL)	7	7	3 tbsp (45 mL)	7	7
Bacon, crisp strips	2 strips	0	0	1½ strips	0	0
	TOTAL CARBS	**32 g**	**31 g**	TOTAL CARBS	**24 g**	**23 g**
	Total carbs minus fiber = NET CARBS ↑			NET CARBS ↑		
	CARB CHOICES (1 carb choice = 15 g net carbs)		2	CARB CHOICES		2

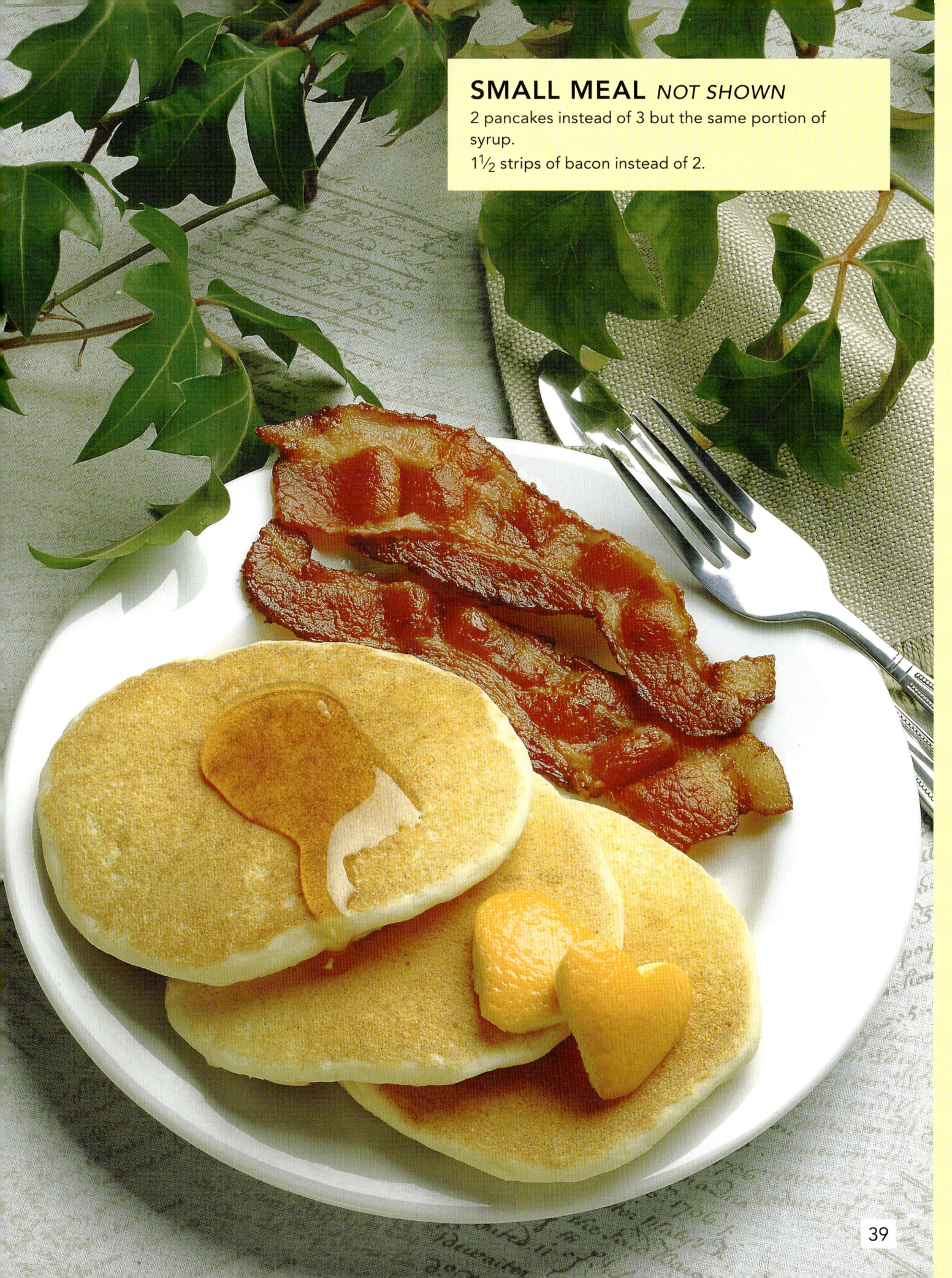

SMALL MEAL *NOT SHOWN*
2 pancakes instead of 3 but the same portion of syrup.
1½ strips of bacon instead of 2.

BREAKFAST MEALS

BREAKFAST 4

Toast & Peanut Butter

○ LOW-CARB SWAP

Swap regular jam:
1 tsp (5 mL)
5 g net carbs

→ For light cream cheese:
½ tbsp (7 mL)
0 g net carbs

HEALTH TIP

Did you know? Jams marked "no sugar added" can have the same amount of carbohydrate as regular jam. Sugar is often added as concentrated fruit juice.

Check labels and choose light jam that has fewer than 10 calories per 1 tsp (5 mL). This would be the same as 30 calories per 1 tbsp (15 mL).

1 tsp (5 mL) of regular jam = 2 tsp (10 mL) of light jam or jelly

Eating breakfast can help improve your blood sugar throughout the day. The breakfast meals in this cookbook have 3 carb choices or less, balanced with protein and fat.

Peanut butter is both a protein and a fat for this breakfast meal.

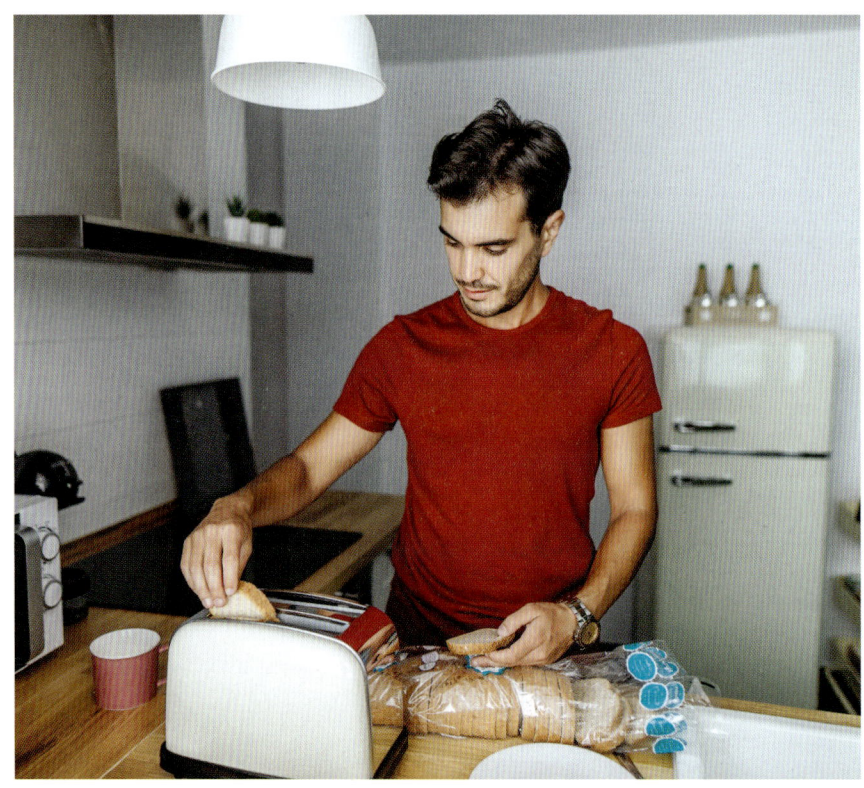

YOUR BREAKFAST MENU	Large Meal (370 calories)	Total Carbs	NET CARBS	Small Meal (250 calories)	Total Carbs	NET CARBS
Whole-grain or whole wheat toast	2 slices	32	27	1 slice	16	13
Peanut butter	1 tbsp (15 mL)	3	2	1 tbsp (15 mL)	3	2
Margarine	1 tsp (5 mL)	0	0	—	—	—
Jam or jelly	1 tsp (5 mL) regular jam, or 2 tsp (10 mL) light jam	5	5	—	—	—
Almond beverage	½ cup (125 mL)	1	1	½ cup (125 mL)	1	1
Apple slices	½ medium apple	11	10	½ medium apple	11	10
	TOTAL CARBS	52 g	45 g	TOTAL CARBS	31 g	26 g
	Total carbs minus fiber = NET CARBS ↑			NET CARBS ↑		
	CARB CHOICES (1 carb choice = 15 g net carbs)		3	CARB CHOICES		2

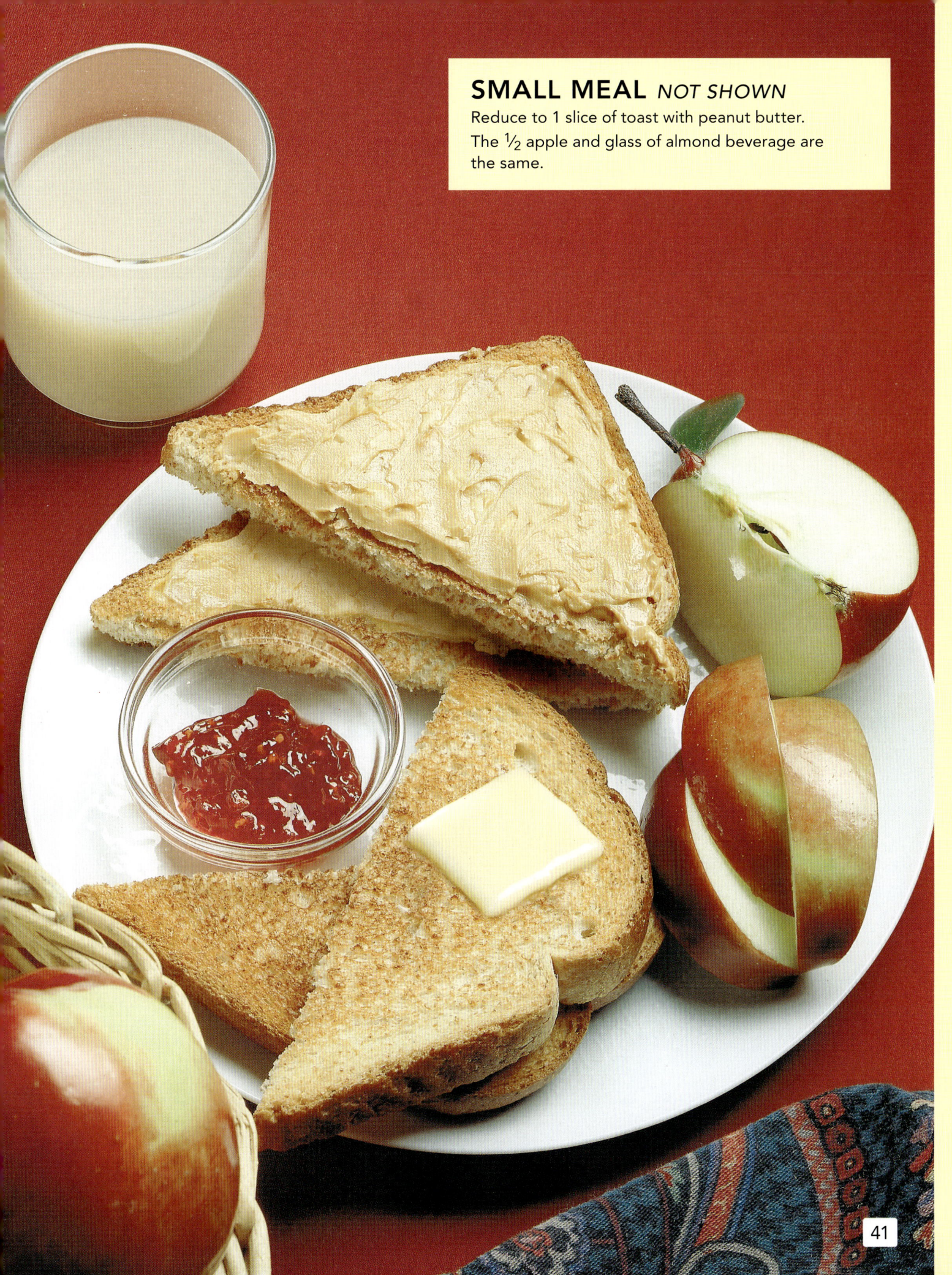

SMALL MEAL *NOT SHOWN*
Reduce to 1 slice of toast with peanut butter. The ½ apple and glass of almond beverage are the same.

BREAKFAST MEALS

BREAKFAST

Spinach & Eggs

Spinach & Eggs

2-egg serving

¼ cup (60 mL) water
2 cups (500 mL) fresh spinach leaves
2 large eggs

1. Pour water into a small nonstick frying pan. Once water is simmering, place spinach in the pan and cover with a lid for 1 minute, until spinach is wilted. Add water if needed to keep spinach moist.
2. Break eggs on top of spinach and cover again with the lid. Let eggs steam for 2 to 3 minutes until they are cooked to your liking.

PER SERVING	
Calories	160
Carbohydrate	3 g
Fiber	1 g
Net Carbs	2 g
Protein	14 g
Fat, total	10 g
Fat, saturated	3 g
Cholesterol	372 mg
Sodium	136 mg

○ LOW-CARB SWAP

There is no swap for this meal as it is only 1 carb for both the large and small meal.

HEALTH TIP

Choose your greens!
Instead of spinach, try arugula, beet tops or kale. If using whole kale, cut out the rough stems.

Fresh Salsa

Makes 1 cup (250 mL)

1 large tomato, finely chopped
2 tbsp (30 mL) fresh cilantro, finely chopped
2 tsp (10 mL) olive oil
1 tbsp (15 mL) onion, finely chopped
⅛ tsp (0.5 mL) salt
¼ tsp (1 mL) black pepper
Juice of 1 lime (or 2 tbsp/30 mL bottled)
Few dashes of hot pepper sauce or ¼ jalapeno pepper, finely chopped

1. In a bowl, combine all ingredients.

PER ¼ CUP (60 ML) SALSA	
Calories	31
Carbohydrate	2 g
Fiber	1 g
Net Carbs	1 g
Protein	1 g
Fat, total	2 g
Fat, saturated	0 g
Cholesterol	0 g
Sodium	76 mg

Cover and refrigerate leftover salsa for up to 3 days.

YOUR BREAKFAST MENU	Large Meal (370 calories)	Total Carbs	NET CARBS	Small Meal (250 calories)	Total Carbs	NET CARBS
Spinach & Eggs	2-egg serving	3	2	2-egg serving	3	2
Whole-grain toast (38 g slice)	1 slice	14	12	1 slice	14	12
Margarine or butter	1 tsp (5 mL)	0	0	—	—	—
Fresh Salsa (or store-bought salsa)	¼ cup (60 mL) (2 tbsp/30 mL if store-bought)	2	1	¼ cup (60 mL) (2 tbsp/30 mL if store-bought)	2	1
Avocado	⅓ medium	4	1	—	—	—
	TOTAL CARBS	23 g	16 g	TOTAL CARBS	19 g	15 g
	Total carbs minus fiber = NET CARBS ↑			NET CARBS ↑		
	CARB CHOICES (1 carb choice = 15 g net carbs)		1	CARB CHOICES		1

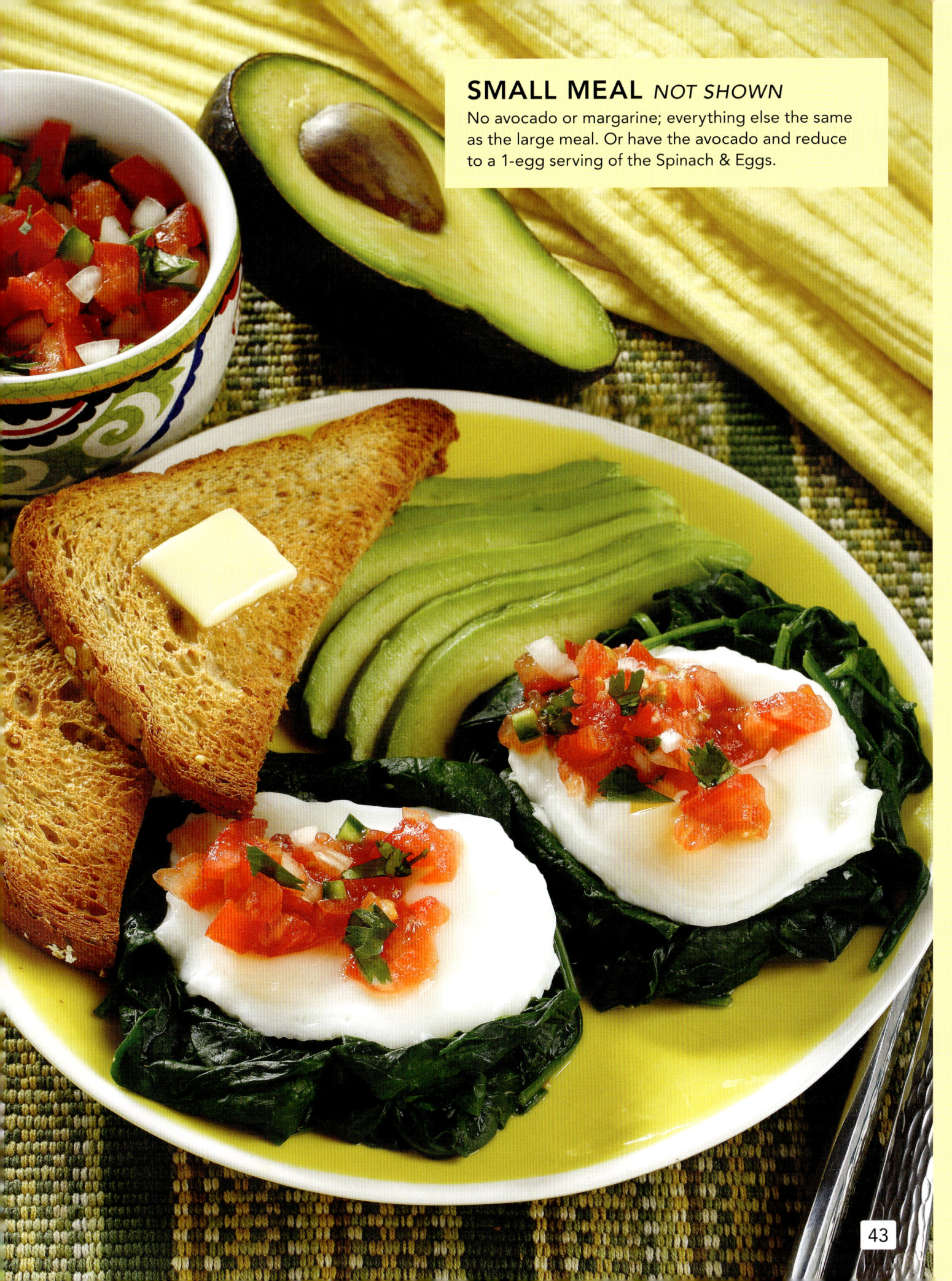

SMALL MEAL *NOT SHOWN*
No avocado or margarine; everything else the same as the large meal. Or have the avocado and reduce to a 1-egg serving of the Spinach & Eggs.

BREAKFAST MEALS

BREAKFAST 6

Muffin & Cheese

Bran Muffins

Makes 12 medium muffins

Preheat oven to 400°F (200°C)

½ cup (125 mL) flour
½ cup (125 mL) ground flaxseed
1½ tsp (7 mL) baking powder
½ tsp (2 mL) baking soda
½ tsp (2 mL) salt
¼ cup (60 mL) unsweetened applesauce
2 tbsp (30 mL) vegetable oil
¼ cup (60 mL) packed brown sugar
¼ cup (60 mL) molasses (or honey)
1 large egg
1 cup (250 mL) skim milk
1 cup (250 mL) wheat bran
½ cup (125 mL) raisins

PER MUFFIN	
Calories	148
Carbohydrate	24 g
Fiber	4 g
Net Carbs	20 g
Protein	4 g
Fat, total	5 g
Fat, saturated	1 g
Cholesterol	18 mg
Sodium	170 mg

1. In a medium bowl, mix flour, ground flaxseed, baking powder, baking soda and salt together.
2. In a large bowl, combine applesauce, oil, brown sugar, molasses and egg. Stir with a wooden spoon until well mixed.
3. Add milk, then add wheat bran to the large bowl.
4. Add flour mixture to the large bowl. Then add raisins. The mixture will be wet.
5. Spoon into a greased nonstick muffin tin. Bake in oven for 20 to 25 minutes. They are ready when a toothpick put into the center of a muffin comes out clean.

◯ LOW-CARB SWAP

LARGE MEAL

Swap Greek yogurt:
½ cup (125 mL)
5 g net carbs

→ For extra cheese: an extra ½ oz (15 g)
0 g net carbs

See Yogurt Swaps, page 278.

RECIPE TIP
HOMEMADE DIET YOGURT

Into plain unsweetened yogurt, blend Crystal Light or Diet Kool-Aid to taste. This adds no extra carbs or calories.

YOUR BREAKFAST MENU	Large Meal (370 calories)	Total Carbs	NET CARBS	Small Meal (250 calories)	Total Carbs	NET CARBS
Bran Muffin	1	24	20	1	24	20
Piece of cheese	1 oz (30 g)	0	0	¾ oz (23 g)	0	0
Greek yogurt, 0 to 2%, flavored, less sugar	½ cup (125 mL)	6	5	—	—	—
Orange	½ medium	8	7	½ medium	8	7
	TOTAL CARBS	38 g	32 g	TOTAL CARBS	32 g	27 g
	Total carbs minus fiber = NET CARBS ↑			NET CARBS ↑		
	CARB CHOICES (1 carb choice = 15 g net carbs)		2	CARB CHOICES		2

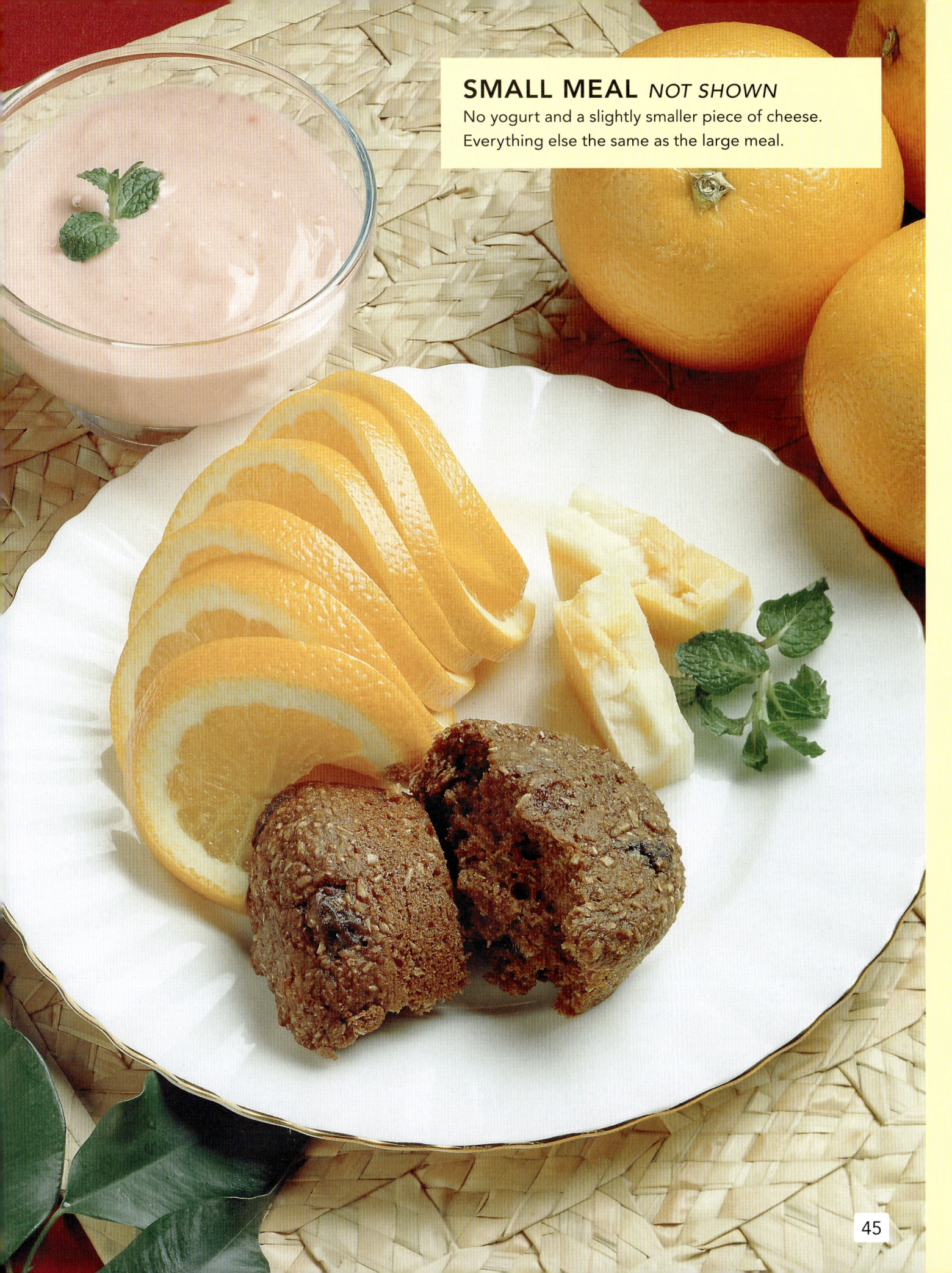

SMALL MEAL *NOT SHOWN*
No yogurt and a slightly smaller piece of cheese. Everything else the same as the large meal.

BREAKFAST MEALS

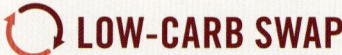

BREAKFAST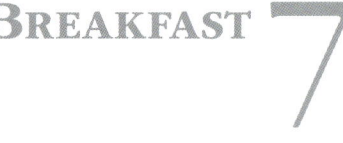

Raisin Toast & Fruit

Choose raisin bread that has 70 calories or less per slice. Or replace two slices of raisin bread with one raisin scone or one hot cross bun.

Grapefruit Treat

Here's a great way to eat half a grapefruit. Sprinkle it with cinnamon or nutmeg and sugar or zero-calorie sweetener, and warm it up for 30 seconds in the microwave.

Grapefruit interactions with some medications

If you are on a cholesterol medication such as a statin that recommends you avoid or limit grapefruit, choose another fruit serving.

Here are a few examples of other fruit servings with similar net carbs. Each of these fruit servings is equal to 1 Carb Choice (see page 10):

- ½ cup (125 mL) unsweetened applesauce
- 2 medium kiwis
- 1 small or ½ large banana
- 1 cup (250 mL) blueberries
- 15 cherries
- 3 guava
- ½ medium mango
- 1 large peach
- 2 medium plums
- 1 cup (250 mL) melon

◯ LOW-CARB SWAP

Swap raisin toast:
1 piece
12 g net carbs

→ For low-carb bread (may also be called keto bread), sprinkled with cinnamon and zero-calorie sweetener:
1 slice
1 to 4 g net carbs

See Bread Swaps, page 274.

WHAT IS LOW-CARB BREAD?

It is a dense bread and may contain flaxseed, nuts or seeds, chickpea flour or almond flour. Check the carbs on the label.

YOUR BREAKFAST MENU	Large Meal (370 calories)	Total Carbs	NET CARBS	Small Meal (250 calories)	Total Carbs	NET CARBS
Raisin toast	2 slices	27	25	1 slice	13	12
Margarine or butter	1½ tsp (7 mL)	0	0	1 tsp (5 mL)	0	0
Jam or jelly	1 tsp (5 mL)	5	5	—	—	—
Gouda cheese	2 cheeses = 1½ oz (40 g)	0	0	1½ cheeses = 1 oz (30 g)	0	0
Grapefruit	½ small	10	8	½ small	10	8
	TOTAL CARBS	**42 g**	**38 g**	TOTAL CARBS	**23 g**	**20 g**
	Total carbs minus fiber = NET CARBS ↑			NET CARBS ↑		
	CARB CHOICES (1 carb choice = 15 g net carbs)		3	CARB CHOICES		1

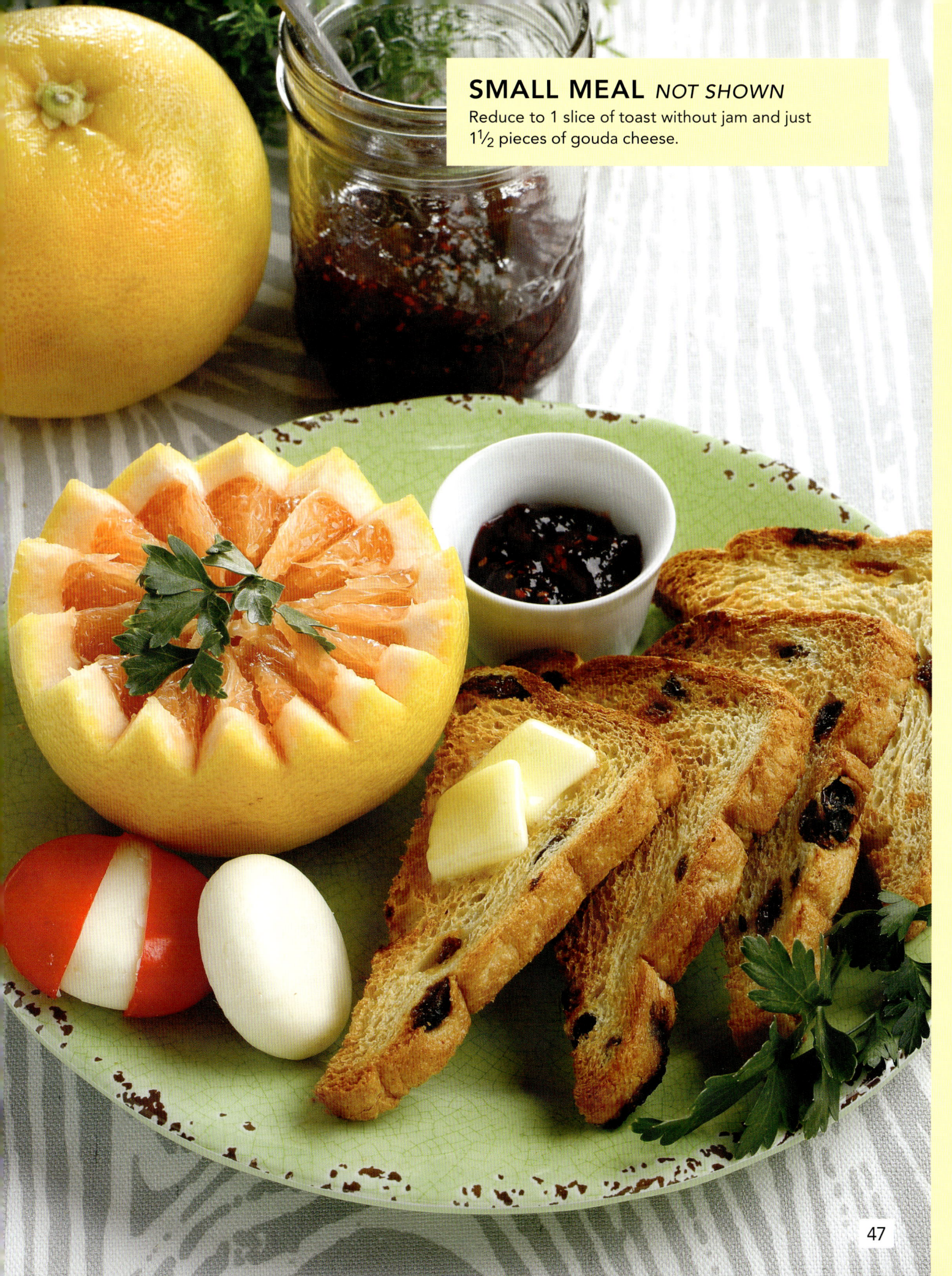

SMALL MEAL *NOT SHOWN*
Reduce to 1 slice of toast without jam and just 1½ pieces of gouda cheese.

BREAKFAST MEALS

BREAKFAST 8

Tuna Scramble

Tuna Scramble

2 large or 3 small servings

- 1 tbsp (15 mL) butter, margarine or oil
- 1 medium 3-inch (7.5 cm) precooked potato, chopped
- 4 green onions, chopped
- 2 tbsp (30 mL) bell pepper, finely chopped
- 2 large eggs
- 1 can of tuna (5 oz/213 g) or ½ can of salmon, drained
- ¼ cup (60 mL) Cheddar cheese, shredded
- Salt and pepper to taste

PER LARGE SERVING	
Calories	342
Carbohydrate	17 g
Fiber	2 g
Net Carbs	15 g
Protein	30 g
Fat, total	16 g
Fat, saturated	8 g
Cholesterol	276 mg
Sodium	359 mg

1. In a nonstick frying pan, melt fat at medium heat.
2. Add potato, green onions and bell pepper and cook until potatoes are lightly browned.
3. In a small bowl, beat eggs with a fork. Mix in tuna and cheese.
4. Add egg mixture to the pan with the vegetables and stir until cooked.

Arugula Salad

1 serving

Over ½ cup (125 mL) of arugula, drizzle a teaspoon (5 mL) of oil and vinegar.

LOW-CARB SWAP

There is no swap for this meal as it is only 1 carb for both the large and small meal.

RECIPE TIP

Quick and easy cooked potatoes for Tuna Scramble

Poke a potato with a fork and microwave for a couple of minutes.

RECIPE TIP

Tuna Scramble without the tuna?

Omit the tuna and use four eggs. This recipe will still make enough for two large meals.

Drink water with all your meals, including breakfast.

YOUR BREAKFAST MENU	Large Meal (370 calories)	Total Carbs	NET CARBS	Small Meal (250 calories)	Total Carbs	NET CARBS
Tuna Scramble	½ of recipe	17	15	⅓ of recipe	11	10
Arugula Salad	1 serving	1	1	1 serving	1	1
Cherry tomatoes (or a couple of tomato slices)	3	1	1	3	1	1
	TOTAL CARBS	19 g	17 g	TOTAL CARBS	13 g	12 g
	Total carbs minus fiber = NET CARBS ↑			NET CARBS ↑		
CARB CHOICES (1 carb choice = 15 g net carbs)		1		CARB CHOICES		1

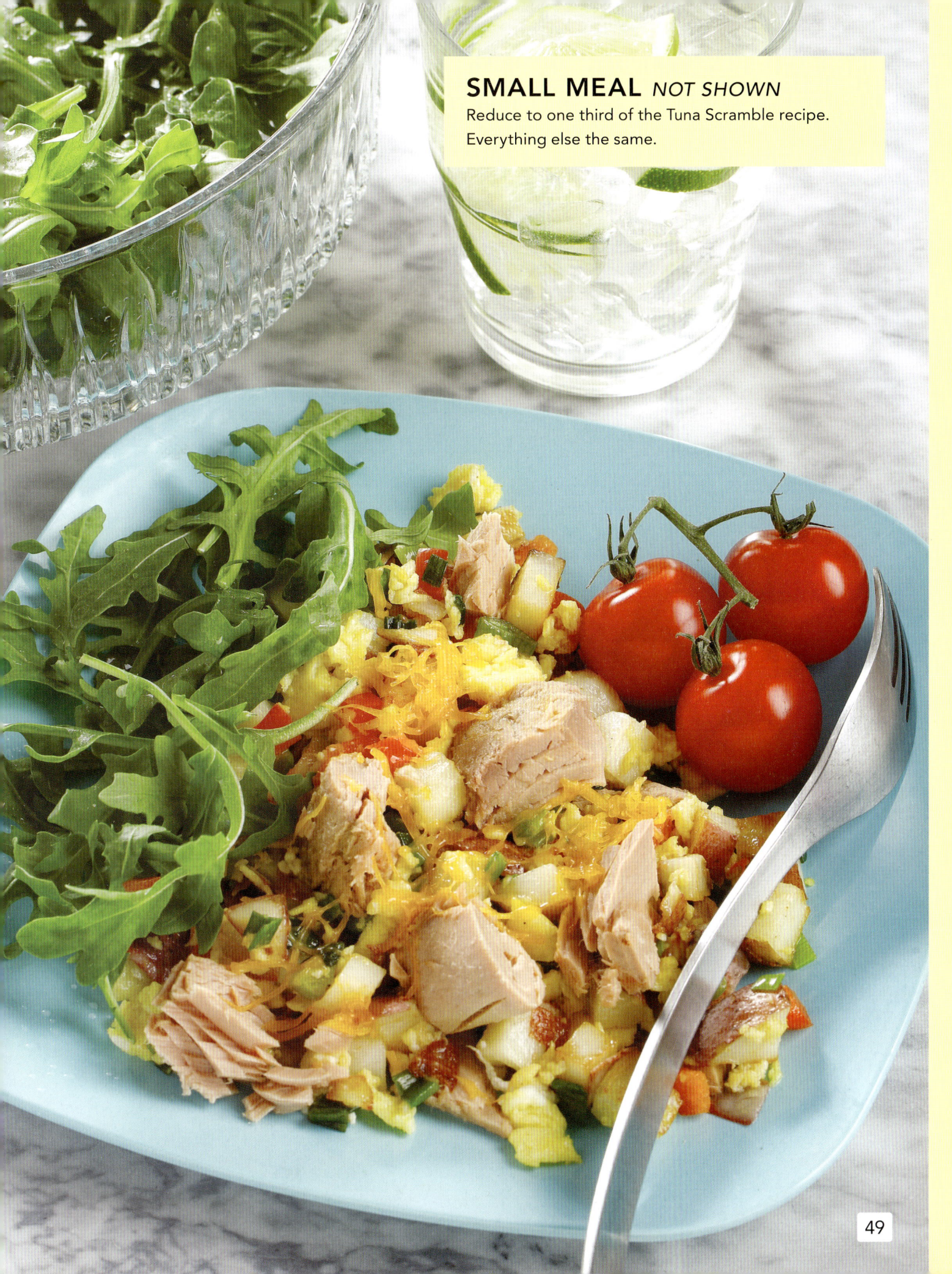

SMALL MEAL *NOT SHOWN*
Reduce to one third of the Tuna Scramble recipe. Everything else the same.

BREAKFAST MEALS

BREAKFAST 9

Homemade Waffles

The number of waffles this recipe makes will depend on the size and shape of your waffle iron. One cup (250 mL) of batter will make four 4-inch (10 cm) waffles or, if you have a 7-inch (18 cm) round waffle iron, two larger waffles.

LOW-CARB SWAP

Swap 1 Homemade waffle:
7 g net carbs
→ For 1 Chaffle:
1 g net carbs
(but double the calories)

See Chaffle recipe on page 259.

HEALTH TIP

Store-bought frozen 4-inch (10 cm) waffles
These waffles have more carbohydrate and less protein than this Homemade Waffle. Two store-bought ones will have **25 g net carbs**.

Low-Carb Homemade Waffle

Makes 1 cup (250 mL) of batter, enough for four 4-inch (10 cm) square waffles

2 tbsp (30 mL) flour
¼ cup (60 mL) skim milk powder
1 tsp (5 mL) baking powder
Dash of salt
⅛ tsp (0.5 mL) nutmeg
2 large eggs
3 tbsp (45 mL) Greek yogurt, 0–2%

1. In a medium bowl, whisk together all ingredients until smooth.
2. Cook the batter according to your waffle iron directions, until lightly browned. Use a well-oiled hot waffle iron.

PER ¼ CUP (60 ML) BATTER (1 SQUARE WAFFLE)	
Calories	81
Carbohydrate	7 g
Fiber	0 g
Net Carbs	7 g
Protein	7 g
Fat, total	3 g
Fat, saturated	1 g
Cholesterol	95 mg
Sodium	167 mg

Extra cooked waffles can be frozen and later reheated from frozen in the toaster.

YOUR BREAKFAST MENU	Large Meal (370 calories)	Total Carbs	NET CARBS	Small Meal (250 calories)	Total Carbs	NET CARBS
Homemade Waffles	Two 4-inch (10 cm)	14	14	Two 4-inch (10 cm)	14	14
Margarine or butter	1 tsp (5 mL)	0	0	—	—	—
Syrup, light (40% less sugar)	3 tbsp (45 mL)	7	7	1½ tbsp (22 mL)	3	3
Berries	½ cup (125 mL)	9	7	½ cup (125 mL)	9	7
Chopped nuts, raw or toasted	2 tbsp (30 mL)	4	2	1 tbsp (15 mL)	2	1
Tea or coffee with single milk, low-calorie sweetener	1 cup (250 mL)	1	1	1 cup (250 mL)	1	1
	TOTAL CARBS	**35 g**	**31 g**	TOTAL CARBS	**29 g**	**26 g**
	Total carbs minus fiber = NET CARBS ↑			NET CARBS ↑		
CARB CHOICES (1 carb choice = 15 g net carbs)		2		CARB CHOICES		2

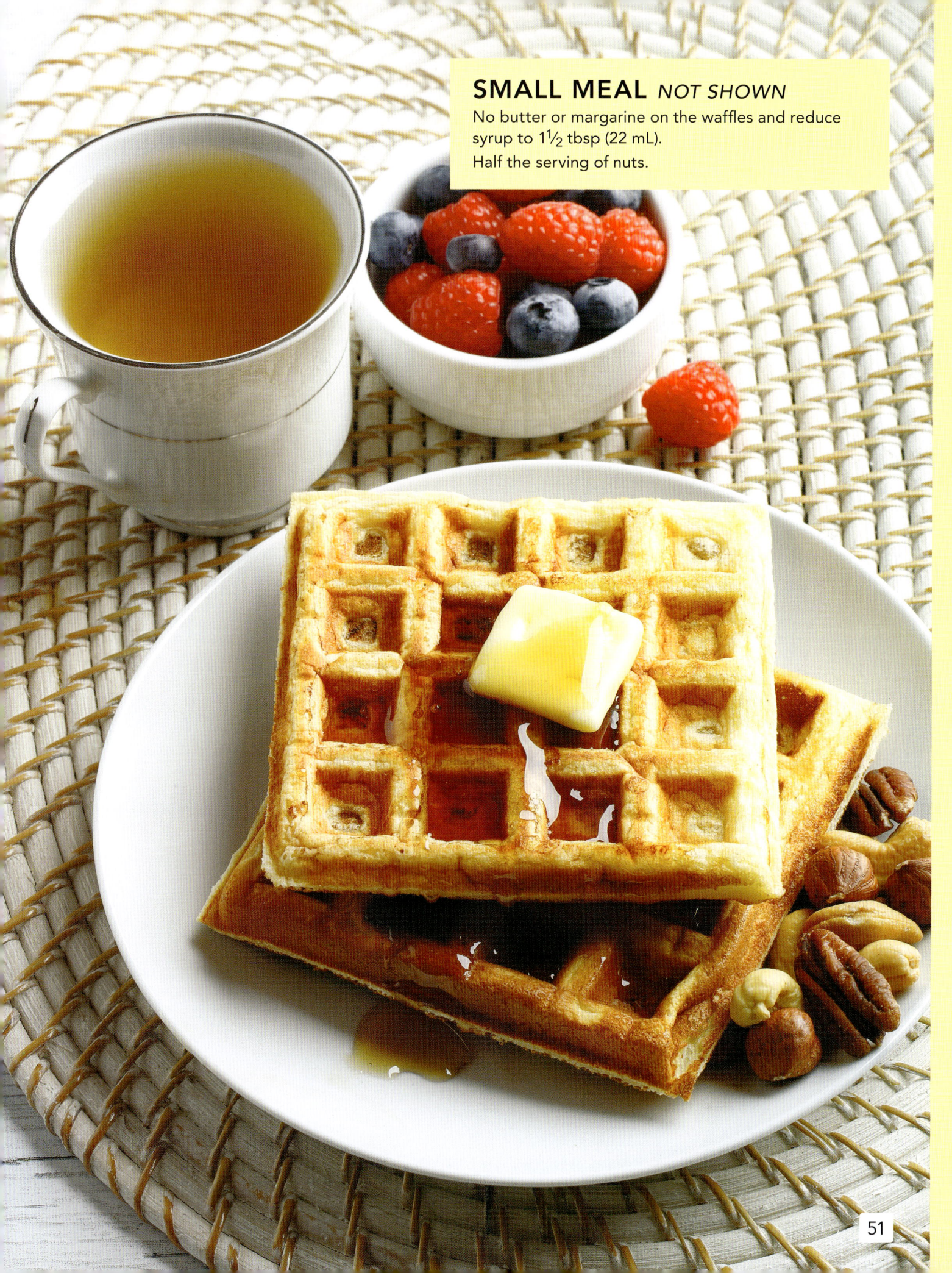

SMALL MEAL *NOT SHOWN*
No butter or margarine on the waffles and reduce syrup to 1½ tbsp (22 mL).
Half the serving of nuts.

BREAKFAST MEALS

BREAKFAST 10 Smoothie & Protein Bar

To go with your smoothie, choose a high-protein (low-carb) bar. See Snack Bar Swaps on page 280.

🔄 LOW-CARB SWAP

Swap high-protein snack bar:
40 g (1.4 oz) bar
10 g net carbs
→ For 80% dark chocolate:
25 g (¾ oz) piece
4 g net carbs

See Snack Bar Swaps, page 280, and Candy Swaps, page 281.

HEALTH TIP

Benefits of soy
Tofu is made from soybeans, which are high in protein. Soybeans contain natural compounds called isoflavones; these can help reduce bad LDL cholesterol and increase good HDL cholesterol.

See page 268 for information about reading a yogurt label.

Tofu Fruit Smoothie
Makes 2 cups (500 mL)

⅔ cup (150 mL) soft or silken tofu

½ cup (125 mL) Greek yogurt, 0–2%, flavored, less sugar

½ cup (125 mL) almond beverage, unsweetened

2 peach halves (fresh or canned, juice-packed) or ½ small banana

1. Place all ingredients in a blender and blend until smooth.

PER 1 CUP (250 ML)	
Calories	97
Carbohydrate	9 g
Fiber	2 g
Net Carbs	7 g
Protein	9 g
Fat, total	3 g
Fat, saturated	0 g
Cholesterol	3 mg
Sodium	70 mg

Spinach Fruit Smoothie
Makes 2 cups (500 mL)

½ cup (125 mL) Greek yogurt, 0–2%, flavored, less sugar

½ cup (125 mL) almond beverage, unsweetened

3 tbsp (45 mL) skim milk powder

½ cup (125 mL) raw spinach or other greens, packed

2 peach halves (fresh or canned, juice-packed) or ½ small banana

1 tsp (5 mL) honey

Dash of cinnamon

1. Place all ingredients in a blender and blend until smooth.

PER 1 CUP (250 ML)	
Calories	94
Carbohydrate	15 g
Fiber	2 g
Net Carbs	13 g
Protein	7 g
Fat, total	1 g
Fat, saturated	0 g
Cholesterol	4 mg
Sodium	108 mg

YOUR BREAKFAST MENU	Large Meal (370 calories)	Total Carbs	NET CARBS	Small Meal (250 calories)	Total Carbs	NET CARBS
Tofu Fruit Smoothie or Spinach Fruit Smoothie	2 cups (500 mL)	28	25	1 cup (250 mL)	14	13
High-protein bar (1.4 oz/40 g); 150–170 calories	1 bar	17	10	1 bar	17	10
	TOTAL CARBS	**45 g**	**35 g**	TOTAL CARBS	**31 g**	**23 g**
	Total carbs minus fiber = NET CARBS ↑			NET CARBS ↑		
	CARB CHOICES (1 carb choice = 15 g net carbs)		2	CARB CHOICES		2

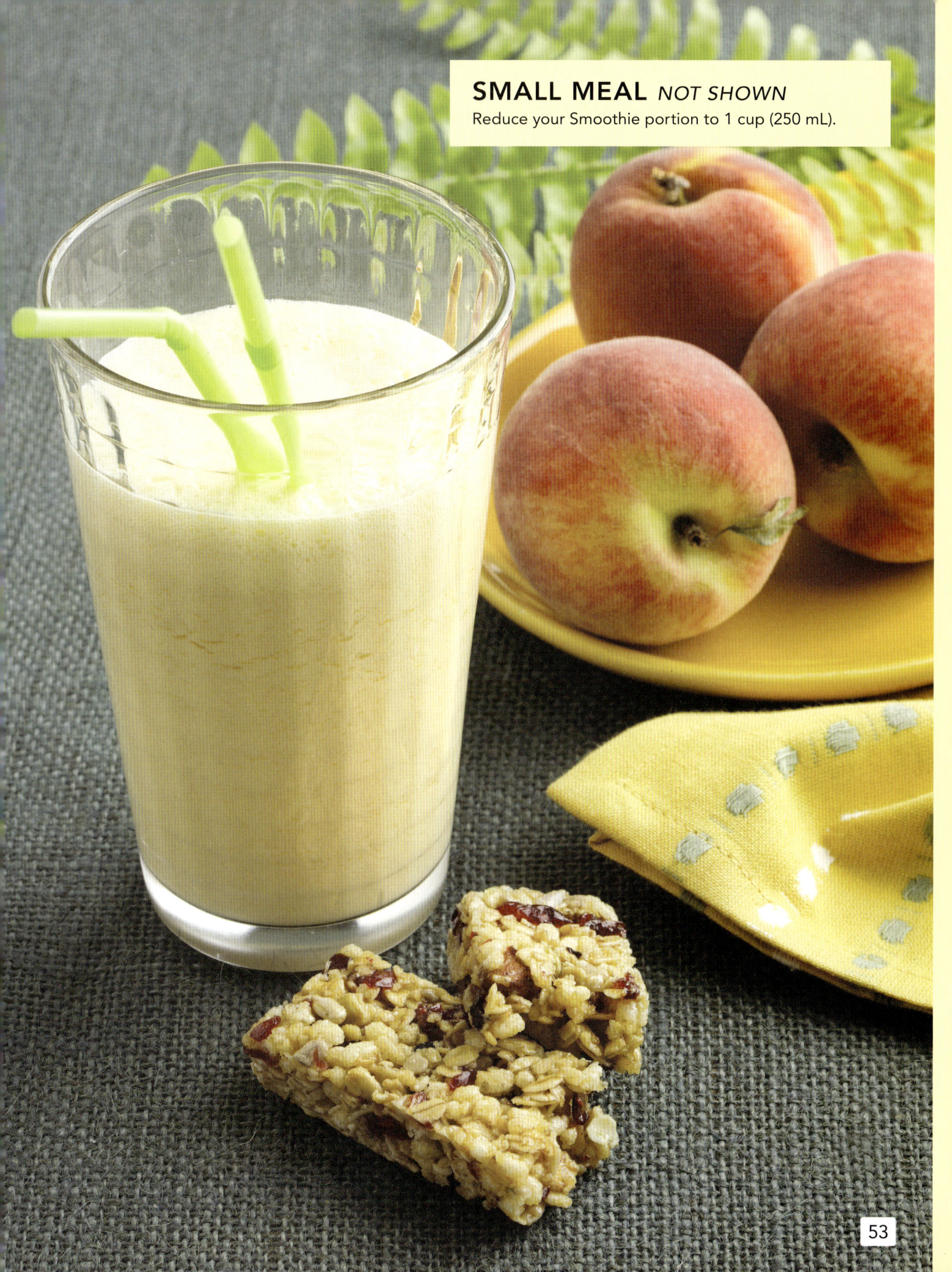

SMALL MEAL *NOT SHOWN*
Reduce your Smoothie portion to 1 cup (250 mL).

BREAKFAST MEALS

BREAKFAST 11

Fiesta Breakfast

Mexican Rice & Beans

Makes just over 2 cups (500 mL)

- 2 tsp (10 mL) olive oil or vegetable oil
- 1 small onion, finely chopped
- 3 cloves garlic, minced
- ½ tsp (2 mL) ground cumin
- ½ tsp (2 mL) dried oregano
- 1 tbsp (15 mL) fresh cilantro, chopped
- ¼ tsp (1 mL) hot pepper flakes
- 1 cup (250 mL) canned black beans, rinsed and drained
- 1 cup (250 mL) long-grain cooked (leftover) rice

1. Add oil to frying pan and heat to sizzling. Then add onions, garlic, cumin, oregano, cilantro and hot pepper flakes. Cook, stirring several times, until onions are soft.
2. Add cooked rice and beans to pan; stir until heated.

PER ¾ CUP (175 ML)	
Calories	195
Carbohydrate	33 g
Fiber	5 g
Net carbs	28 g
Protein	7 g
Fat, total	4 g
Fat, saturated	1 g
Cholesterol	0 mg
Sodium	204 mg

Cinnamon Coffee

Makes 1 serving

- 1 cup (250 mL) almond beverage, unsweetened
- 1 tsp (5 mL) instant coffee
- ¼ tsp (1 mL) cinnamon
- Zero-calorie sweetener, to taste

1. In your coffee mug, add the almond beverage, coffee and cinnamon.
2. Microwave until hot, about 2 minutes. Stir and add sweetener.

PER 1 CUP (250 ML)	
Calories	34
Carbohydrate	2 g
Fiber	1 g
Net carbs	1 g
Protein	1 g
Fat, total	3 g
Fat, saturated	0 g
Cholesterol	0 mg
Sodium	131 mg

⊙ LOW-CARB SWAP

LARGE MEAL

Swap Mexican Rice & Beans:
¾ cup (175 mL)
28 g net carbs

→ For Mexican Rice & Beans made with a cup of cooked couscous instead of rice:
¾ cup (175 mL)
16 g net carbs

SMALL MEAL

Swap Mexican Rice & Beans: ½ cup (125 mL)
19 g net carbs

→ For Mexican Rice & Beans made with a cup of cooked couscous instead of rice:
½ cup (125 mL)
11 g net carbs

See Rice Swaps, page 276.

YOUR BREAKFAST MENU	Large Meal (370 calories)	Total Carbs	NET CARBS	Small Meal (250 calories)	Total Carbs	NET CARBS
Mexican Rice & Beans	¾ cup (175 mL)	33	**28**	½ cup (125 mL)	22	**19**
Scrambled egg	2 large	0	**0**	1 large	0	**0**
Salsa	2 tbsp (30 mL)	2	**1**	2 tbsp (30 mL)	2	**1**
Sliced cucumbers	6 slices	1	**1**	6 slices	1	**1**
Cinnamon Coffee	1 cup (250 mL)	2	**1**	1 cup (250 mL)	2	**1**
	TOTAL CARBS	**38 g**	**31 g**	TOTAL CARBS	**27 g**	**22 g**
	Total carbs minus fiber = NET CARBS ↑				NET CARBS ↑	
	CARB CHOICES (1 carb choice = 15 g net carbs)		2		CARB CHOICES	1

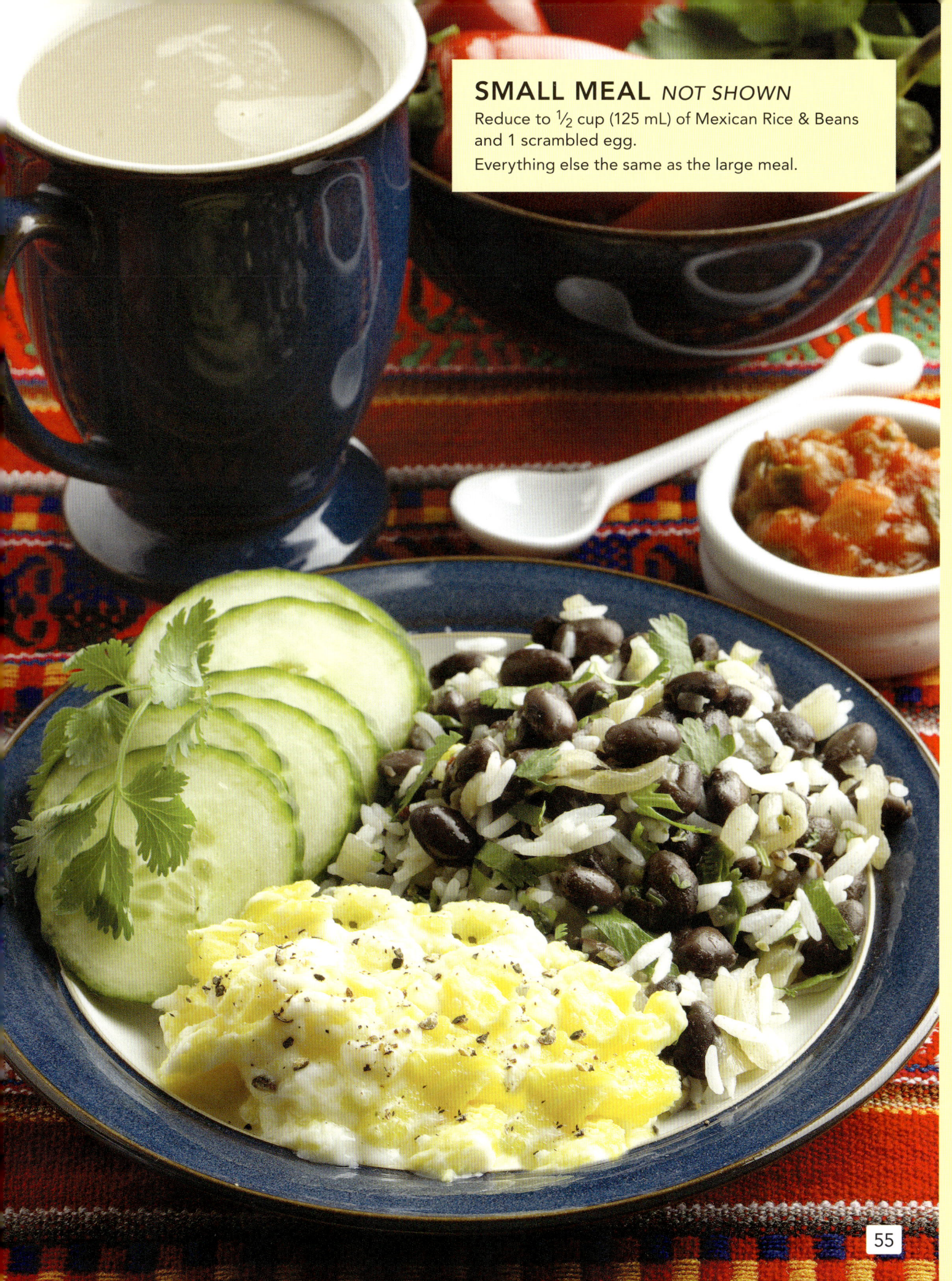

SMALL MEAL *NOT SHOWN*
Reduce to ½ cup (125 mL) of Mexican Rice & Beans and 1 scrambled egg.
Everything else the same as the large meal.

BREAKFAST MEALS

BREAKFAST 12

Fast-Food Breakfast

There are not many breakfast menu items in a fast-food restaurant or coffee shop that fit into a lower-carb diabetes meal plan. This English muffin with cheese and egg, shown in the photograph, does fit. However, there are no options for fruit or vegetables to make this a healthy, balanced meal.

Beware of supersizing: Check online nutrient information for any other restaurant breakfast item you want to choose.

HEALTH TIP
One store-bought or restaurant muffin can have 500 calories, which is a lot more than the large meal.

◯ LOW-CARB SWAP RECIPE: Homemade Low-Carb Egg Muffin

LARGE MEAL
Swap fast-food English egg muffin with cheese and bacon/ham:
28 g net carbs

→ For Homemade Low-Carb Egg Muffin:
2 g net carbs

SMALL MEAL
Swap fast-food English egg muffin with cheese:
27 g net carbs

→ For Homemade Low-Carb Egg Muffin (omit either the fried egg or shredded cheese):
2 g net carbs

Makes 1 serving

FOR THE MUFFIN:
2 tbsp (30 mL) almond flour
¼ tsp (1 mL) baking powder
Dash of salt
1 large egg
1 tbsp (15 mL) melted butter

FOR THE TOPPING:
1 fried egg
2 tbsp (30 mL) cheese, shredded

1. In a microwaveable bowl (4 to 6 inches/10 to 15 cm across), combine the muffin ingredients.
2. Microwave on high for 1 minute, or until fluffy and dry.
3. Fry the egg in a greased nonstick pan. Top the cooked muffin with the shredded cheese and fried egg.

1 SERVING
Calories 381
Total carbs 4 g
Net carbs 2 g

YOUR BREAKFAST MENU	Large Meal (370 calories)	Total Carbs	NET CARBS	Small Meal (250 calories)	Total Carbs	NET CARBS
Restaurant Meal (as shown in photo)	English egg muffin with cheese and bacon/ham	30	28	English egg muffin with cheese	29	27
Coffee or tea	Medium (15 oz/455 mL) with 2 milks	6	6	Medium (15 oz/455 mL) black or small with 1 milk	0	0
	TOTAL CARBS	36 g	34 g	TOTAL CARBS	29 g	27 g
	Total carbs minus fiber = NET CARBS ↑			NET CARBS ↑		
	CARB CHOICES (1 carb choice = 15 g net carbs)		2	CARB CHOICES		2

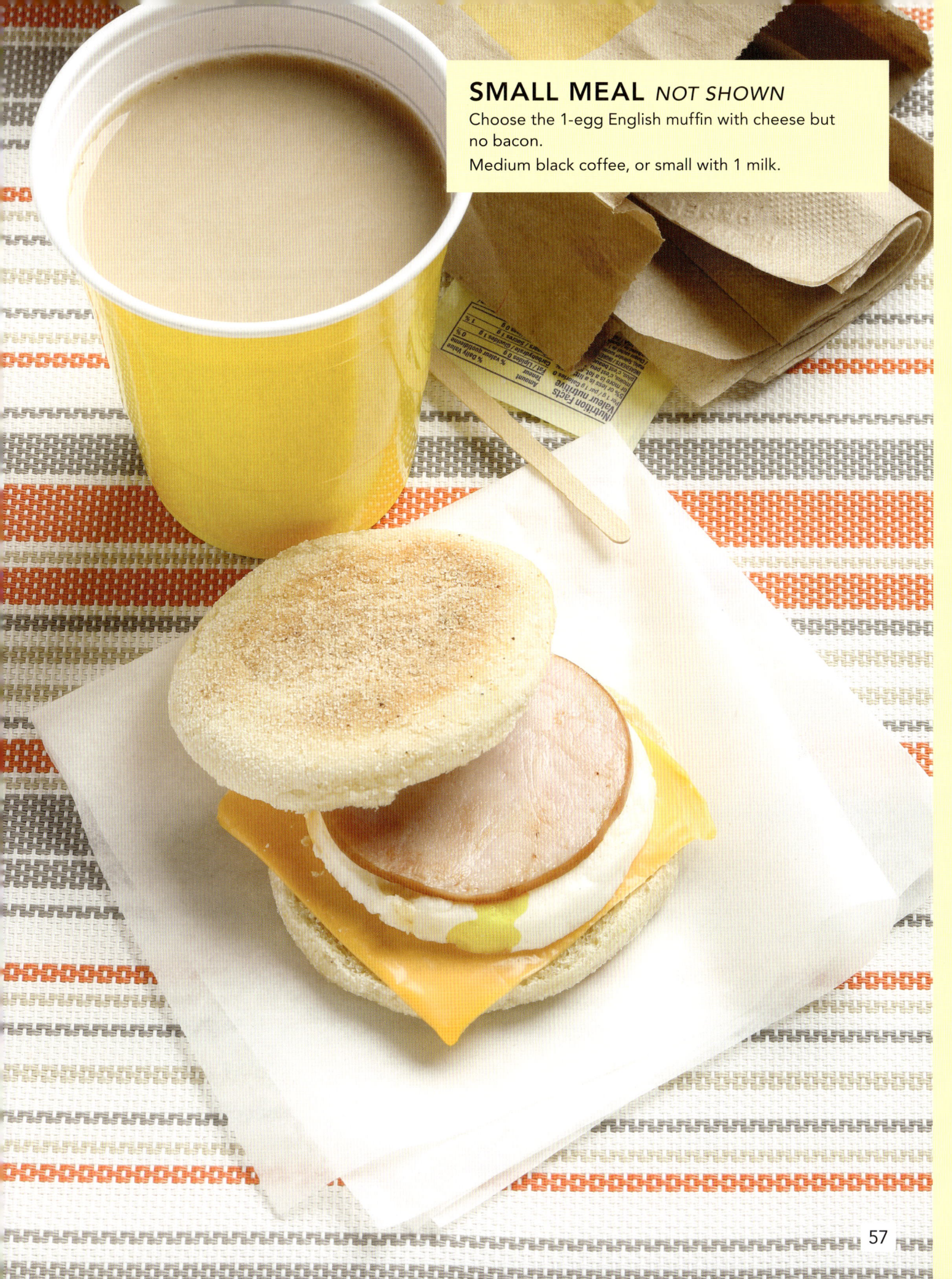

SMALL MEAL *NOT SHOWN*
Choose the 1-egg English muffin with cheese but no bacon.
Medium black coffee, or small with 1 milk.

BREAKFAST MEALS

BREAKFAST 13

Granola Combo

Crunchy Nut Granola

Makes 7 cups (1.75 L)

Preheat oven to 350°F (180°C)

¾ cup (175 mL) shelled sunflower seeds or pumpkin seeds
¾ cup (175 mL) sweetened flaked shredded coconut
¼ cup (60 mL) wheat germ
¼ cup (60 mL) ground flaxseed
1 cup (250 mL) almonds, walnuts or pecans, sliced or chopped
2 cups (500 mL) large-flake old-fashioned rolled oats
⅓ cup (75 mL) vegetable oil
⅓ cup (75 mL) corn syrup
2 tsp (10 mL) vanilla extract (or half almond extract or coconut extract)
½ cup (125 mL) round oat or crisp rice cereal
½ cup (125 mL) raisins or other dried fruit, chopped

1. In a large bowl, mix sunflower seeds, coconut, wheat germ, ground flaxseed, nuts and oats.
2. In a small bowl, combine oil, corn syrup and extract flavoring. Add and mix well into dry ingredients.
3. Place granola on a greased rimmed baking sheet. Bake on middle rack for 20 to 30 minutes, or until slightly toasted. *Stir every 10 minutes.*
4. Once toasted, remove from the oven. Immediately transfer to a metal bowl or pot so the granola won't stick to the pan. Once cooled, add cereal and raisins. Store in an airtight container.

PER ¼ CUP (60 ML)
Calories	137
Carbohydrate	14 g
Fiber	2 g
Net carbs	12 g
Protein	3 g
Fat, total	9 g
Fat, saturated	2 g
Cholesterol	0 mg
Sodium	19 mg

⬤ LOW-CARB SWAP

LARGE MEAL

Swap Greek yogurt, flavored and less sugar:
¾ cup (175 mL)
8 g net carbs

→ For sour cream:
⅓ cup (75 mL)
5 g net carbs

OR

→ For cream cheese or mascarpone cheese:
2 tbsp (30 mL)
1 to 3 g net carbs

SMALL MEAL

Swap Greek yogurt, flavored and less sugar:
½ cup (125 mL)
5 g net carbs

→ For sour cream:
¼ cup (60 mL)
4 g net carbs

OR

→ For cream cheese or mascarpone cheese:
1½ tbsp (22 mL)
1 to 2 g net carbs

YOUR BREAKFAST MENU	Large Meal (370 calories)	Total Carbs	NET CARBS	Small Meal (250 calories)	Total Carbs	NET CARBS
Berries and chopped fruit (fresh or frozen)	1½ cups (375 mL)	20	15	1 cup (250 mL)	15	12
Greek yogurt, 0–2%, flavored, less sugar	¾ cup (175 mL)	9	8	½ cup (125 mL)	6	5
Crunchy Nut Granola	⅓ cup (75 mL)	18	15	¼ cup (60 mL)	14	12
Tea or coffee	1 cup (250 mL)	1	1	1 cup (250 mL)	1	1
	TOTAL CARBS	48 g	39 g	TOTAL CARBS	36 g	30 g
	Total carbs minus fiber = NET CARBS ↑			NET CARBS ↑		
	CARB CHOICES (1 carb choice = 15 g net carbs)		3	CARB CHOICES		2

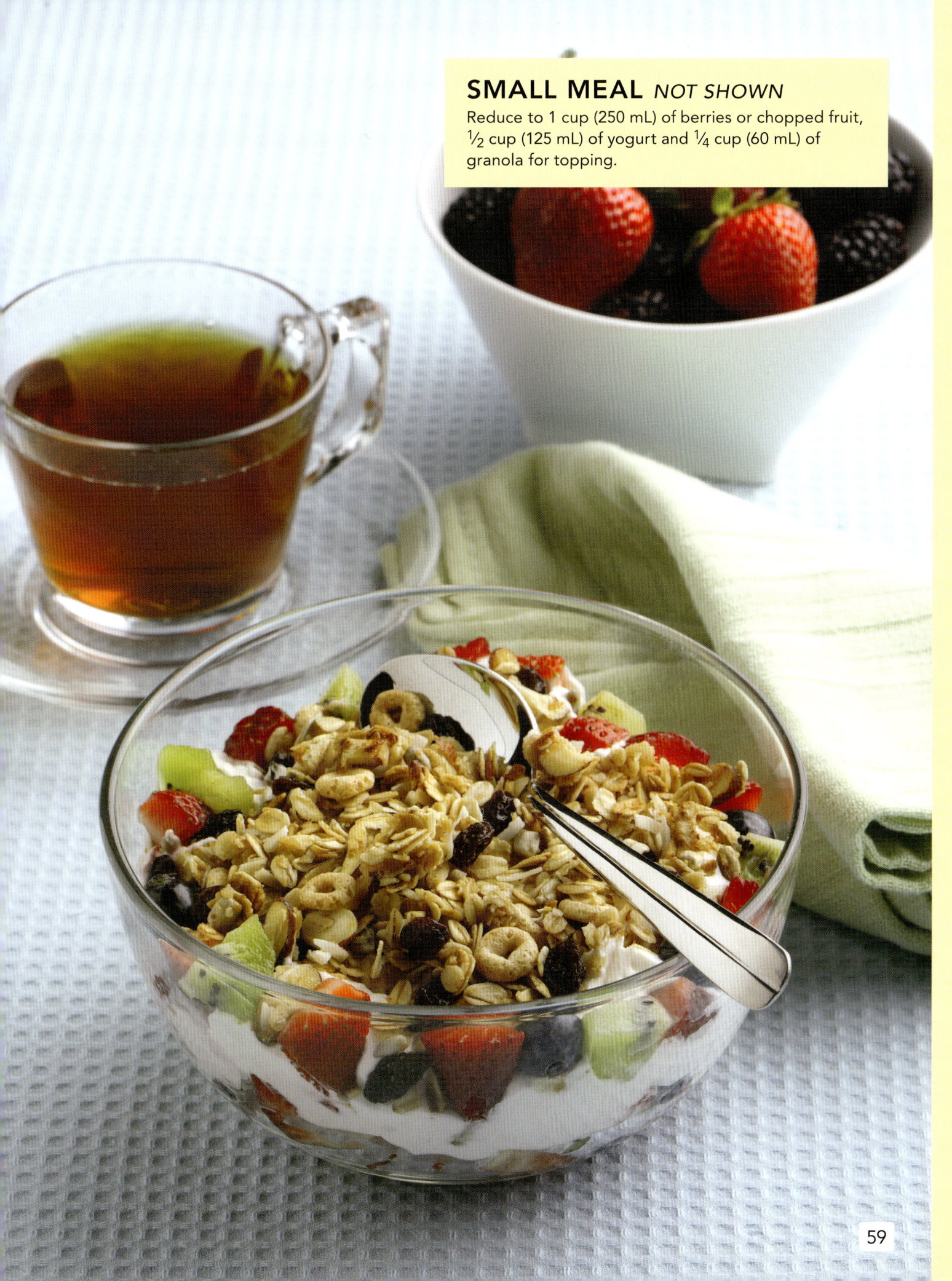

SMALL MEAL NOT SHOWN
Reduce to 1 cup (250 mL) of berries or chopped fruit, ½ cup (125 mL) of yogurt and ¼ cup (60 mL) of granola for topping.

BREAKFAST MEALS

BREAKFAST 14

⊙ LOW-CARB SWAP

Go crustless. In the recipe, grease your casserole and omit the bread crumbs from the recipe. Instead, add 2 extra eggs for the filling (4 eggs total in the recipe) to make up the calories.

LARGE MEAL
Swap Prairie Quiche with bread crumb crust:
Half of recipe
18 g net carbs

→ For crustless version:
   Half of recipe
   6 g net carbs

SMALL MEAL
Swap Prairie Quiche with bread crumb crust:
Third of recipe
12 g net carbs

→ For crustless version:
   Third of recipe
   4 g net carbs

Prairie Quiche

Prairie Quiche has a bread crumb crust, which is much lower in calories, carbs and fat than a traditional pastry crust. This quiche takes about 45 minutes to prepare and bake.

Prairie Quiche

Makes 2 large or 3 small servings

Preheat oven to 400°F (200°C)

1 tsp (5 mL) margarine or butter, to generously grease the casserole

⅓ cup (75 mL) dry bread crumbs

2 large eggs

2 slices raw bacon, fat partly trimmed off, chopped, or 2 tbsp (30 mL) real bacon bits

⅓ cup (75 mL) skim milk

¾ cup (175 mL) bell pepper, chopped

Black pepper, to taste

½ cup (125 mL) cheese, shredded

PER ½ QUICHE	
Calories	337
Carbohydrate	19 g
Fiber	2 g
Net carbs	17 g
Protein	20 g
Fat, total	20 g
Fat, saturated	9 g
Cholesterol	223 mg
Sodium	554 mg

1. Grease the sides and bottom of a 6-inch (15 cm) casserole dish with the 1 teaspoon (5 mL) of margarine or butter. Spread bread crumbs on the bottom of the dish.
2. In a bowl, combine eggs, chopped bacon or bacon bits, milk, bell pepper and black pepper. Pour on top of bread crumbs. Top with shredded cheese.
3. Bake for 25 minutes, or until egg is cooked.
4. Once cooked, remove from the oven and let sit for 5 minutes. Gently remove slices with an egg turner.

Serve a small glass of orange, apple, grapefruit or cranberry juice with the Prairie Quiche. Juice is an excellent source of vitamin C but has little of the fiber found in fresh fruit (see page 36).

YOUR BREAKFAST MENU	Large Meal (370 calories)	Total Carbs	NET CARBS	Small Meal (250 calories)	Total Carbs	NET CARBS
Prairie Quiche	½ of the recipe	19	17	⅓ of the recipe	13	12
Orange juice, unsweetened	½ cup (125 mL)	13	13	½ cup (125 mL)	13	13
	TOTAL CARBS	32 g	30 g	TOTAL CARBS	26 g	25 g
	Total carbs minus fiber = NET CARBS ↑			NET CARBS ↑		
	CARB CHOICES (1 carb choice = 15 g net carbs)		2	CARB CHOICES		2

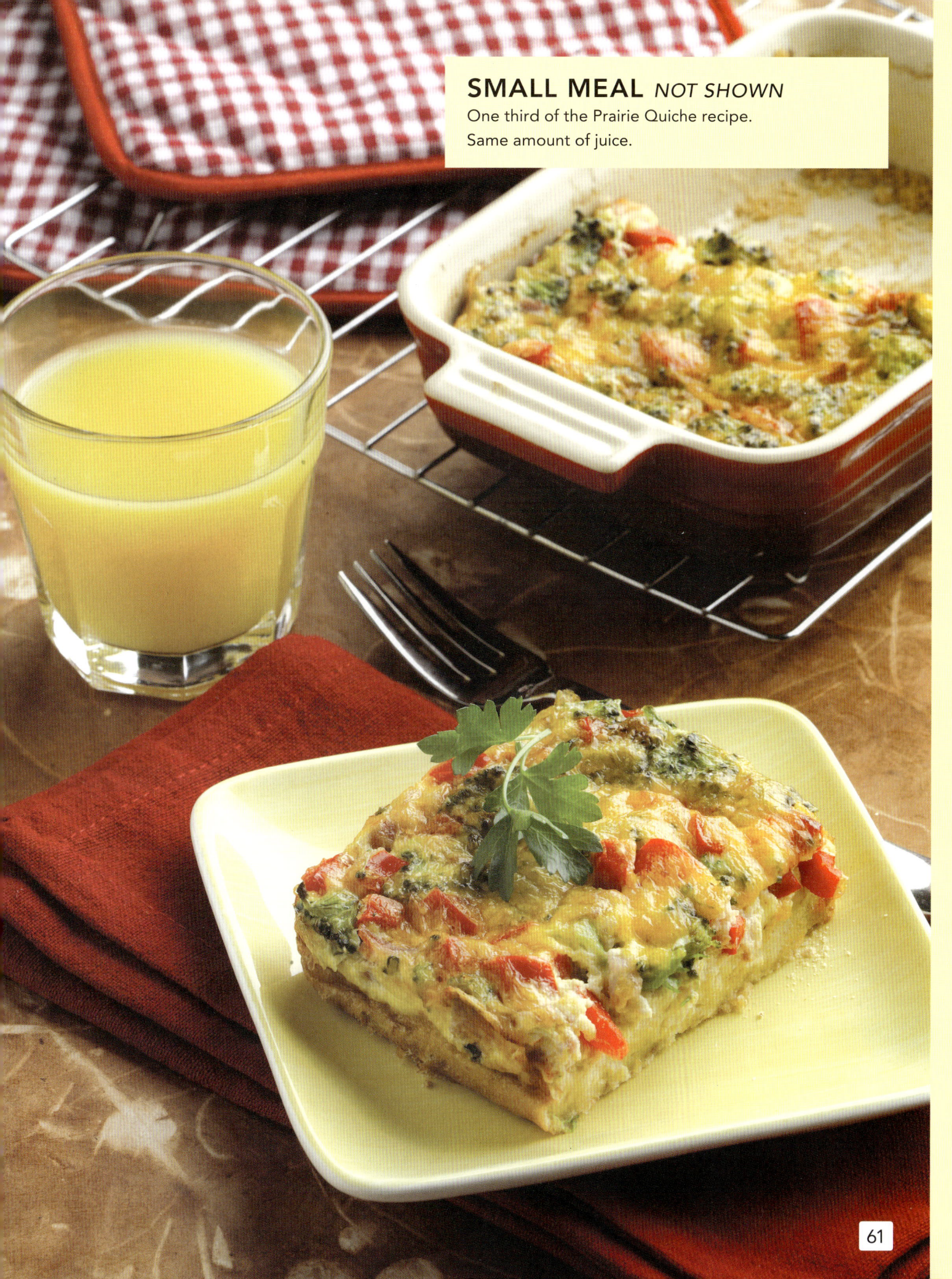

SMALL MEAL *NOT SHOWN*
One third of the Prairie Quiche recipe.
Same amount of juice.

BREAKFAST MEALS

Breakfast 15

Irish Currant Cake

Irish Currant Cake

Makes 10 slices

Preheat oven to 350°F (180°C)

1 cup (250 mL) flour
1 cup (250 mL) almond flour
1½ tsp (7 mL) baking powder
½ tsp (2 mL) baking soda
½ tsp (2 mL) salt
⅓ cup (75 mL) sugar
¾ cup (175 mL) dried currants
1 large egg
1 cup (250 mL) buttermilk (if you don't have buttermilk, start with 2 tbsp/30 mL vinegar and add skim or 1% milk to make up 1 cup/250 mL)
¼ cup (60 mL) butter, melted

1. In a large bowl, mix together flours, baking powder, baking soda, salt and sugar. Sift out any lumps.
2. Add currants to the dry ingredients and toss until they are well coated in flour.
3. In a small bowl, beat egg with a fork. Stir in the buttermilk and melted butter.
4. Add this milk mixture to the dry ingredients and blend until all the flour is mixed in.
5. Turn batter into a greased 10-inch (25 cm) cast iron pan, or a 9- by 5-inch (2 L) loaf pan or an 8-inch (20 cm) square baking pan.
6. Bake for 30 to 40 minutes, until golden brown. Cool slightly, slice and serve warm.

PER SLICE	
Calories	229
Carbohydrate	27 g
Fiber	2 g
Net carbs	25 g
Protein	6 g
Fat, total	12 g
Fat, saturated	4 g
Cholesterol	32 mg
Sodium	306 mg

◯ LOW-CARB SWAP

You can replace part of the sugar with a calorie-free sweetener in the Irish Currant Cake.

Note: Any cake made with less sugar will not rise as high.

Swap Irish Currant Cake:
1 slice
25 g net carbs
→ For Irish Currant Cake made with 3 tbsp (45 mL) zero-calorie sweetener plus 3 tbsp (45 mL) sugar instead of ⅓ cup (75 mL) sugar:
1 slice
22 g net carbs

YOUR BREAKFAST MENU	Large Meal (370 calories)	Total Carbs	NET CARBS	Small Meal (250 calories)	Total Carbs	NET CARBS
Irish Currant Cake	1 slice	27	**25**	1 slice	27	**25**
Piece of cheese	1 oz (30 g)	0	**0**	—	0	**0**
Papaya with lime juice (or other ½ fruit)	½ small	7	**6**	½ small	7	**6**
Tea or coffee	1 cup (250 mL)	1	**1**	1 cup (250 mL)	1	**1**
	TOTAL CARBS	35 g	**32 g**	TOTAL CARBS	35 g	**32 g**
	Total carbs minus fiber = NET CARBS ↑			NET CARBS ↑		
	CARB CHOICES (1 carb choice = 15 g net carbs)		**2**	CARB CHOICES		**2**

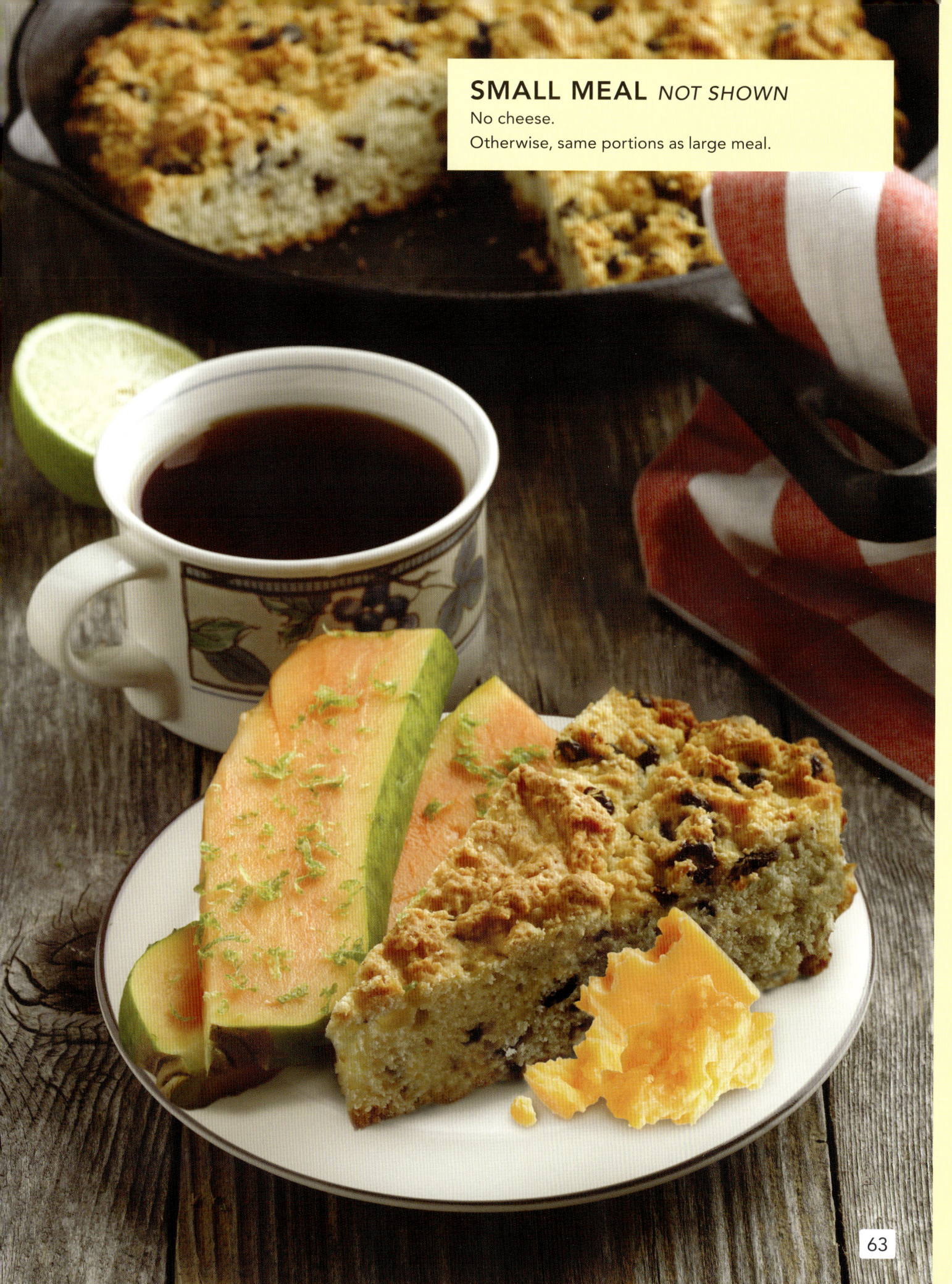

SMALL MEAL *NOT SHOWN*
No cheese.
Otherwise, same portions as large meal.

63

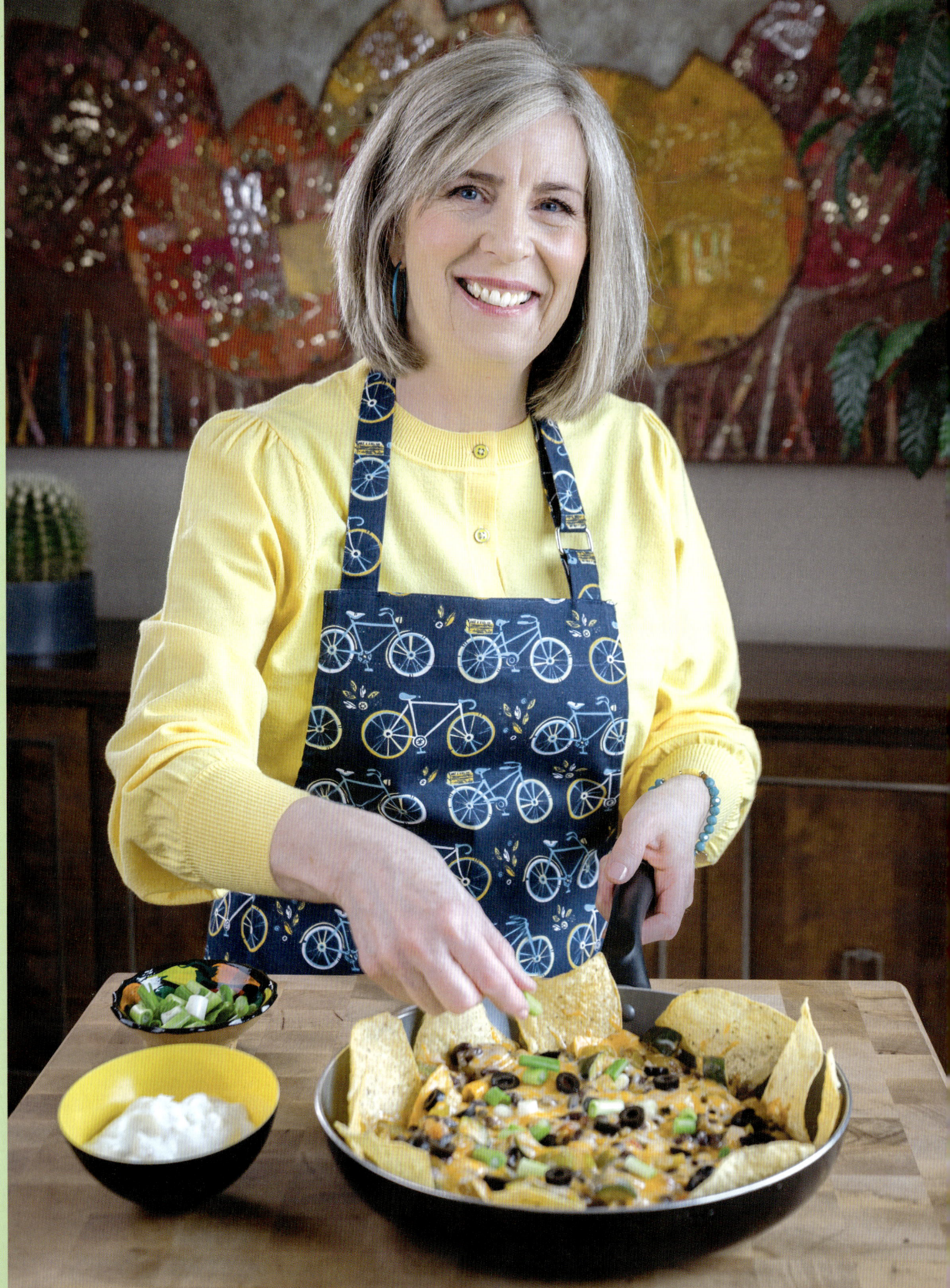

Lunch Meals

- Each large lunch has **520 calories** and 3–4 Carb Choices
  Total carbs: 78 g or less | Net carbs: 66 g or less
- Each small lunch has **400 calories** and 2–3 Carb Choices
  Total carbs: 59 g or less | Net carbs: 50 g or less

1. Beef Dip Sandwich 66
2. Beans & Toast 68
3. Chicken Soup & Bagel 70
4. Toasted Cheese & Tomato Sandwich 72
5. Cold Plate with Soup 74
6. Fried Peanut Butter & Banana Sandwich 76
7. Pita Sandwich 78
8. Chef's Salad 80
9. French Onion Soup 82
10. Quesadilla 84
11. Tuna Sandwich 86
12. Cheese & Crackers 88
13. Avocado Salad & Bruschetta 90
14. Crab Cakes 92
15. Nachos in a Pan 94

ALL MEAL PHOTOS ARE LIFE-SIZE

LUNCH MEALS

LUNCH 1

Beef Dip Sandwich

Life-size photos are the LARGE MEALS

◯ LOW-CARB SWAP

Swap bread for a bell pepper. Cut the pepper in half; remove the seeds but not the stem. Then fill each half with the meat, gravy and cheese and grill under the broiler until cheese is melted.

LARGE MEAL

Swap multigrain bread: 3 slices
41 g net carbs
→ For bell pepper:
   2 halves
   8 g net carbs

SMALL MEAL

Swap multigrain bread: 2 slices
27 g net carbs
→ For bell pepper:
   2 halves
   8 g net carbs

HEALTH TIP
Use fresh roast beef. Processed deli roast beef is high in salt.

Imagine warm roast beef with cheese tucked into multigrain bread, grilled until the cheese melts, then it's ready to dip. Yum! Be sure to look for "Au Jus Gravy Mix" for dipping.

Making the Beef Dip Sandwich

- Make the gravy according to directions on the package. A 26 g package will make 2 cups (500 mL) of gravy.
- Warm up leftover roast beef (see Dinner 4) in a frying pan or microwave.
- Arrange the roast beef with the cheese of your choice on the bread.
- Add pan-fried onions, horseradish or mustard, all optional.
- Grill the sandwich on the second-highest oven rack under the broiler for 30 seconds each side.

Cut the sandwich in half or quarters, dip in the gravy and enjoy!

YOUR LUNCH MENU	Large Meal (520 calories)	Total Carbs	NET CARBS	Small Meal (400 calories)	Total Carbs	NET CARBS
Beef Dip Sandwich	1½ sandwiches			1 sandwich		
• Multigrain bread (30 g per slice)	3 slices bread	49	41	2 slices bread	32	27
• Beef, thinly sliced	3 oz (90 g)	0	0	2 oz (60 g)	0	0
• Cheese, mozzarella	1 ounce (30 g)	1	1	1 ounce (30 g)	1	1
• Au jus gravy	¼ cup (60 mL)	2	2	¼ cup (60 mL)	2	2
Radishes	3	0	0	3	0	0
Cantaloupe, chopped	1 cup (250 mL)	12	11	1 cup (250 mL)	12	11
Soda water with lime	12 oz	0	0	12 oz	0	0
	TOTAL CARBS	**64 g**	**55 g**	TOTAL CARBS	**47 g**	**41 g**
	Total carbs minus fiber = NET CARBS ↑			NET CARBS ↑		
	CARB CHOICES (1 carb choice = 15 g net carbs)		4	CARB CHOICES		3

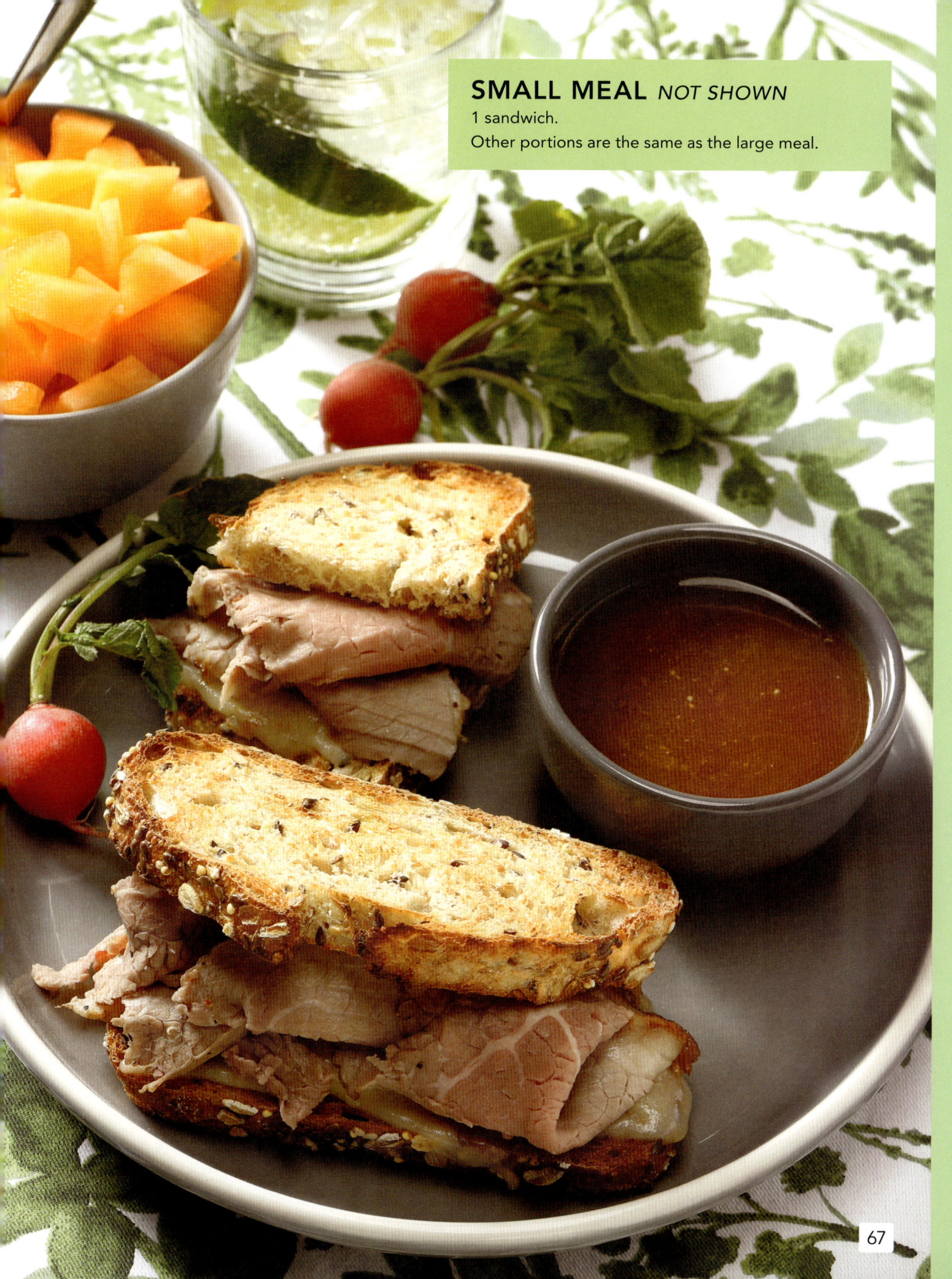

SMALL MEAL *NOT SHOWN*
1 sandwich.
Other portions are the same as the large meal.

LUNCH MEALS

LUNCH 2

Beans & Toast

Baked beans go so well with toast, egg and crunchy, crisp celery.

🔴 LOW-CARB SWAP RECIPE: Low-Carb Egg Bread

As an option ahead of time, make Low-Carb Egg Bread. It has the same calories as regular bread but a lot less carbs. You're going to love it.

Swap rye bread:
1 slice
13 g net carbs
→ For Low-Carb Egg Bread:
1 piece
1 g net carbs

See Bread Swaps, page 274.

Makes 8 pieces
Preheat oven to 300°F (150°C)

4 large eggs, room temperature
Dash of salt
¼ tsp (1 mL) cream of tartar
¼ cup/2 oz (60 mL) light cream cheese (¼ of an 8 oz block), room temperature
2 tbsp (30 mL) almond flour

1 PIECE	
Calories	65
Total carbs	1 g
Net carbs	1 g

1. Separate egg yolks into one bowl and place egg whites into a second bowl of glass or metal.
2. Add the salt and cream of tartar to the egg whites. Beat with an electric mixer until soft peaks form.
3. Add the cream cheese and almond flour to the egg yolks. Beat with the electric mixer until smooth.
4. Fold egg white mixture into the egg yolk mixture.
5. Cover a rimmed baking sheet with parchment paper. Spoon the egg bread mixture onto the paper and spread it out with a spatula.
6. Bake for 30 minutes, or until golden.
7. Cool and cut into 8 pieces. Refrigerate extras.

YOUR LUNCH MENU	Large Meal (520 calories)	Total Carbs	NET CARBS	Small Meal (400 calories)	Total Carbs	NET CARBS
Canned baked beans	1 cup (250 mL)	54	44	½ cup (125 mL)	27	22
Toast, light rye	1 slice	15	13	1 slice	15	13
Margarine	1 tsp (5 mL)	0	0	1 tsp (5 mL)	0	0
Egg, fried	1	0	0	1	0	0
Oil, butter or margarine for frying egg	1 tsp (5 mL)	0	0	—	—	—
Celery sticks	2 stalks	3	2	2 stalks	3	2
Greek yogurt, 0–2%, flavored, less-sugar	½ cup (125 mL)	6	5	½ cup (125 mL)	6	5
	TOTAL CARBS	**78 g**	**64 g**	TOTAL CARBS	**51 g**	**42 g**
	Total carbs minus fiber = NET CARBS ↑			NET CARBS ↑		
	CARB CHOICES (1 carb choice = 15 g net carbs)		4	CARB CHOICES		3

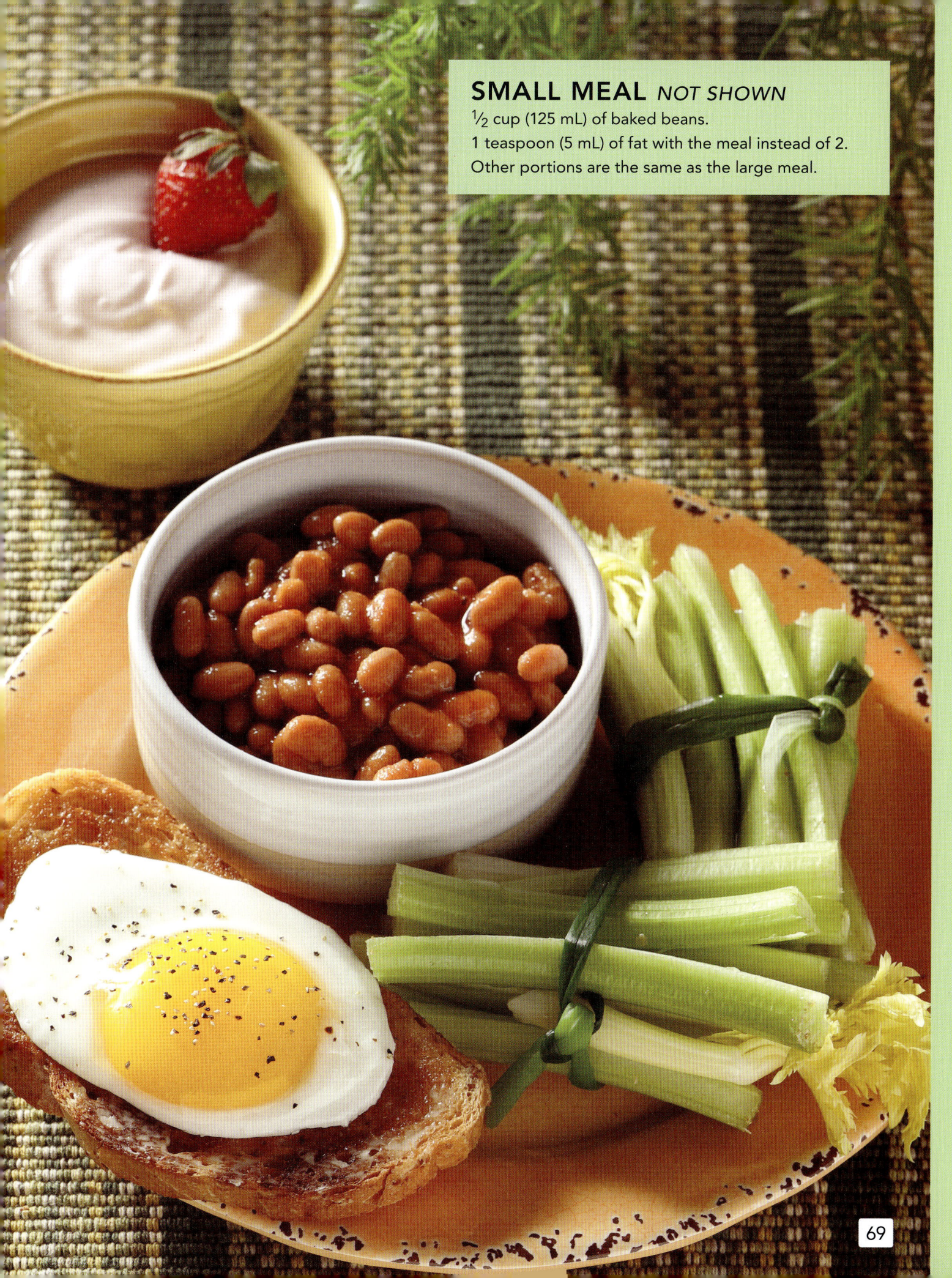

SMALL MEAL *NOT SHOWN*
½ cup (125 mL) of baked beans.
1 teaspoon (5 mL) of fat with the meal instead of 2.
Other portions are the same as the large meal.

LUNCH MEALS

Lunch 3

Chicken Soup & Bagel

🔴 LOW-CARB SWAP

Two slices of Mug Bread (recipe on page 259) have fewer carbs than the bagel but have double the calories because of the extra fat and protein.

LARGE MEAL
Swap the bagel:
30 g net carbs
→ For 2 slices Mug Bread:
3 g net carbs

SMALL MEAL
Swap half the bagel:
15 g net carbs
→ For 1 slice Mug Bread:
2 g net carbs

See Mug Bread recipe on page 259.

The bagel in this meal is a small one, a 3-inch (7.5 cm) bagel weighing 2 oz (60 g), and it equals two slices of bread. More standard-size bagels are larger and can equal four or more slices of bread.

The bagel is served with light cream cheese, salmon, tomato and onion. For a change, try smoked salmon (lox). Serve with Chicken Rice Soup.

Chicken Rice Soup

Makes 7½ cups (1.9 L)

2 medium carrots, chopped
1 medium onion, chopped
2 stalks celery, chopped
¼ cup (60 mL) rice (uncooked)
1 package (2 oz/60 g) dried chicken noodle soup mix
½ tsp (2 mL) dried dill
6 cups (1.5 L) water

1. In a medium pot, add all ingredients.
2. Cover and gently boil for about 20 minutes, until carrots are cooked. Stir occasionally.

PER 1½ CUP (375 ML)	
Calories	101
Carbohydrate	20 g
Fiber	2 g
Net carbs	18 g
Protein	3 g
Fat, total	2 g
Fat, saturated	0 g
Cholesterol	9 mg
Sodium	474 mg

YOUR LUNCH MENU	Large Meal (520 calories)	Total Carbs	NET CARBS	Small Meal (400 calories)	Total Carbs	NET CARBS
Chicken Rice Soup	1½ cups (375 mL)	20	18	1½ cups (375 mL)	20	18
Soda crackers	2	4	4	—	—	—
Bagel	1 (or 2 slices bread)	31	30	½ (or 1 slice bread)	16	15
Light cream cheese (20%)	2 tbsp (30 mL)	1	1	2 tbsp (30 mL)	1	1
Canned red salmon	¼ cup (60 mL)	0	0	¼ cup (60 mL)	0	0
Tomato	½ medium	2	1	½ medium	2	1
Sliced onion	2 slices	2	2	2 slices	2	2
Orange	1 small	12	10	1 small	12	10
	TOTAL CARBS	73 g	66 g	TOTAL CARBS	53 g	47 g
	Total carbs minus fiber = NET CARBS ↑			NET CARBS ↑		
	CARB CHOICES (1 carb choice = 15 g net carbs)		4	CARB CHOICES		3

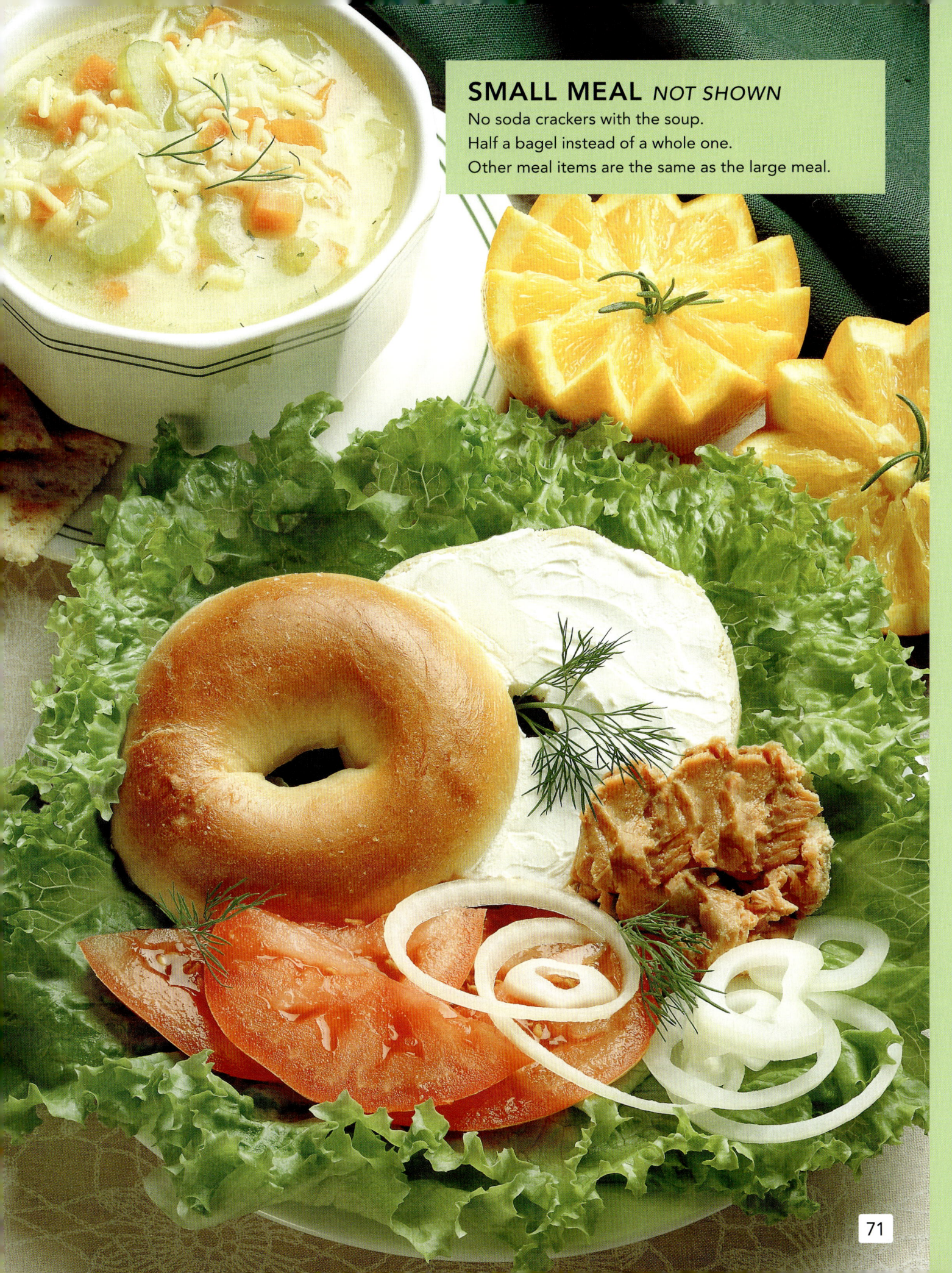

SMALL MEAL *NOT SHOWN*
No soda crackers with the soup.
Half a bagel instead of a whole one.
Other meal items are the same as the large meal.

LUNCH MEALS

LUNCH 4

Toasted Cheese & Tomato Sandwich

Try this healthy low-fat coleslaw that celebrates the flavors of the vegetables.

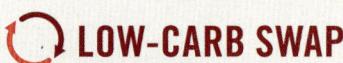 **LOW-CARB SWAP**

LARGE MEAL
Swap whole wheat bread:
3 slices
42 g net carbs
→ For low-carb bread (may also be called keto bread), see page 46:
3 slices
6 g net carbs

SMALL MEAL
Swap whole wheat bread:
2 slices
27 g net carbs
→ For low-carb bread:
2 slices
4 g net carbs

See Bread Swaps, page 274.

Coleslaw

Makes 6½ cups (1.6 L)

4 cups (1 L) cabbage, finely shredded
4 medium carrots, grated
4 stalks celery, finely chopped
1 small onion, finely chopped, or 2 green onions, chopped
¼ cup (60 mL) light mayonnaise
1 tbsp (15 mL) sugar
¼ cup (60 mL) vinegar
¼ tsp (1 mL) garlic powder
Salt and pepper, to taste

1. In a large bowl, combine carrots, celery and onion.
2. In a small bowl, mix mayonnaise, sugar, vinegar, garlic powder, salt and pepper. Add to cabbage. Mix well.
3. Cover and put in the fridge. This will keep well for one week.

PER ½ CUP (125 ML)
Calories 37
Carbohydrate 5 g
Fiber 1 g
Net carbs 4 g
Protein 1 g
Fat, total 2 g
Fat, saturated 0 g
Cholesterol 2 mg
Sodium 55 mg

YOUR LUNCH MENU	Large Meal (520 calories)	Total Carbs	NET CARBS	Small Meal (400 calories)	Total Carbs	NET CARBS
Toasted cheese & tomato sandwich	1½ sandwiches			1 sandwich		
• bread (whole wheat)	3 slices	49	42	2 slices	32	27
• cheese	1½ slices	2	2	1 slice	2	2
• tomato	1 large	5	3	1 medium	5	3
• lettuce	1 to 2 leaves	0	0	1 to 2 leaves	0	0
• light mayonnaise	2 tsp (10 mL)	1	1	2 tsp (10 mL)	1	1
Coleslaw (or raw veggies)	½ cup (125 mL)	5	4	½ cup (125 mL)	5	4
Cherries	½ cup (125 mL)	8	7	½ cup (125 mL)	8	7
Skim or 1% milk	½ cup (125 mL)	6	6	½ cup (125 mL)	6	6
	TOTAL CARBS	76 g	65 g	TOTAL CARBS	59 g	50 g
	Total carbs minus fiber = NET CARBS ↑			NET CARBS ↑		
	CARB CHOICES (1 carb choice = 15 g net carbs)		4	CARB CHOICES		3

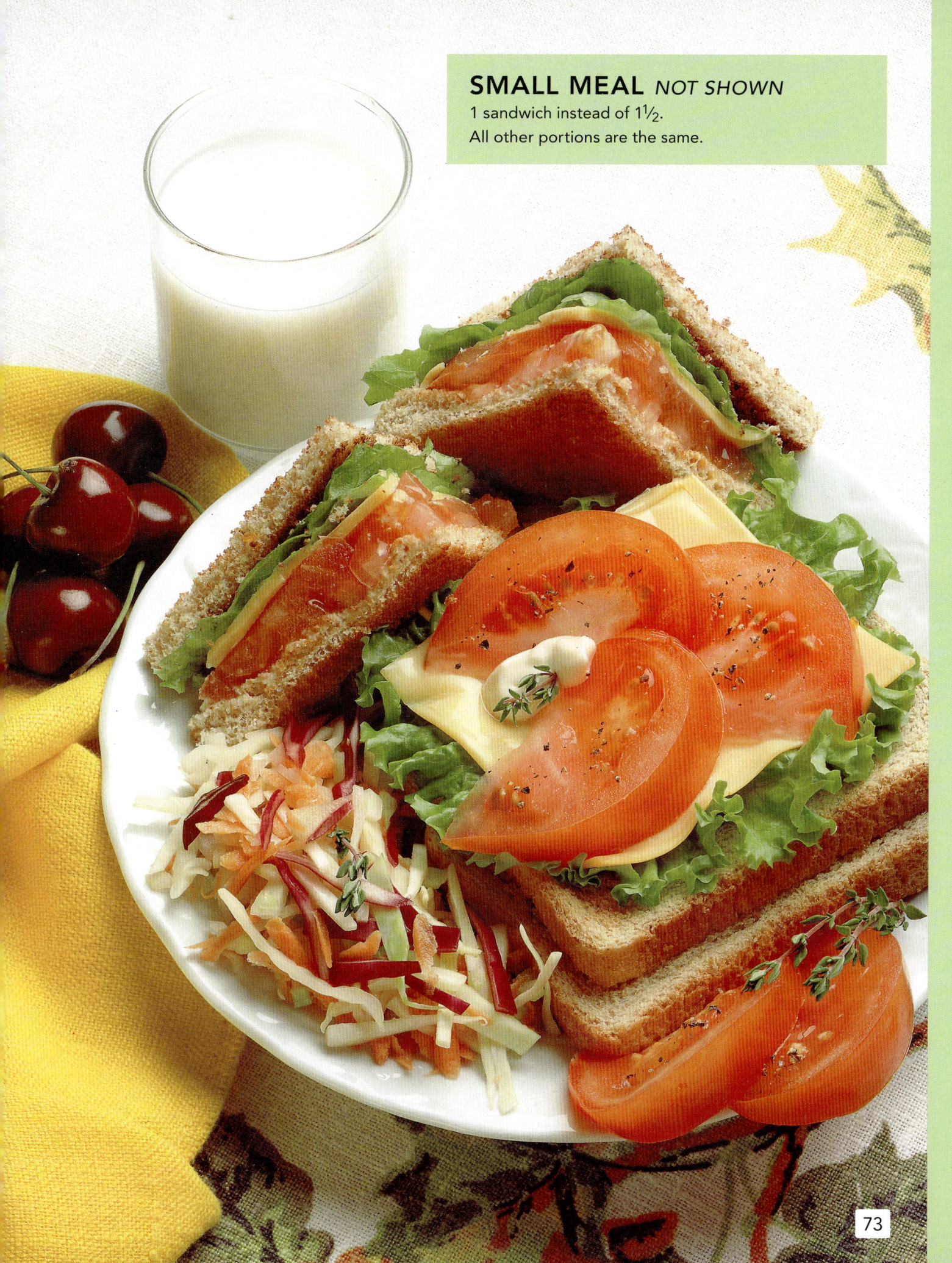

SMALL MEAL *NOT SHOWN*
1 sandwich instead of 1½.
All other portions are the same.

LUNCH MEALS

LUNCH 5

Cold Plate with Soup

Cold plates don't require any cooking. This one is full of vegetables served with cottage cheese and canned fruit.

Instant cup-of-soup is simple and quick to prepare but tends to be salty. Use a sieve or a spoon to remove half the salty spice mix and keep the dehydrated vegetables with the noodles. Add a 14 g serving package of instant cup-of-soup to 1 cup (250 mL) of boiling water.

○ **LOW-CARB SWAP**

Swap whole wheat bun with butter:
14 g net carbs
→ For extra cottage cheese:
Plus ½ cup (125 mL)
4 g net carbs

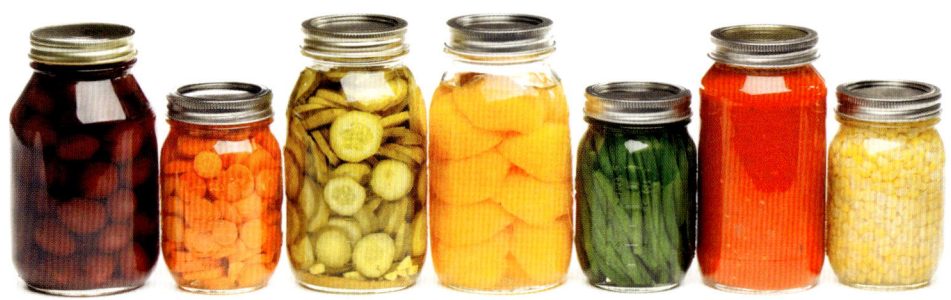

Canned peaches and pickles are two of many home-canning options.

YOUR LUNCH MENU	Large Meal (520 calories)	Total Carbs	NET CARBS	Small Meal (400 calories)	Total Carbs	NET CARBS
Reduced-Salt Instant Cup-of-Soup	1 cup (250 mL)	6	6	1 cup (250 mL)	6	6
Cold Plate						
• 2% cottage cheese	1 cup (250 mL)	7	7	¾ cup (175 mL)	5	5
• peaches, canned or fresh	2 halves	17	15	2 halves	17	15
• dill pickle	1 medium	3	2	1 medium	3	2
• lettuce	5 large leaves	1	1	5 large leaves	1	1
• tomato	1 medium	4	3	1 medium	4	3
• green onions	4	4	2	4	4	2
• whole wheat bun (small)	1	16	14	1	16	14
• margarine or butter	1 tsp (5 mL)	0	0	1 tsp (5 mL)	0	0
• arrowroot biscuits	3	12	12	—	—	—
	TOTAL CARBS	**70 g**	**62 g**	TOTAL CARBS	**56 g**	**48 g**
	Total carbs minus fiber = NET CARBS ↑			NET CARBS ↑		
	CARB CHOICES (1 carb choice = 15 g net carbs)		4	CARB CHOICES		3

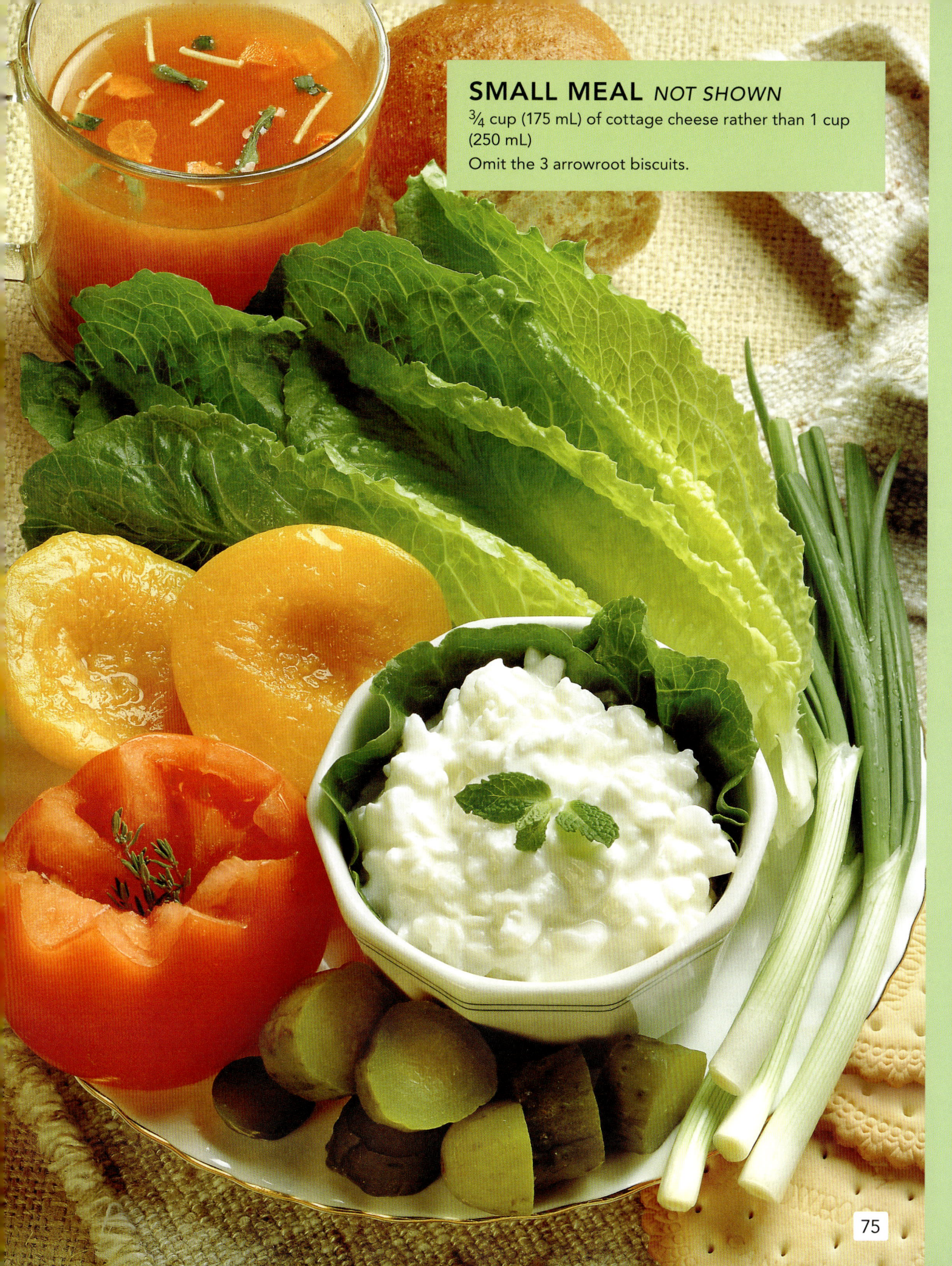

SMALL MEAL *NOT SHOWN*
¾ cup (175 mL) of cottage cheese rather than 1 cup (250 mL)
Omit the 3 arrowroot biscuits.

LUNCH MEALS

LUNCH 6

Fried Peanut Butter & Banana Sandwich

◯ LOW-CARB SWAP

If you love the crunch and tang of raw onions, try pairing them with peanut butter. See Low-Carb Swap below. Raw onions are also extremely rich in disease-fighting antioxidants.

Swap banana in peanut butter sandwich:
½ banana
11 g net carbs
→ For red or white onion:
Several slices
3 g net carbs

HEALTH TIP

Always have water with your meals.

This warm, gooey peanut butter and banana fried sandwich takes ordinary up a notch or two. Spread peanut butter on bread and add sliced banana. The margarine or butter goes on the outside of the bread. Fry your sandwich on both sides at medium heat.

Some of us find carrots are hard to eat when raw. These thin-cut carrots are much easier to eat. Carrots are full of vitamin A that boosts your immune system.

RECIPE TIP

A shredded carrot can be warmed up in the frying pan used to fry the sandwich. Then serve it with a few raisins (no more than 10) and a dusting of cinnamon. Like carrot cake without the cake!

Serve vegetables with every lunch meal

This will help you get your necessary servings every day. Choose a range of colors for best health: you'll get a healthy variety of vitamins, minerals and antioxidants.

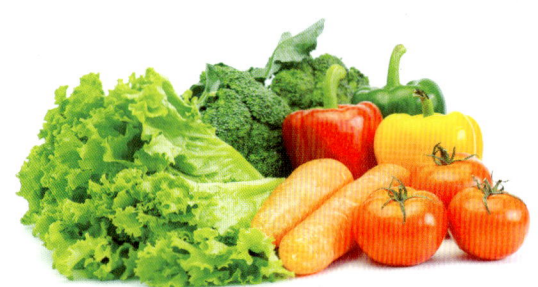

YOUR LUNCH MENU	Large Meal (520 calories)	Total Carbs	NET CARBS	Small Meal (400 calories)	Total Carbs	NET CARBS
Fried Peanut Butter & Banana Sandwich	1 sandwich			1 sandwich		
• whole-grain bread	2 slices	32	28	2 slices	32	28
• margarine or butter	2 tsp (10 mL)	0	0	1 tsp (5 mL)	0	0
• peanut butter	2 tbsp (30 mL)	6	4	1½ tbsp (22 mL)	5	3
• small banana	½	12	11	½	12	11
Carrot sticks	1 medium carrot	8	6	1 medium carrot	8	6
	TOTAL CARBS	58 g	49 g	TOTAL CARBS	57 g	48 g
Total carbs minus fiber = NET CARBS ↑				NET CARBS ↑		
CARB CHOICES (1 carb choice = 15 g net carbs)			3	CARB CHOICES		3

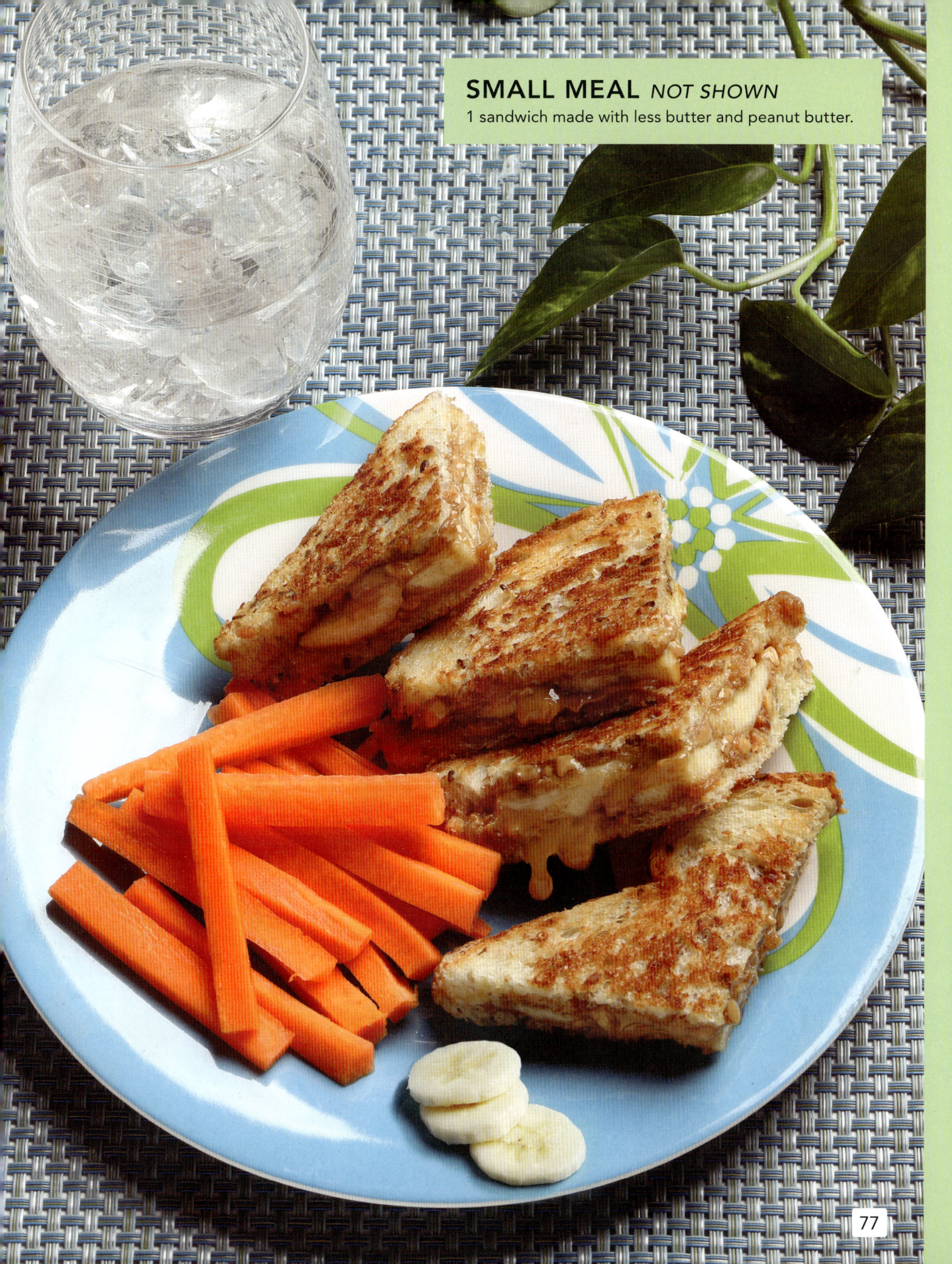

SMALL MEAL *NOT SHOWN*
1 sandwich made with less butter and peanut butter.

LUNCH MEALS

LUNCH 7

Pita Sandwich

Stuff the pita with:
- Lettuce, spinach, arugula or other greens
- Bean sprouts or alfalfa sprouts
- Grated carrots
- Chopped bell peppers, all colors
- Tomatoes, cucumber or zucchini

Protein options instead of ham and cheese:
- ½ cup (125 mL) tuna or salmon, drained
- ½ cup (125 mL) 2% cottage cheese
- 3 oz (85 g) firm tofu, chopped
- 2 tbsp (30 mL) peanut butter
- ⅓ cup (75 mL) hummus
- ½ small avocado, sliced (avocado has no protein but is high in healthy fat)

Portions are for the large meal.

⟳ LOW-CARB SWAP

Swap 2 gingersnap cookies:
11 g net carbs
→ For extra shredded cheese in pita: 2 extra tbsp (30 mL)
0 g net carbs

TWO MORE SWAP OPTIONS

1) Look for low-carb pitas. They have about **22 g net carbs** instead of **32 g net carbs**.

2) Swap the pita for 2 slices Low-Carb Egg Bread (page 68), with just **2 g net carbs**.

YOUR LUNCH MENU	Large Meal (520 calories)	Total Carbs	NET CARBS	Small Meal (400 calories)	Total Carbs	NET CARBS
Pita	1 (6-inch/15 cm)	33	32	½ (6-inch/15 cm)	17	16
• lettuce	¼ cup (60 mL), chopped	0	0	¼ cup (60 mL), chopped	0	0
• tomato	½ medium	2	1	½ medium	2	1
• bean sprouts	¼ cup (60 mL)	1	1	¼ cup (60 mL)	1	1
• carrots	½ small	2	1	½ small	2	1
• green pepper	2 tbsp (30 mL), chopped	1	1	2 tbsp (30 mL), chopped	1	1
• ham, lean	1 oz (30 g)	0	0	1 oz (30 g)	0	0
• Cheddar cheese	¼ cup (1 oz/60 mL), shredded	0	0	¼ cup (1 oz/60 mL), shredded	0	0
Plum	2 medium	15	13	1 medium	8	7
Skim or 1% milk	½ cup (125 mL)	6	6	½ cup (125 mL)	6	6
Gingersnap cookies	2	11	11	2	11	11
	TOTAL CARBS	71 g	66 g	TOTAL CARBS	48 g	44 g
	Total carbs minus fiber = NET CARBS ↑			NET CARBS ↑		
	CARB CHOICES (1 carb choice = 15 g net carbs)		4	CARB CHOICES		3

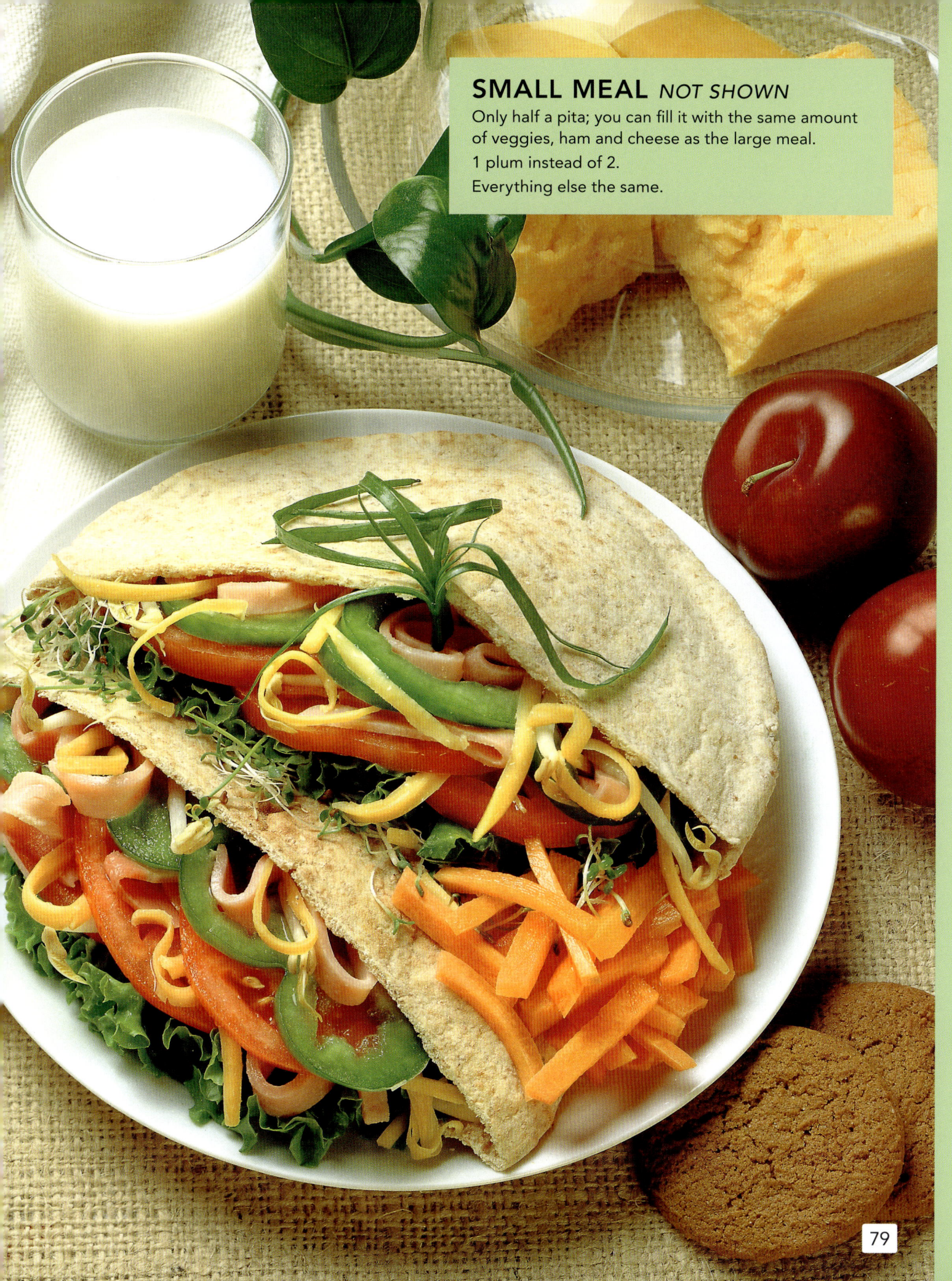

SMALL MEAL *NOT SHOWN*
Only half a pita; you can fill it with the same amount of veggies, ham and cheese as the large meal.
1 plum instead of 2.
Everything else the same.

LUNCH MEALS

LUNCH 8

Chef's Salad

You can prepare Chef's Salad differently every day of the week with whatever vegetables and proteins you have on hand.

RECIPE TIP

Citrus Vinaigrette

2 servings, about 1½ tbsp (22 mL) each

In a small dish, add 1 tbsp (15 mL) each of oil, vinegar and lemon juice and 1 tsp (5 mL) each of mustard and zero-calorie sweetener. Mix with a fork.

Chef's Salad

Makes 2 servings

- 2 cups (500 mL) lettuce, chopped
- 2 medium tomatoes, sliced
- Other vegetables, such as onions, bell peppers, celery, radishes or carrots
- 1 apple, sliced
- 2 slices (2 oz/60 g) sliced cooked chicken, meat or fish, or cheese
- 2 large eggs, hard boiled and sliced
- 2 tbsp (30 mL) croutons

1. Toss vegetables and apple. Place the meat or cheese and egg on top. Add croutons.

For the large meal, have a serving of soup with your salad. Make your cream soup with water or unsweetened nut beverage; it will still be creamy and smooth.

PER SERVING	
Calories	204
Carbohydrate	19 g
Fiber	5 g
Net carbs	14 g
Protein	17 g
Fat, total	8 g
Fat, saturated	2 g
Cholesterol	213 mg
Sodium	117 mg

LOW-CARB SWAP

Swap the bun:
14 g net carbs

→ For an extra egg or extra ounce (30 g) of chicken added to the Chef's Salad:
0 g net carbs

See Bread Swaps, page 274.

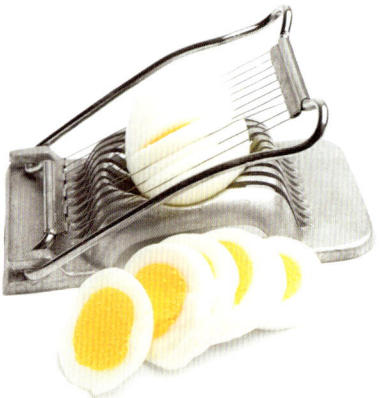

YOUR LUNCH MENU	Large Meal (520 calories)	Total Carbs	NET CARBS	Small Meal (400 calories)	Total Carbs	NET CARBS
Chef's Salad	1 serving (½ recipe)	19	14	1 serving (½ recipe)	19	14
Citrus Vinaigrette or 1 tbsp (15 mL) light salad dressing	1½ tbsp (22 mL)	2	0	1½ tbsp (22 mL)	2	0
Bun, white	1 small	15	14	1 small	15	14
Margarine or butter	1 tsp (5 mL)	0	0	1 tsp (5 mL)	0	0
Cream of mushroom, celery or tomato soup (made with water)	1 cup (250 mL)	8	8	—	—	—
Wheat crackers	2 halves	5	5	—	—	—
	TOTAL CARBS	49 g	41 g	TOTAL CARBS	36 g	28 g
	Total carbs minus fiber = NET CARBS ↑			NET CARBS ↑		
	CARB CHOICES (1 carb choice = 15 g net carbs)		3	CARB CHOICES		2

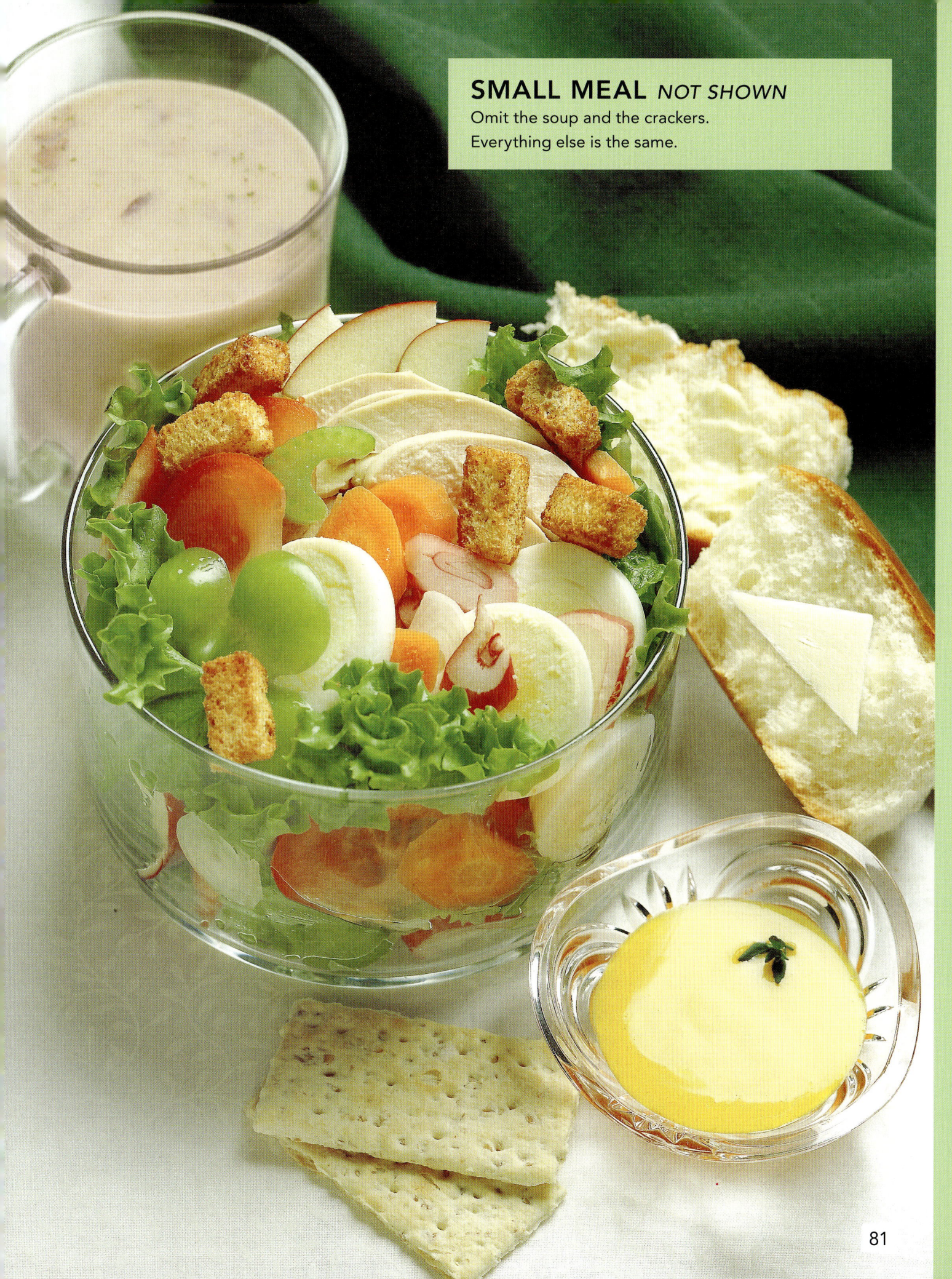

SMALL MEAL *NOT SHOWN*
Omit the soup and the crackers.
Everything else is the same.

LUNCH MEALS

LUNCH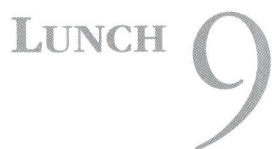

French Onion Soup

French Onion Soup is ready in 15 minutes and is true comfort food.

An even faster way to make this soup is to use 1 package of dried onion soup mix. This package will replace the bouillon mix and the two onions.

French Onion Soup

Makes 4 servings

- 3 packets (each 0.2 oz/4.5 g) reduced-salt beef bouillon mix
- 4 cups (1 L) water
- 2 medium onions, thinly sliced
- 4 slices white bread, toasted
- 4 oz (125 g) Swiss or mozzarella cheese (this is equal to 4 slices of cheese, each 4 inches/10 cm square)

PER SERVING	
Calories	218
Carbohydrate	23 g
Fiber	2 g
Net carbs	21 g
Protein	11 g
Fat, total	9 g
Fat, saturated	5 g
Cholesterol	27 mg
Sodium	621 mg

1. In a pot, add bouillon mix, water and sliced onions. Bring to a boil. Turn down heat and simmer for 15 minutes, until onions are soft.
2. Pour soup into four oven-safe bowls.
3. Cut dry toast into cubes. Put 1 full slice of cubed toast onto each bowl of soup. Place a slice of Swiss cheese on the bread.
4. Broil in the oven until the cheese bubbles.

If you don't have oven-safe bowls, you can broil the cheese on the bread ahead of time, then cube it and place on top of the hot soup.

HEALTH TIP
For a low-salt diet
Use 3 cups (750 mL) of no-salt-added beef broth (or homemade no-salt-added broth) to replace the bouillon and water.

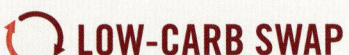 **LOW-CARB SWAP**

FOR THE LARGE MEAL
Swap the bread and butter:
1 slice and 1 tsp (5 mL) margarine/butter
13 g net carbs

→ For extra cheese: An extra ounce (30 g) of cheese added to your bowl of French Onion Soup
1 g net carbs

YOUR LUNCH MENU	Large Meal (520 calories)	Total Carbs	NET CARBS	Small Meal (400 calories)	Total Carbs	NET CARBS
French Onion Soup	1 serving	23	21	1 serving	23	21
Tossed salad	Medium	3	2	Medium	3	2
Oil and vinegar dressing	1 tbsp (15 mL)	0	0	1 tbsp (15 mL)	0	0
Rye bread	1 slice	15	13	—	—	—
Margarine or butter	1 tsp (5 mL)	0	0	—	—	—
Pear	1 medium	26	21	1 medium	26	21
	TOTAL CARBS	**67 g**	**57 g**	TOTAL CARBS	**52 g**	**44 g**
	Total carbs minus fiber = NET CARBS ↑			NET CARBS ↑		
	CARB CHOICES (1 carb choice = 15 g net carbs)		4	CARB CHOICES		3

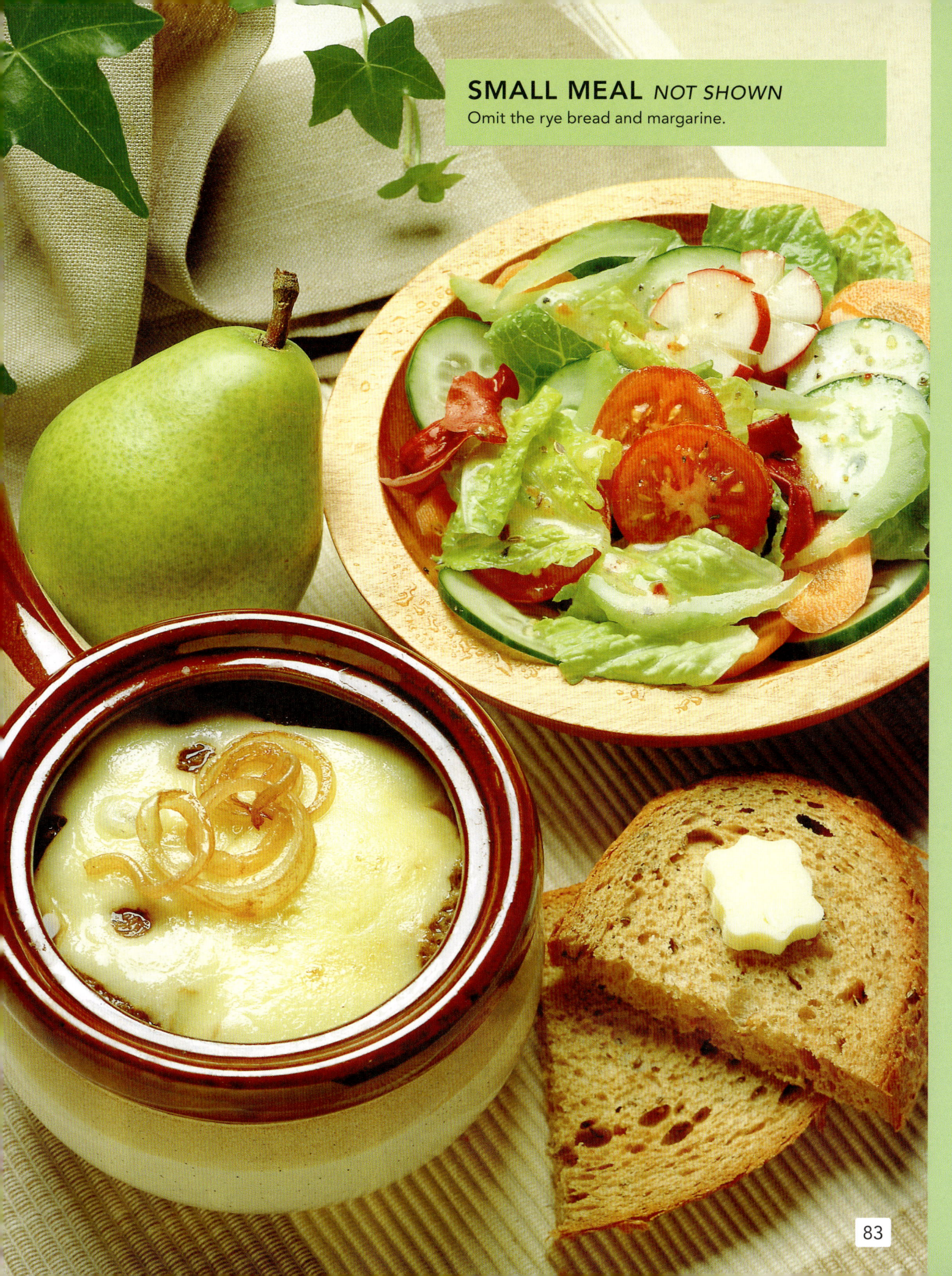

SMALL MEAL *NOT SHOWN*
Omit the rye bread and margarine.

LUNCH MEALS

LUNCH 10

Quesadilla

This quesadilla is a flour tortilla folded in half and lightly fried, with a combination of food in the middle.

🟠 LOW-CARB SWAP

Swap the chocolate pudding, no sugar added:
½ cup (125 mL)
13 g net carbs

→ For dark chocolate (80% cocoa):
10 g (about 1 piece)
2 g net carbs

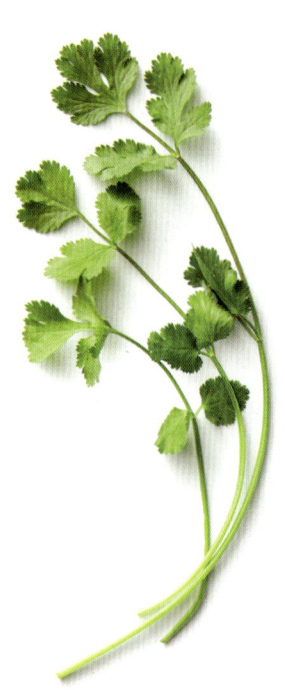

Quesadilla

Each quesadilla:

- 1 8-inch (20 cm) flour tortilla
- 2 tbsp (30 mL) shredded cheese
- 1 oz (30 g) cooked chicken or meat, sliced or cut into small pieces
- 1 tbsp (15 mL) salsa (or several slices of fresh tomato)
- Low-carb add-ins, see below
- 1 tsp (5 mL) margarine, olive oil or other vegetable oil

1. Cover half of the tortilla with cheese, meat, salsa and any low-carb add-ins. Fold the top half over.
2. Lightly coat your tortilla with margarine or oil (use a pastry brush).
3. In a frying pan, cook over low to medium heat until lightly browned on both sides.
4. Remove from pan and cut in half or quarters. Serve with sour cream or Greek yogurt on the side.

Low-carb add-ins: a couple of slices of avocado, a few olives, sliced onions, banana peppers or jalapeno peppers (fresh or pickled), chopped fresh parsley or cilantro, or shredded lettuce or other greens.

PER QUESADILLA	
Calories	302
Carbohydrate	31 g
Fiber	2 g
Net carbs	29 g
Protein	15 g
Fat, total	12 g
Fat, saturated	3 g
Cholesterol	31 mg
Sodium	516 mg

YOUR LUNCH MENU	Large Meal (520 calories)	Total Carbs	NET CARBS	Small Meal (400 calories)	Total Carbs	NET CARBS
Quesadilla	1½	46	43	1	31	29
Sour cream, 5%	1½ tbsp (22 mL)	2	2	1 tbsp (15 mL)	1	1
Raw vegetables	1 cup (250 mL)	5	3	1 cup (250 mL)	5	3
Chocolate pudding, no sugar added	3¾ oz (106 g) container	13	13	3¾ oz (106 g) container	13	13
	TOTAL CARBS	66 g	61 g	TOTAL CARBS	50 g	46 g
	Total carbs minus fiber = NET CARBS ↑			NET CARBS ↑		
	CARB CHOICES (1 carb choice = 15 g net carbs)		4	CARB CHOICES		3

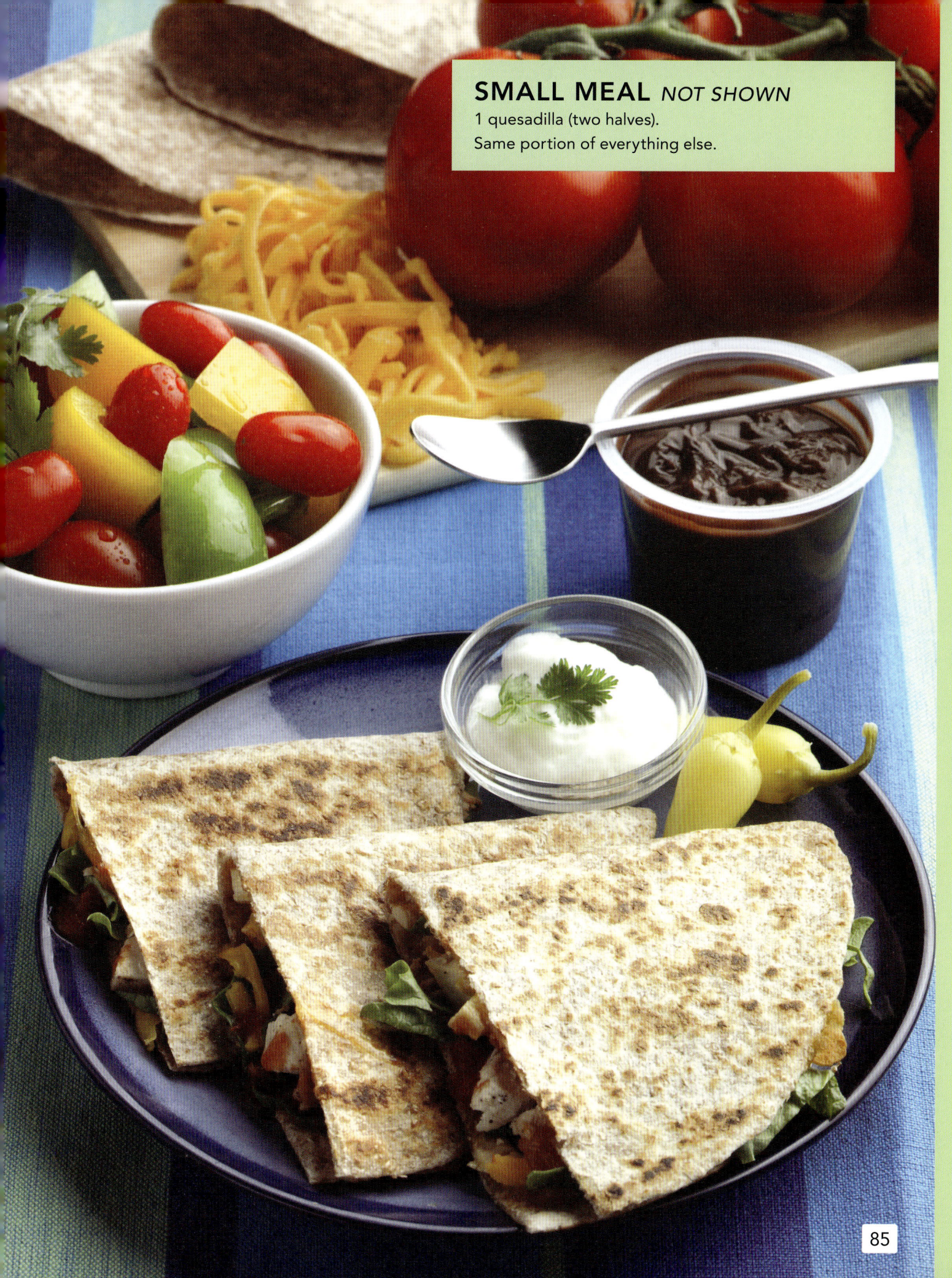

SMALL MEAL *NOT SHOWN*
1 quesadilla (two halves).
Same portion of everything else.

LUNCH MEALS

LUNCH 11

Tuna Sandwich

Aside from tasting good, fish has two amazing benefits to help build a healthy, functioning human body. First, fish is the best source of the most important omega-3 fats, called DHA and EPA. And second, fish is an excellent dietary source of vitamin D.

The American Heart Association and Health Canada recommend that we eat two servings of fish every week. To help meet the recommendation, this cookbook has six fish or seafood dinners, three lunch meals and one breakfast that serve fish, plus several snack ideas found at the back of the book.

A tuna sandwich is a smart way to eat one serving of fish. Canned salmon, sardines and herring are also excellent choices. Pickled herring is a favorite Scandinavian fish option for an open-faced sandwich.

If you love avocado, then mash 3 tbsp (45 mL) of avocado to put in your sandwich instead of the 1½ tbsp (22 mL) of mayonnaise. In these portions, it has similar calories and similar carbs.

Low-carb add-ins for your fish sandwich: chopped celery, chopped or thinly sliced dill pickles, sliced onion, alfalfa sprouts or sliced olives.

RECIPE TIP
Flavored tunas
One small tin (3 oz/85 g) of flavored tuna is equal to half a can of regular tuna. If the tuna is canned in oil, you don't need to add any mayonnaise.

◯ LOW-CARB SWAP

Swap milk:
½ cup (125 mL)
6 g net carbs
→ For unsweetened almond, coconut or cashew beverage:
1 cup (250 mL)
0–3 g net carbs

See Milk Swaps, page 28.

YOUR LUNCH MENU	Large Meal (520 calories)	Total Carbs	NET CARBS	Small Meal (400 calories)	Total Carbs	NET CARBS
Tuna sandwich	1½ sandwiches			1 sandwich		
• bread, whole-grain or whole wheat	3 slices	47	40	2 slices	31	26
• tuna, canned in water, drained	⅔ of a 6 oz (170 g) can	0	0	⅔ of a 6 oz (170 g) can	0	0
• light mayonnaise	1½ tbsp (22 mL)	1	1	1½ tbsp (22 mL)	1	1
• alfalfa sprouts and chopped celery	As desired	1	0	As desired	1	0
Skim or 1% milk	½ cup (125 mL)	6	6	½ cup (125 mL)	6	6
Apple	1 small	15	13	1 small	15	13
	TOTAL CARBS	70 g	60 g	TOTAL CARBS	54 g	46 g
	Total carbs minus fiber = NET CARBS ↑			NET CARBS ↑		
	CARB CHOICES (1 carb choice = 15 g net carbs)		4	CARB CHOICES		3

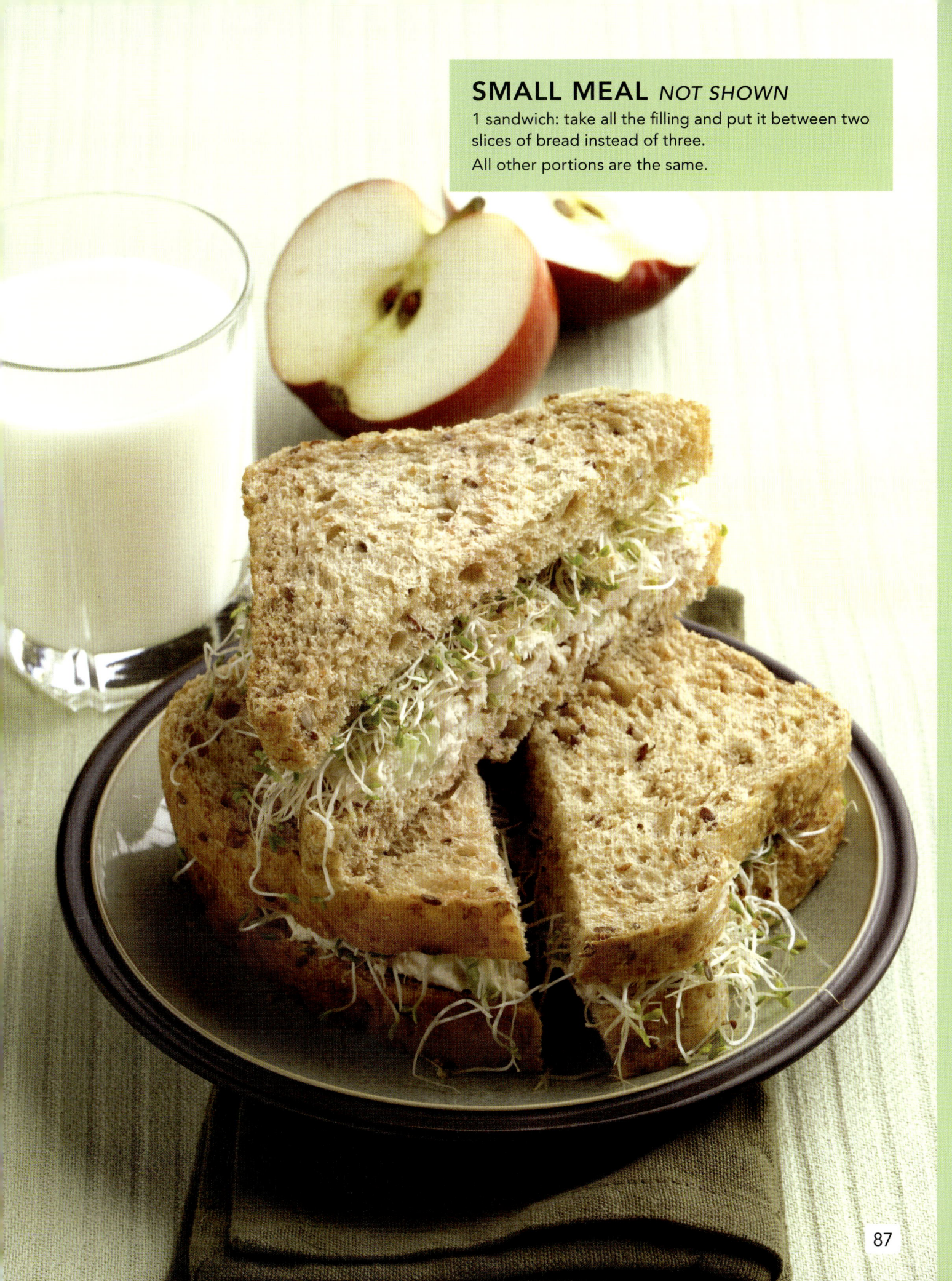

SMALL MEAL *NOT SHOWN*
1 sandwich: take all the filling and put it between two slices of bread instead of three.
All other portions are the same.

LUNCH MEALS

LUNCH 12

Cheese & Crackers

Cheese and crackers can be a hearty and nutritious lunch when combined with nuts and fruit. Nuts give protein and heart-healthy fats, both of which help to reduce hunger pangs later in the day.

In the menu box below, the cheese is a weight amount and the crackers are by calorie count. Check "Nutrition Facts" on labels for portion size and number of crackers.

This lunch is complemented with a cup of hot sugar-free iced tea. Try this – it is surprisingly good. Spoon 1 serving of sugar-free iced tea mix into your mug and add boiling water.

◯ LOW-CARB SWAP

This meal is a nutritious balance and already low-carb with just 3 carb choices in the large meal and 2 in the small meal.

If you want to make a cracker swap, see the Bread Swaps chart on page 274.

RECIPE TIP

Add grated lemon or lime rind to the fruit pieces to boost flavor.

You can also add a spoonful of yogurt.

HEALTH TIP
Food groups for good health
- VEGETABLES AND FRUITS: Provide fiber, vitamins, minerals and antioxidants.
- GRAINS AND STARCHES: Provide fiber, a natural laxative that helps prevent colon cancer and lower blood pressure and blood sugar.
- CALCIUM-RICH FOODS: Important for bones and teeth and is found in milk and milk products and added to plant-based beverages.
- PROTEINS: Includes animal proteins such as lean meats, eggs, fish and dairy and high-fiber vegetable proteins such as beans, lentils, nuts and seeds.
- HEALTHY FATS: Found in vegetable oils, avocados, olives, nuts and seeds. Fish is the best source of omega-3 fats, which are healthy for your brain, blood vessels and eyes.

YOUR LUNCH MENU	Large Meal (520 calories)	Total Carbs	NET CARBS	Small Meal (400 calories)	Total Carbs	NET CARBS
Cheese	1½ oz (45 g)	1	1	1½ oz (45 g)	1	1
Crackers, whole wheat or whole-grain	160-calorie portion	29	24	110-calorie portion	21	17
Fruit pieces	1½ cups (375 mL)	30	24	1 cup (250 mL)	16	11
Nuts	75-calorie portion (8 pecan halves)	2	1	75-calorie portion (8 pecan halves)	2	1
Sugar-free iced tea	1 cup (250 mL)	0	0	1 cup (250 mL)	0	0
	TOTAL CARBS	**62 g**	**50 g**	TOTAL CARBS	**40 g**	**30 g**
	Total carbs minus fiber = NET CARBS ↑			NET CARBS ↑		
	CARB CHOICES (1 carb choice = 15 g net carbs)		3	CARB CHOICES		2

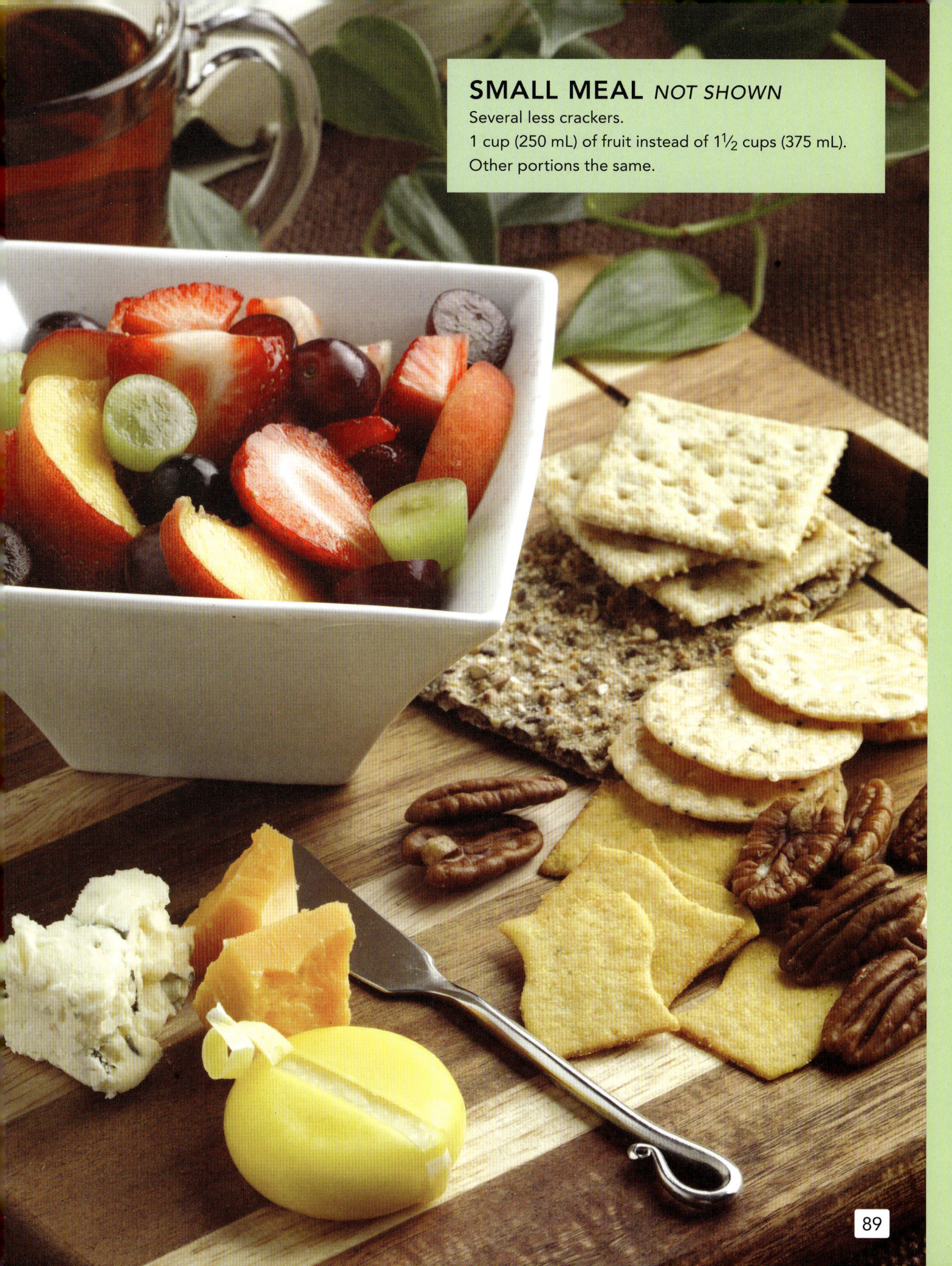

SMALL MEAL *NOT SHOWN*
Several less crackers.
1 cup (250 mL) of fruit instead of 1½ cups (375 mL).
Other portions the same.

LUNCH MEALS

LUNCH 13

Avocado Salad & Bruschetta

HEALTH TIP

Avocados are low in carbohydrates. They have healthy monounsaturated fat – the kind that helps lower the bad LDL cholesterol in your blood.

⊙ LOW-CARB SWAP

This meal is already low-carb, but if you would like a further swap, try this:

LARGE MEAL
Swap French baguette:
6 slices
24 g net carbs
→ For zucchini:
  6 slices
  2 g net carbs

SMALL MEAL
Swap French baguette:
3 slices
12 g net carbs
→ For zucchini:
  3 slices
  1 g net carbs

Avocado Salad

Makes 2 servings

2 cups (500 mL) lettuce pieces
1 medium tomato, cut in wedges
1 medium apple, sliced
1 avocado, sliced
¼ cup (60 mL) shredded cheese
Grated lime rind and a drizzle of lime juice

1. Combine all ingredients.

PER ½ RECIPE	
Calories	269
Carbohydrate	22 g
Fiber	8 g
Net carbs	14 g
Protein	7 g
Fat, total	19 g
Fat, saturated	5 g
Cholesterol	10 mg
Sodium	140 mg

This is a low-fat version of a traditional Italian bruschetta.

Bruschetta

For each slice:

½-inch (1 cm) slice of French baguette
1 tsp (5 mL) salsa or pasta sauce
1 to 2 tsp (5 to 10 mL) of toppings such as sliced olives or capers, pickled garlic or artichoke hearts, or chopped fresh or dried herbs, such as cilantro, basil or chives
2 tsp (10 mL) thinly sliced, crumbled or shredded cheese

1. To each slice of bread add the salsa, toppings of your choice and cheese.
2. Grill the bread slices until the cheese is melted.

PER SLICE	
Calories	40
Carbohydrate	5 g
Fiber	0 g
Net carbs	5 g
Protein	2 g
Fat, total	2 g
Fat, saturated	1 g
Cholesterol	2 mg
Sodium	123 mg

YOUR LUNCH MENU	Large Meal (520 calories)	Total Carbs	NET CARBS	Small Meal (400 calories)	Total Carbs	NET CARBS
Avocado Salad	1 serving	22	14	1 serving	22	14
Light salad dressing	1½ tbsp (22 mL)	4	4	1 tbsp (15 mL)	3	3
Bruschetta	6 baguette slices	29	27	3 baguette slices	14	13
	TOTAL CARBS	55 g	45 g	TOTAL CARBS	39 g	30 g
	Total carbs minus fiber = NET CARBS ↑			NET CARBS ↑		
	CARB CHOICES (1 carb choice = 15 g net carbs)		3	CARB CHOICES		2

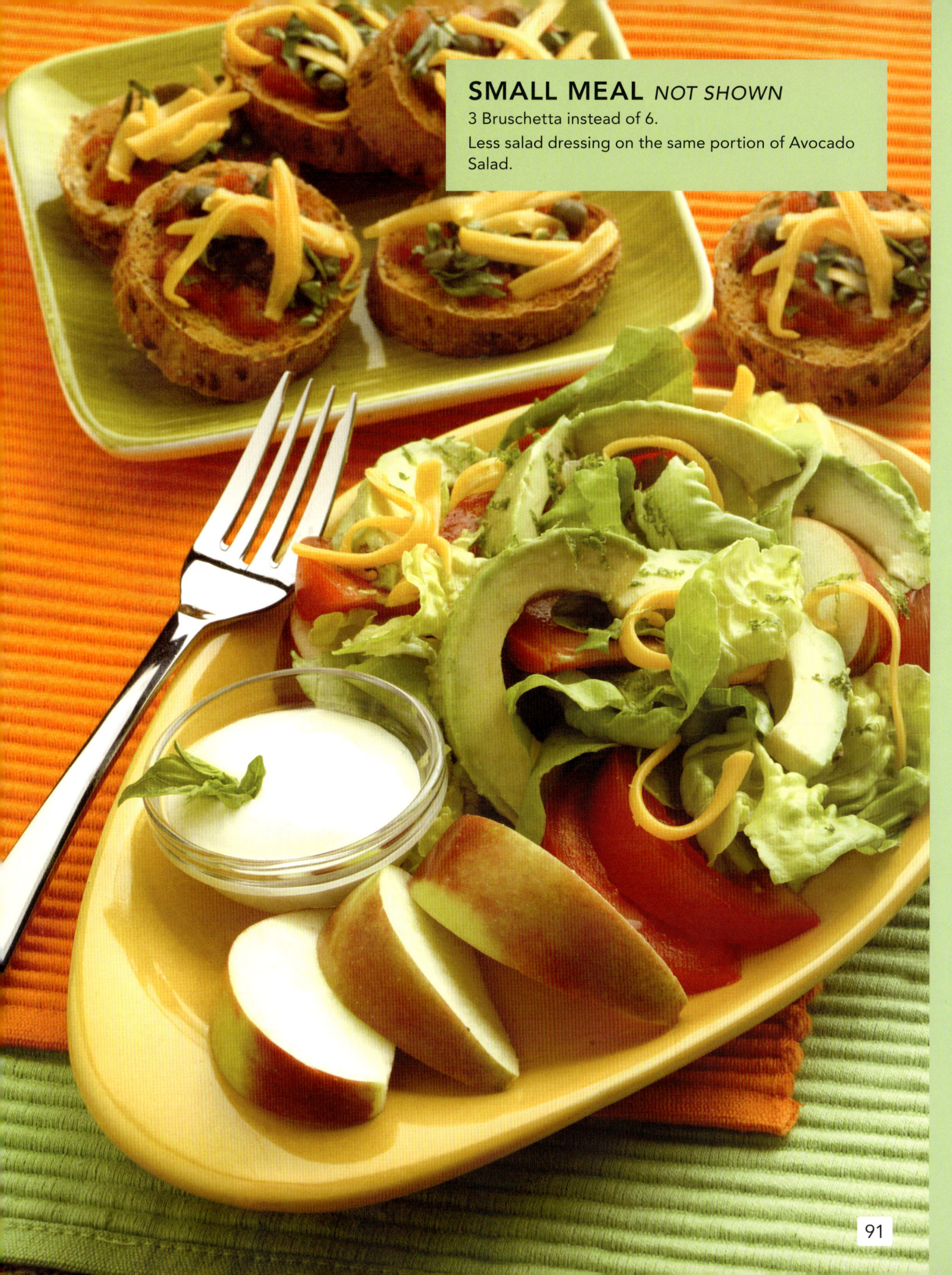

SMALL MEAL *NOT SHOWN*
3 Bruschetta instead of 6.
Less salad dressing on the same portion of Avocado Salad.

LUNCH MEALS

LUNCH 14

Crab Cakes

Maryland Crab Cakes

Makes 6 crab cakes

Preheat oven to 450°F (230°C)

1 large egg
¼ cup (60 g) light mayonnaise
2 tsp (10 mL) prepared or Dijon mustard
2 tsp (10 mL) Worcestershire sauce
1 tsp (5 mL) Old Bay seasoning
  (or ¼ tsp/1 mL each paprika and celery salt)
1 tbsp (15 mL) fresh parsley, chopped (or 2 tsp/10 mL dried)
1 tsp (5 mL) lemon juice, fresh
1 lb (500 g) fresh chunky crab meat (fresh crab is essential for best flavor; 2 cans of drained salmon are a good, less expensive alternative to fresh crab)
⅔ cup (150 mL) soda cracker crumbs
2 tbsp (30 mL) butter, melted

1. In a large bowl, whisk together egg, mayonnaise, mustard, Worcestershire sauce, Old Bay, parsley and lemon juice. Add crab meat and cracker crumbs and gently fold together using a spatula or large spoon.
2. Cover tightly and refrigerate for at least 30 minutes to chill the mixture, then it can be shaped.
3. Butter the baking sheet. Portion the mixture into 6 on the sheet and form into cakes. Brush each lightly with the remaining melted butter.
4. Bake for 12 to 14 minutes or until lightly browned. Drizzle each with fresh lemon juice and serve warm.

PER CRAB CAKE	
Calories	166
Carbohydrate	7 g
Fiber	0 g
Net Carbs	6 g
Protein	14 g
Fat, total	9 g
Fat, saturated	4 g
Cholesterol	10 mg
Sodium	469 mg

RECIPE TIP

Grilled Vegetables

In a bowl, place the corn pieces and a cup of low-carb vegetables (see page 134). Toss with 1 tablespoon (15 mL) of oil or butter, and sprinkle with dried oregano. Grill in the oven with the crab cakes, on their own baking sheet, until tender.

◯ LOW-CARB SWAP

Swap ½ cob of corn:
17 g net carbs
→ For an extra ½ Maryland Crab Cake: (For a total of 1½ crab cakes)
3 g net carbs

This swap has about the same calories with fewer carbs.

YOUR LUNCH MENU	Large Meal (520 calories)	Total Carbs	NET CARBS	Small Meal (400 calories)	Total Carbs	NET CARBS
Maryland Crab Cakes	1 crab cake	7	6	1 crab cake	7	6
Cocktail sauce	2 tbsp (30 mL)	10	9	1 tbsp (15 mL)	5	5
Grilled corn	1 medium cob	38	34	½ medium cob	19	17
Grilled vegetables	1 cup (250 mL)	5	4	1 cup (250 mL)	5	4
Oil or butter (for grilled vegetables)	1 tbsp (15 mL)	0	0	1 tbsp (15 mL)	0	0
	TOTAL CARBS	60 g	53 g	TOTAL CARBS	36 g	32 g
	Total carbs minus fiber = NET CARBS ↑			NET CARBS ↑		
	CARB CHOICES (1 carb choice = 15 g net carbs)		4	CARB CHOICES		2

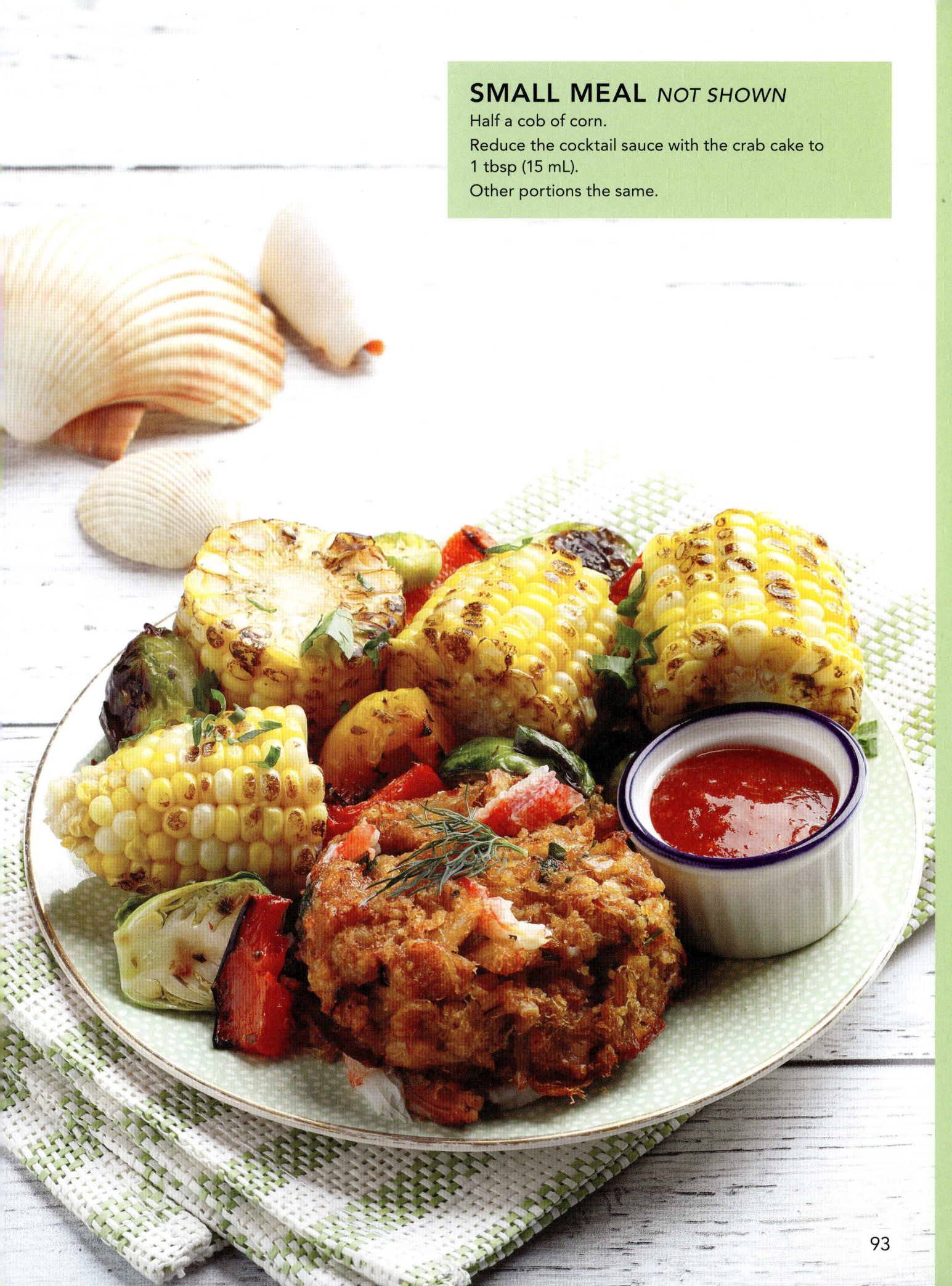

SMALL MEAL *NOT SHOWN*
Half a cob of corn.
Reduce the cocktail sauce with the crab cake to 1 tbsp (15 mL).
Other portions the same.

LUNCH MEALS

LUNCH 15

Nachos in a Pan

All the favorite nacho ingredients with fewer carbs.

Nachos in a Pan

Makes 3 large or 4 small servings

2 tsp (10 mL) vegetable oil

1 medium green pepper (1 cup/250 mL), chopped

1 small zucchini (1 cup/250 mL), chopped

1 cup (250 mL) canned chili beans in chili sauce (undrained)

½ cup (125 mL) salsa, thick and chunky

30 tortilla chips (90 g)

1½ cups (375 mL) cheese (such as mozzarella, Monterey Jack or Cheddar, or a combination), shredded

2 tbsp (30 mL) olives, sliced

2 green onions, sliced

PER SMALL SERVING	
Calories	330
Carbohydrate	28 g
Fiber	6 g
Net Carbs	22 g
Protein	15 g
Fat, total	19 g
Fat, saturated	8 g
Cholesterol	23 mg
Sodium	898 mg

RECIPE TIP

A cold non-alcohol beer pairs nicely with this pan-cooked meal. An alternative beverage is soda water mixed with apple juice. Serve either drink with a slice of lime.

LOW-CARB SWAP

Swap 1 bottle non-alcohol beer:
10–13 g carbs

→ For 1 bottle non-alcohol, low-carb beer
2–5 g carbs

See Beer Swaps, page 282.

1. Heat oil in a 12-inch (30 cm) nonstick frying pan over medium heat. Add chopped pepper and zucchini and stir-fry for 5 minutes, or until vegetables are crisp-tender.
2. Stir in beans and salsa and simmer, stirring for several minutes to cook off some of the juice.
3. Remove mixture from frying pan and place in a bowl. Wipe out juices in pan with a spatula.
4. Place tortilla chips in a single layer in the skillet and up the edges. Pour vegetable and bean mixture onto chips. The tortilla chips will form a soft layer on the bottom. Top with cheese, sliced olives and green onions.
5. Cover the pan with a lid and cook over medium heat for 3 minutes, or until cheese is melted.

YOUR LUNCH MENU	Large Meal (520 calories)	Total Carbs	NET CARBS	Small Meal (400 calories)	Total Carbs	NET CARBS
Cheese and Bean Nachos	⅓ of the pan	37	29	¼ of the pan	28	22
Sour cream, 5%	2 tbsp (30 mL)	2	2	2 tbsp (30 mL)	2	2
Non-alcohol beer (or soda water with ½ cup/125 mL apple juice)	12 oz (330 mL)	13	13	12 oz (330 mL)	13	13
	TOTAL CARBS	**52 g**	**44 g**	TOTAL CARBS	**43 g**	**37 g**
	Total carbs minus fiber = NET CARBS ↑			NET CARBS ↑		
	CARB CHOICES (1 carb choice = 15 g net carbs)		3	CARB CHOICES		2

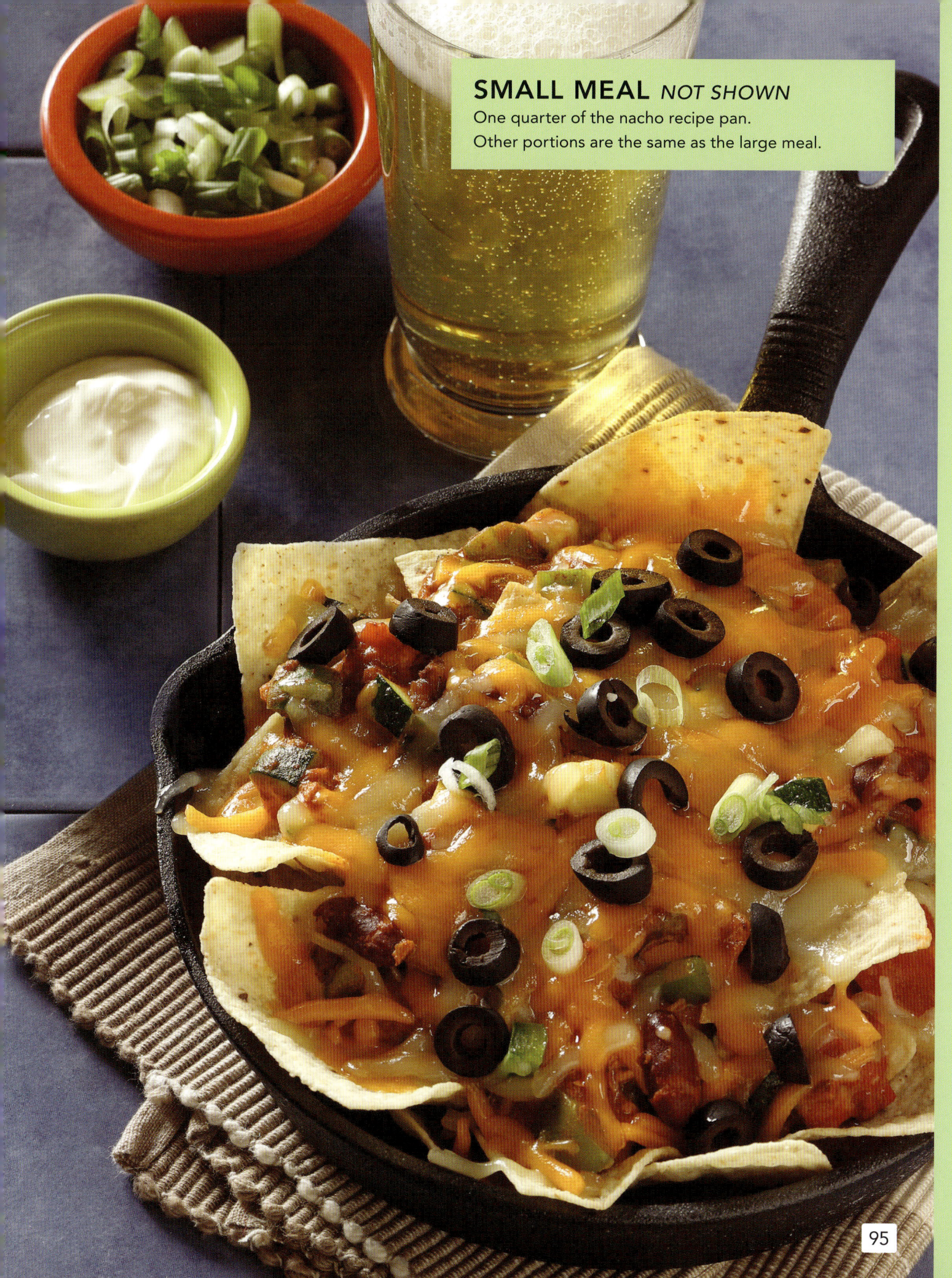

SMALL MEAL *NOT SHOWN*
One quarter of the nacho recipe pan.
Other portions are the same as the large meal.

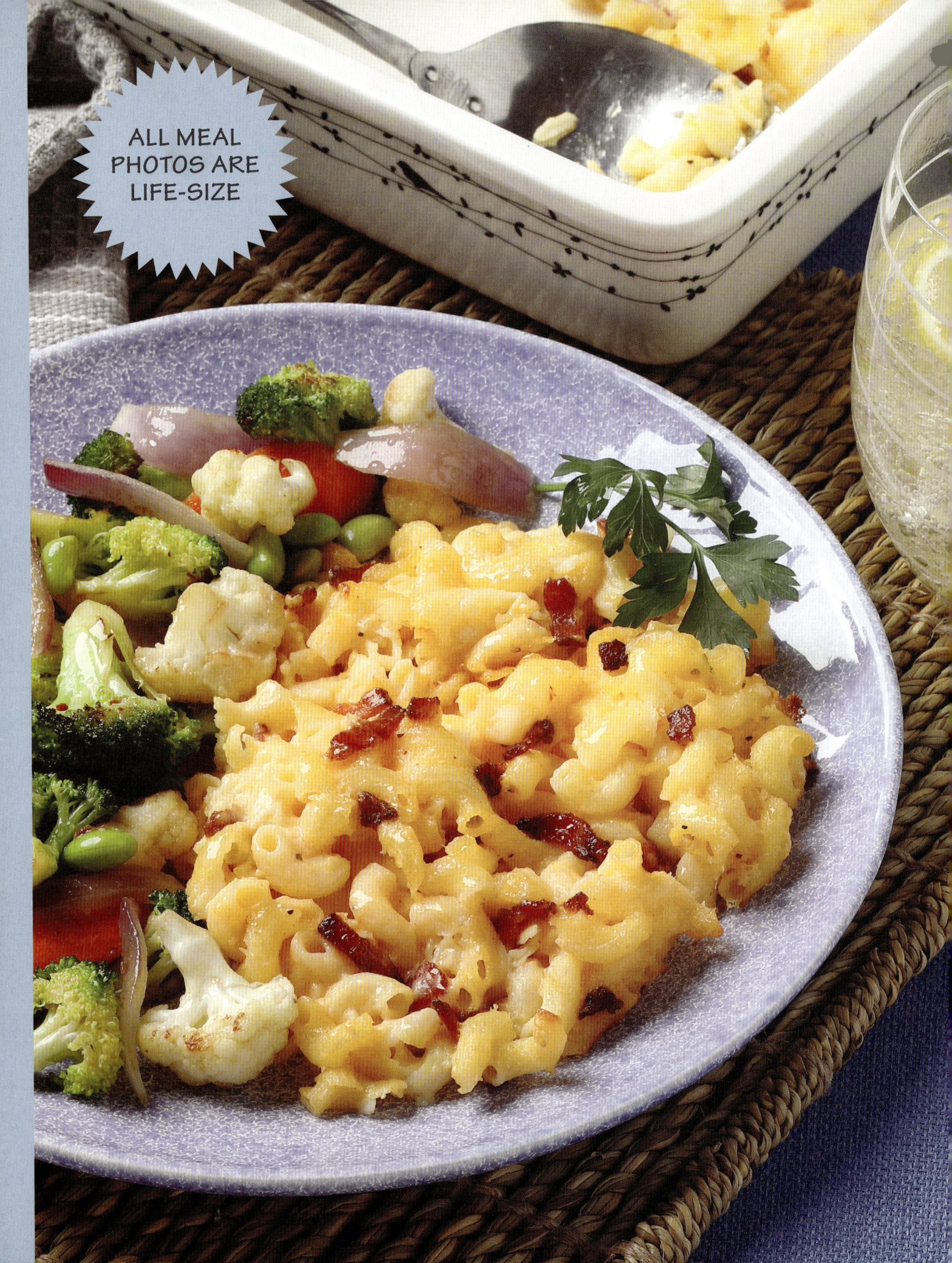

ALL MEAL PHOTOS ARE LIFE-SIZE

Dinner Meals

- Each large dinner has 730 calories and 4–5 Carb Choices
  Total carbs: 90 g or less | net carbs: 75 g or less
- Each small dinner has 550 calories and 3–4 Carb Choices
  Total carbs: 70 g or less | net carbs: 55 g or less

1. Baked Chicken & Potato 98
2. Spaghetti & Meat Sauce 102
3. Fish with Rice 106
4. Roast Beef 110
5. Cold Plate Dinner 114
6. Hamburger Soup & Bannock 118
7. Beans & Wieners 122
8. Steak & Potato 126
9. Cheese Omelet 130
10. Ham & Sweet Potato 134
11. Beef Stew 138
12. Fish & Chips 142
13. Sausages & Cornbread 146
14. Chili Con Carne 150
15. Perogies 154
16. Hamburger with Potato Salad 158
17. Roast Turkey Dinner 162
18. Mac & Cheese 166
19. Pork Chop & Applesauce 170
20. Tacos 174
21. Caribbean Chicken Roti 178
22. Liver & Onions 182
23. Sun Burgers 186
24. Salmon Potato Dish 190
25. Hamburger Casserole 194
26. Pizza 198
27. Fast-Food Dinner 202
28. Stir-Fry 206
29. Denver Sandwich & Soup 210
30. Shish Kebabs 214
31. Tandoori Chicken & Rice 218
32. Swiss Steak 222
33. Thai Chicken 226
34. Poached Salmon with Dill 230
35. Sub Sandwich 234
36. Beef Parmesan 238
37. Santa Fe Salad 242
38. Pork Chop Casserole 246
39. Shrimp Linguine 250
40. Chicken Cordon Bleu 254

DINNER MEALS

DINNER 1

Baked Chicken & Potato

RECIPE TIP

Five Spice Blend
Makes 2 tbsp

2 tsp (10 mL) oregano

1 tsp (5 mL) each of:
- thyme
- paprika
- black pepper
- chili powder

Put spices in a jar and shake. Sprinkle on the skinless chicken.

Your Dinner Menu: See blue menu box at bottom of next page and photo on page 100–101.

Baked chicken: Choose chicken breasts as shown in the photo or chicken legs (skin removed). Sprinkle Five Spice Blend (see sidebar) on the chicken. Bake the chicken at 350° (180°C) for about an hour. Or grill on the barbecue. Chicken is cooked when the juice has no trace of pink, or the internal temperature reads 170°F (75°C).

Baked potatoes: Wash potatoes and poke with a fork. Bake in the oven with the chicken until cooked inside.

Vegetables: Choose frozen or fresh mixed vegetables, and enjoy raw radishes and celery.

Butterscotch Pudding: See page 99 for recipe.

⭕ LOW-CARB SWAP RECIPE: Roasted Rutabaga

LARGE MEAL

Swap roasted potato:
1½ medium (1½ cups/375 mL)
50 g net carbs

→ For roasted rutabaga:
1½ cups (375 mL)
27 g net carbs

→ For roasted turnip:
1½ cups (375 mL)
19 g net carbs

SMALL MEAL

For roasted potato:
1 medium (1 cup/250 mL)
32 g net carbs

→ For roasted rutabaga:
1 cup (250 mL)
18 g net carbs

→ For roasted turnip:
1 cup (250 mL)
9 g net carbs

See Potato Swaps, page 275.

Makes 2 cups (500 mL) cooked

Preheat oven to 425°F (220°C)

Roasted rutabaga has a firm texture similar to potato and has a mild, sweet flavour. Roasted turnips are even lower in carbs than roasted rutabaga, but you may find turnip strong tasting.

1 5-inch (12.5 cm) rutabaga, cut in 1-inch (2.5 cm) pieces (4 cups/1 L raw chopped)

1 tbsp (15 mL) olive or vegetable oil

Salt and pepper to taste

1. Place peeled and chopped rutabaga into a large bowl.
2. Toss rutabaga with oil and salt and pepper.
3. Spread out evenly on greased baking sheet.
4. Bake for 30 to 45 minutes until the rutabaga pieces are tender. Turn once or twice during cooking for even roasting.

1 CUP	
Calories	166
Total carbs	25 g
Net carbs	18 g

DINNER MEALS

Butterscotch Pudding

Makes four (½-cup/125 mL) servings

1 package instant pudding: "fat-free" butterscotch (made with low-calorie sweetener)

1¾ cups (375 mL) cold soy beverage

1. Follow instructions on the box but substitute 1¾ cup (375 mL) soy beverage for the 2 cups (500 mL) of milk.

PER ½ CUP (125 ML)	
Calories	69
Carbohydrate	9 g
Fiber	1 g
Net carbs	8 g
Protein	3 g
Fat, total	2 g
Fat, saturated	1 g
Cholesterol	0 mg
Sodium	366 mg

RECIPE TIP

If you like coconut, add 2 tbsp (30 mL) of dried, shredded, unsweetened coconut into the pudding after you are finished mixing. This will add only 29 calories and 1 g net carbs per serving.

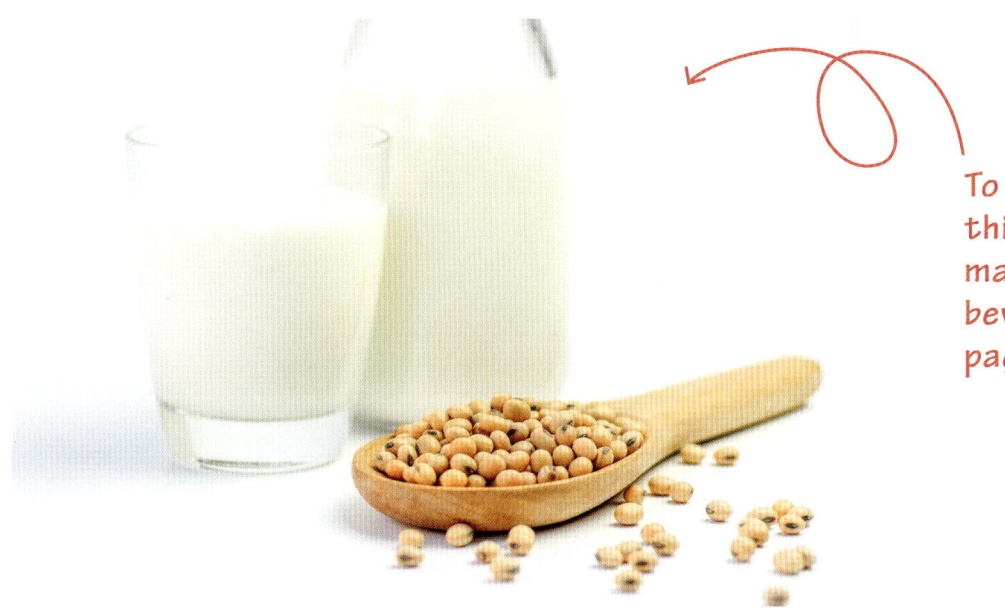

To reduce carbs, this pudding is made with soy beverage (see page 28).

YOUR DINNER MENU	Large Meal (730 calories)	Total Carbs	NET CARBS	Small Meal (550 calories)	Total Carbs	NET CARBS
Baked chicken	1½ breasts (5 oz/150 g, cooked)	0	0	1½ breasts (5 oz/150 g, cooked)	0	0
Baked potato, with skin	1½ medium (1½ cups/375 mL)	55	50	1 medium (1 cup/250 mL)	35	32
Margarine or butter	2 tsp (10 mL)	0	0	—	—	—
Sour cream, 5%	2 tbsp (30 mL)	2	2	2 tbsp (30 mL)	2	2
Mixed vegetables	1 cup (250 mL)	10	6	1 cup (250 mL)	10	6
Radishes	4	1	0	4	1	0
Celery	1 stalk	1	1	1 stalk	1	1
Butterscotch Pudding	½ cup (125 mL)	9	8	½ cup (125 mL)	9	8
	TOTAL CARBS	78 g	67 g	TOTAL CARBS	58 g	49 g
	Total carbs minus fiber = NET CARBS ↑			NET CARBS ↑		
	CARB CHOICES (1 carb choice = 15 g net carbs)	4		CARB CHOICES	3	

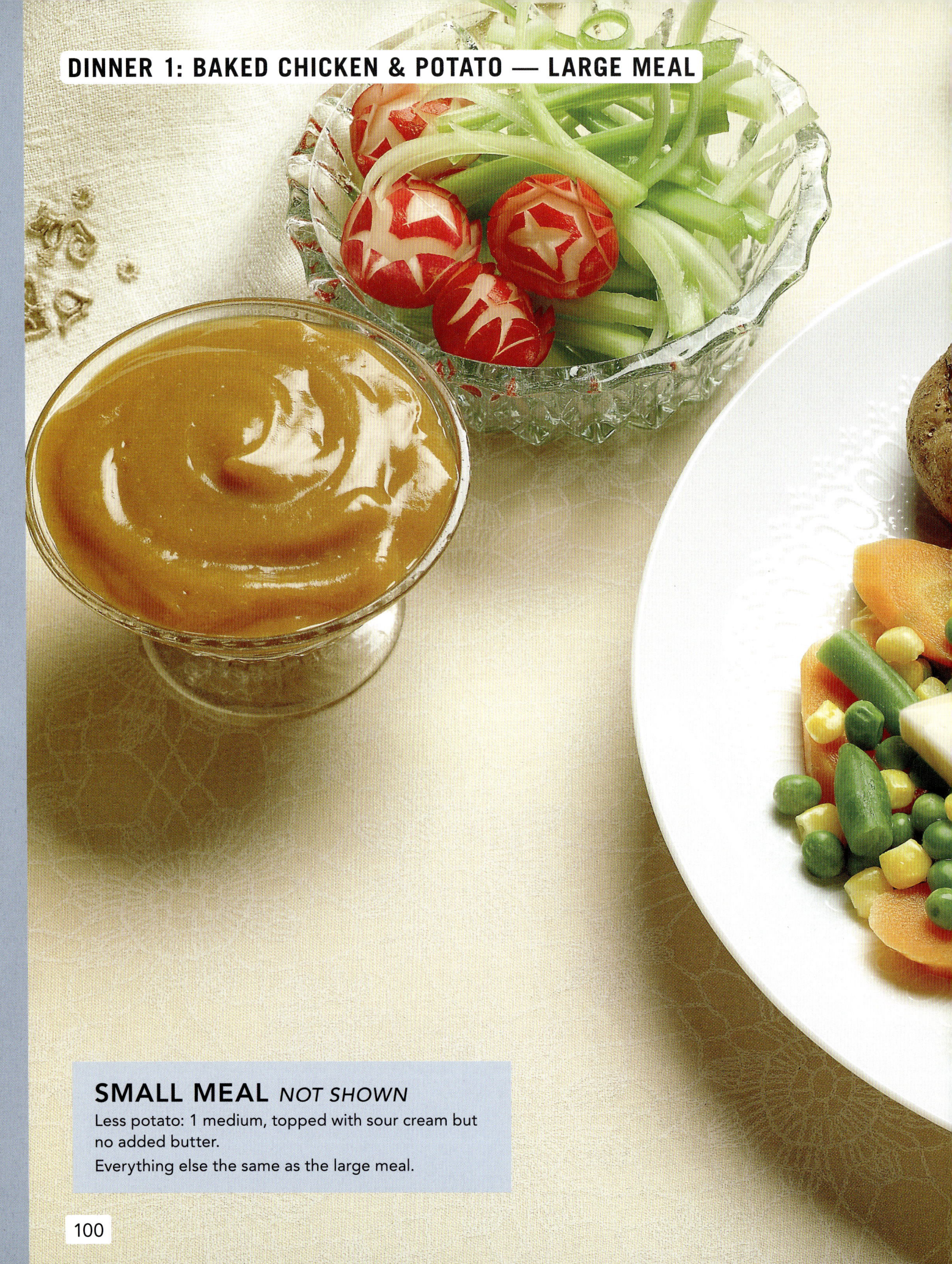

DINNER 1: BAKED CHICKEN & POTATO — LARGE MEAL

SMALL MEAL *NOT SHOWN*

Less potato: 1 medium, topped with sour cream but no added butter.

Everything else the same as the large meal.

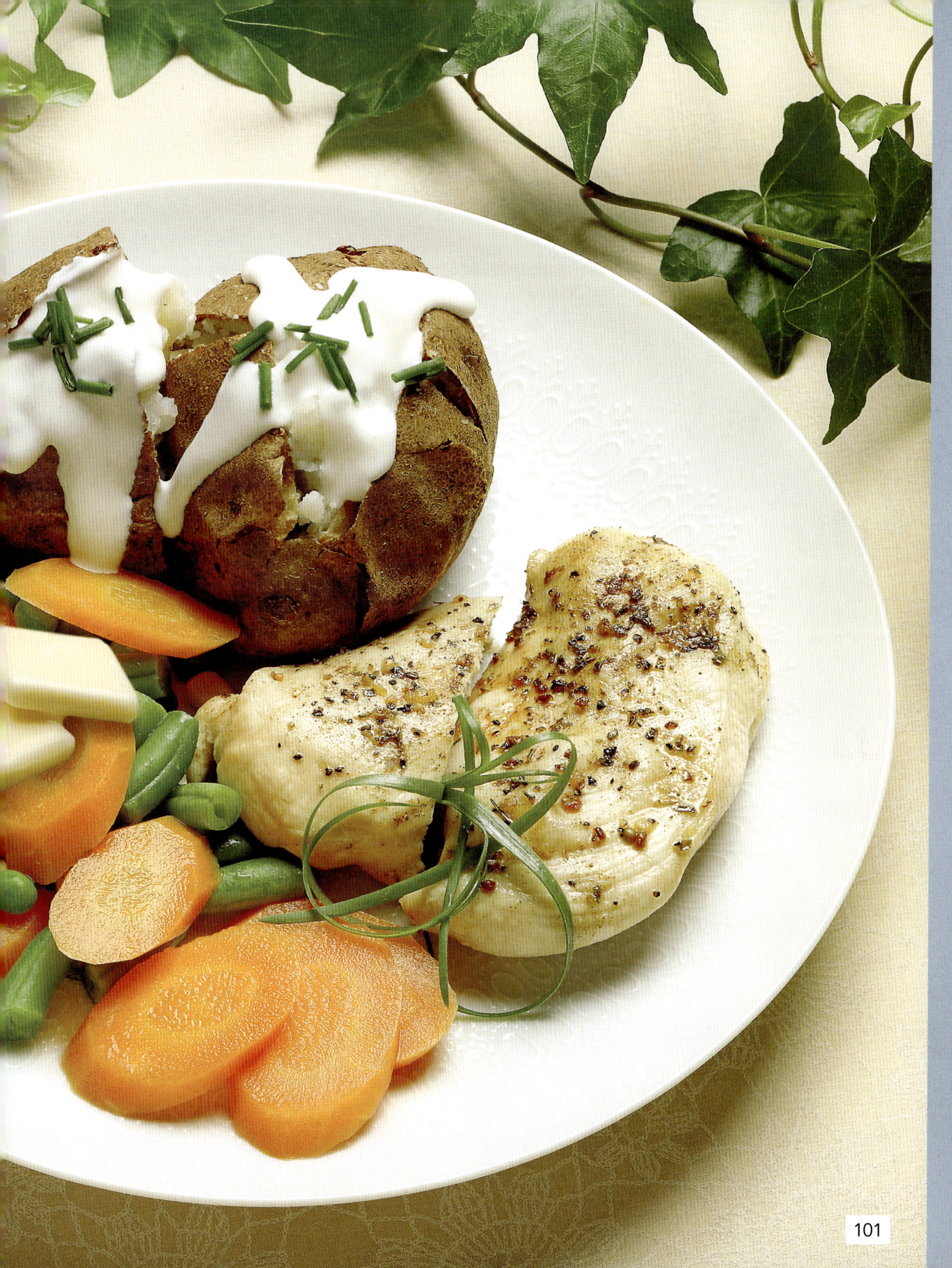

DINNER MEALS

DINNER 2

Spaghetti & Meat Sauce

Spaghetti and meat sauce is an easy-to-make favorite.

If you would like a glass of red or white wine with your meal, a 5 oz (140 mL) glass of red table wine has 125 calories, 4 g net carbs and 12% alcohol.

Spaghetti Meat Sauce

Makes 8 cups (2 L) of sauce

1 lb (500 g) lean ground beef
1 medium onion, chopped
28 oz (796 mL) can tomatoes
1 cup (250 mL) water
1 small tin (5½ oz/156 mL) tomato paste
1 tsp (5 mL) garlic powder or 4 cloves garlic, chopped
3 bay leaves (remove before serving)
1 tsp (5 mL) chili powder
2 tsp (10 mL) dried oregano
2 tsp (10 mL) dried basil
½ tsp (2 mL) paprika
¼ tsp (1 mL) ground cinnamon
¼ tsp (1 mL) ground cloves
2 cups (500 mL) chopped vegetables, such as green pepper, celery or mushrooms

PER 1 CUP (250 ML)	
Calories	153
Carbohydrate	14 g
Fiber	3 g
Net carbs	11 g
Protein	13 g
Fat, total	6 g
Fat, saturated	2 g
Cholesterol	30 mg
Sodium	224 mg

1. Brown the ground beef. Drain off as much fat as you can.
2. Add the rest of the ingredients.
3. Bring to a boil, then turn down heat. Cover and simmer for about 1 hour. Stir every now and then so the sauce doesn't stick. Add extra water if it gets too thick.
4. Serve over hot spaghetti with grated Parmesan cheese.

Dessert

Light gelatin is a carb-free dessert that pairs well with a pasta meal. It takes only a few minutes to make, but it must be left in the fridge for about 2 hours to set. Follow the package directions.

RECIPE TIP

Meatless Spaghetti Sauce

Do not include the meat (omit step 1).

Include other proteins:

- 5 tbsp (75 mL) cheese, shredded
- Or 3 tbsp (45 mL) seeds or nuts

These proteins can be sprinkled on the sauce just before eating. Use less for the small meal.

Portion of dry spaghetti to cooked

60 g (2 oz) of dry spaghetti equals about 1 cup (250 mL) cooked spaghetti.

LOW-CARB SWAP RECIPE: Vegetable Noodles

LARGE MEAL

Swap cooked spaghetti:
1¼ cups (300 mL)
47 g net carbs

→ For whole wheat spaghetti:
1¼ cups (300 mL)
43 g net carbs

→ For zucchini noodles:
1¼ cups (300 mL)
5 g net carbs

SMALL MEAL

Swap cooked spaghetti:
¾ cup (175 mL)
28 g net carbs

→ For whole wheat spaghetti:
¾ cup (175 mL)
26 g net carbs

→ For zucchini noodles:
¾ cup (175 mL)
3 g net carbs

See Pasta Swaps, page 275.

Make zucchini noodles with a cheese grater

Start with the whole zucchini with the skin on. Use the side of the grater with the large holes and make long strokes along these holes to create lovely zucchini noodles (zoodles). Discard the zucchini center with the seeds.

A spiralizer (see photo below) has options for quickly making different types of vegetable noodles (such as zucchini or butternut squash noodles).

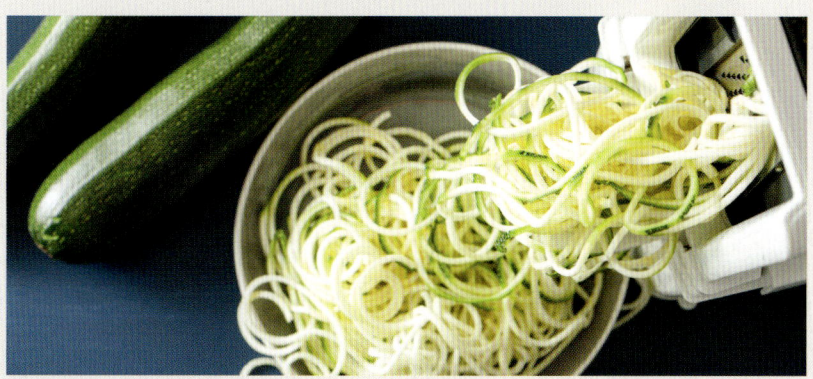

How to cook vegetable noodles

In a teaspoon of oil on medium heat, quickly fry and move the noodles around for no more than a minute. Vegetable noodles will get mushy if overcooked.

YOUR DINNER MENU	Large Meal (730 calories)	Total Carbs	NET CARBS	Small Meal (550 calories)	Total Carbs	NET CARBS
Spaghetti, cooked	1¼ cups (300 mL)	50	47	¾ cups (175 mL)	30	28
Meat sauce	1½ cups (375 mL)	20	16	1½ cups (375 mL)	20	16
Parmesan cheese	2 tbsp (30 mL)	1	1	1 tbsp (15 mL)	1	1
Cooked carrots	½ cup (125 mL)	8	6	½ cup (125 mL)	8	6
Margarine or butter	1 tsp (5 mL)	0	0	—	—	—
Salad	Medium	3	2	Medium	3	2
Oil and vinegar dressing (half oil, half vinegar)	1 tbsp (15 mL)	0	0	1 tbsp (15 mL)	0	0
Almond beverage	1 cup (250 mL)	1	0	1 cup (250 mL)	1	0
Light gelatin	½ cup (125 mL)	0	0	½ cup (125 mL)	0	0
	TOTAL CARBS	83 g	72 g	TOTAL CARBS	63 g	53 g
Total carbs minus fiber = NET CARBS ↑				NET CARBS ↑		
CARB CHOICES (1 carb choice = 15 g net carbs)			5	CARB CHOICES		4

DINNER 2: SPAGHETTI & MEAT SAUCE — LARGE MEAL

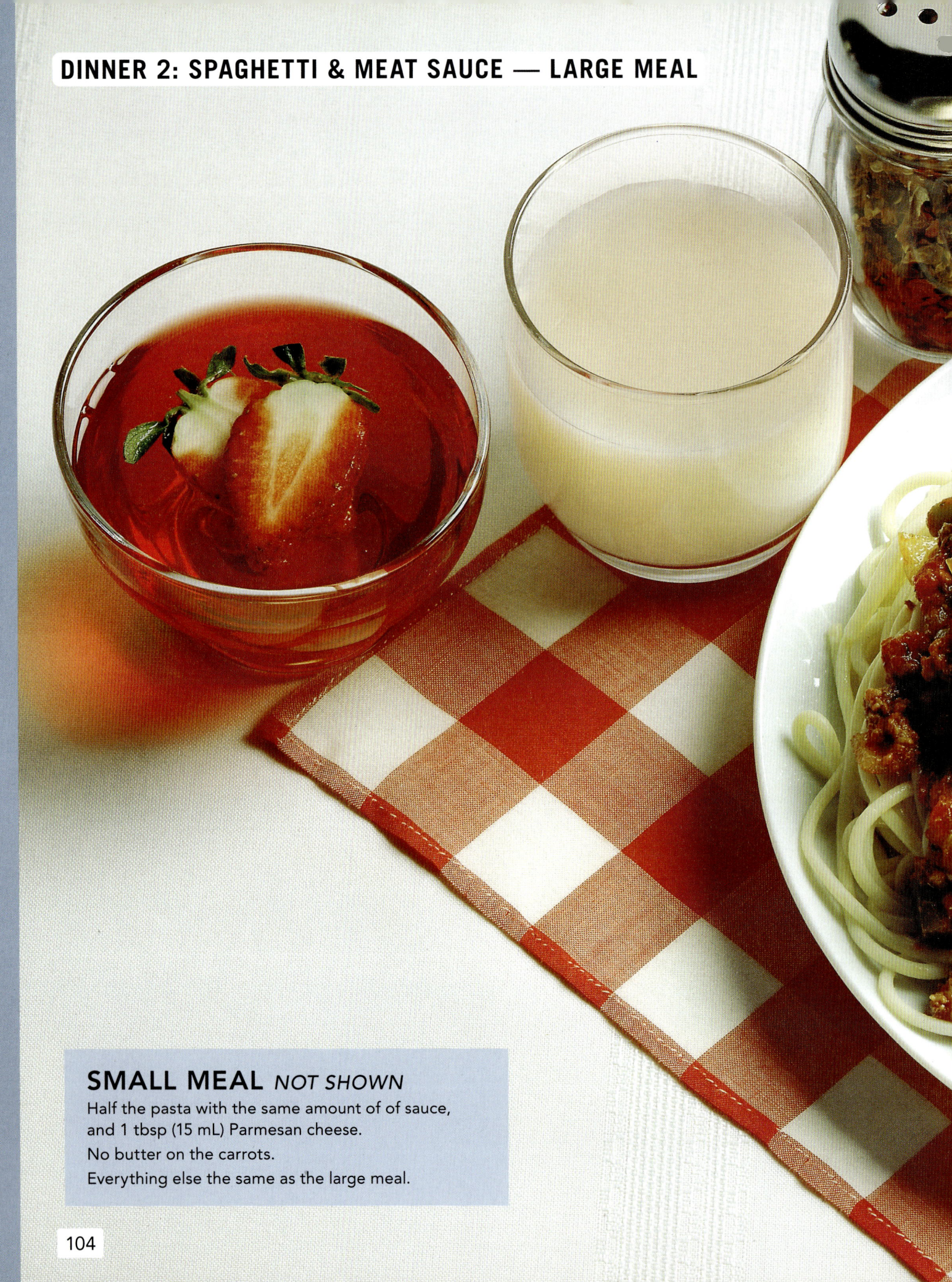

SMALL MEAL *NOT SHOWN*

Half the pasta with the same amount of of sauce, and 1 tbsp (15 mL) Parmesan cheese.

No butter on the carrots.

Everything else the same as the large meal.

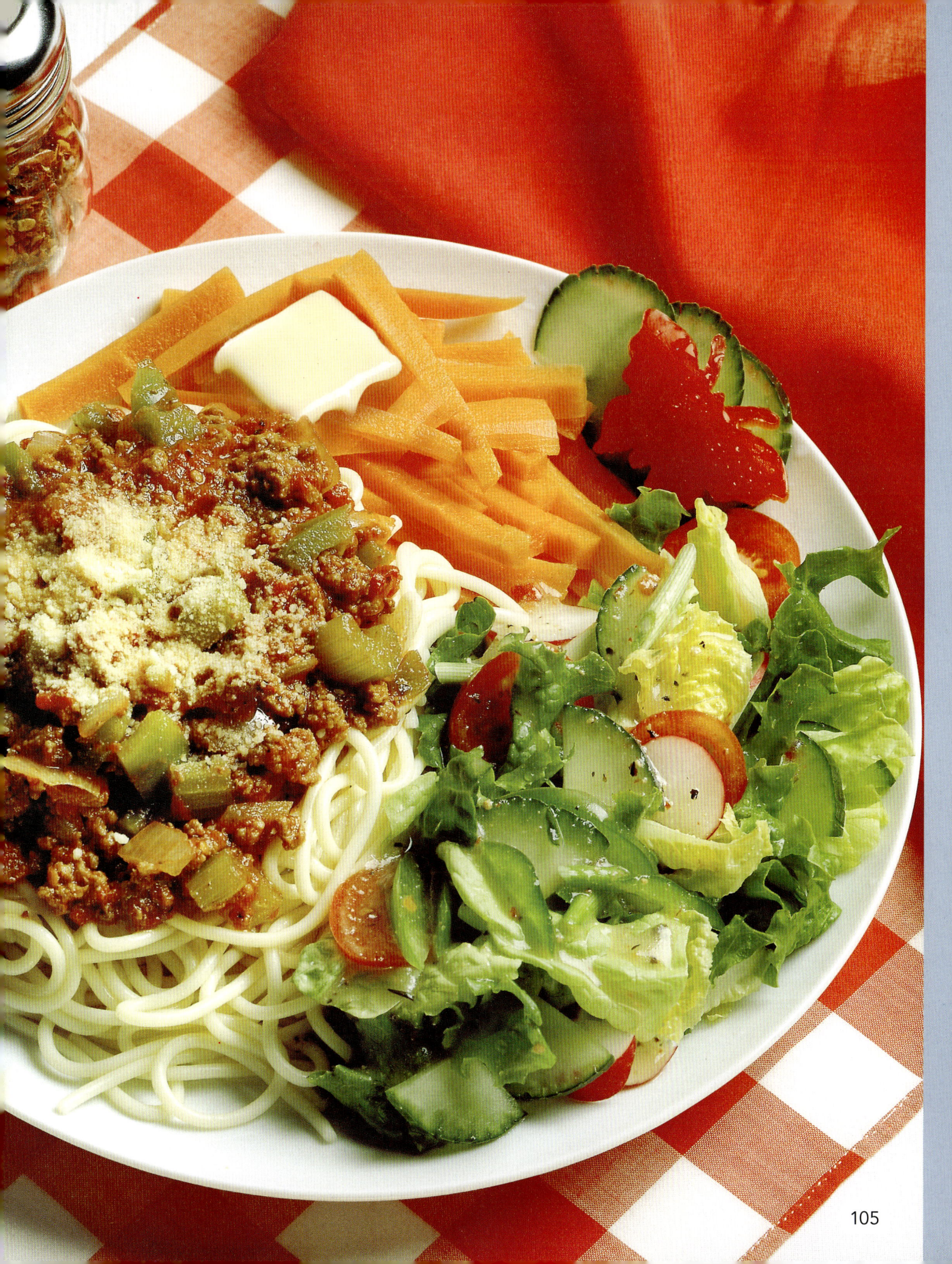

DINNER MEALS

DINNER 3

Fish with Rice

How to Cook Fish

Fish can be pan fried or poached, broiled or baked in the oven at 350°F to 400°F (180°C to 200°C) for 10 to 15 minutes. These spices go well with fish: basil, Cajun spice, curry, dill, oregano, parsley, thyme or Old Bay Seasoning. The secret to great-tasting fish is: do not overcook it. Fish is cooked when it flakes easily.

HEALTH TIP

Low-fat fish:
- bass
- cod
- haddock
- perch
- pickerel (walleye)
- pike
- red snapper
- sole
- tilapia

High-fat fish:
This fish is highest in the healthy omega-3 fats but also higher in calories.
- herring
- mackerel
- salmon
- sardines
- trout
- tuna

Rice

Cook brown rice according to directions on the package, omitting the salt. If you have wild rice, add ¼ cup (60 mL) into the pot: this small amount will cook in the same time as the brown rice. The carbohydrates listed in the menu are for this brown rice and wild rice mixture.

Riced cauliflower (see Low-Carb Swap) is sold in the frozen vegetable section. This cauliflower has been chopped into rice-sized pieces.

Vegetables

This meal is served with peas, a sweet vegetable and yellow or green beans, which are less sweet. See page 134 for a list of low-carb vegetables.

◯ LOW-CARB SWAP

LARGE MEAL
Swap cooked brown rice:
1 cup (250 mL)
42 g net carbs
→ For riced cauliflower:
1 cup (250 mL)
3 g net carbs

SMALL MEAL
Swap cooked brown rice:
½ cup (125 mL)
21 g net carbs
→ For riced cauliflower:
½ cup (125 mL)
2 g net carbs

See Rice Swaps, page 276.

DINNER MEALS

Fruit Milkshake

Makes 2 cups (500 mL)

1 cup (250 mL) skim milk

½ cup (125 mL) frozen raspberries or other frozen berries

1 tbsp (15 mL) zero-calorie sweetener

1. Pour milk in a blender. Place in your freezer for 30 minutes. If doubling the recipe, freeze for an hour.
2. Take blender out of the freezer. Add fruit and zero-calorie sweetener. Mix in blender for 30 seconds, until thick and frothy. Serve right away.

PER 1 CUP (250 ML)	
Calories	52
Carbohydrate	8 g
Fiber	0 g
Net carbs	8 g
Protein	5 g
Fat, total	0 g
Fat, saturated	0 g
Cholesterol	2 mg
Sodium	52 mg

⟳ LOW-CARB SWAP

FRUIT MILKSHAKE RECIPE

Swap 1 cup (250 mL) of milkshake made with skim milk
8 g net carbs

→ For 1 cup (250 mL) of milkshake made with unsweetened almond beverage
2 g net carbs

See Milk Swaps, page 28.

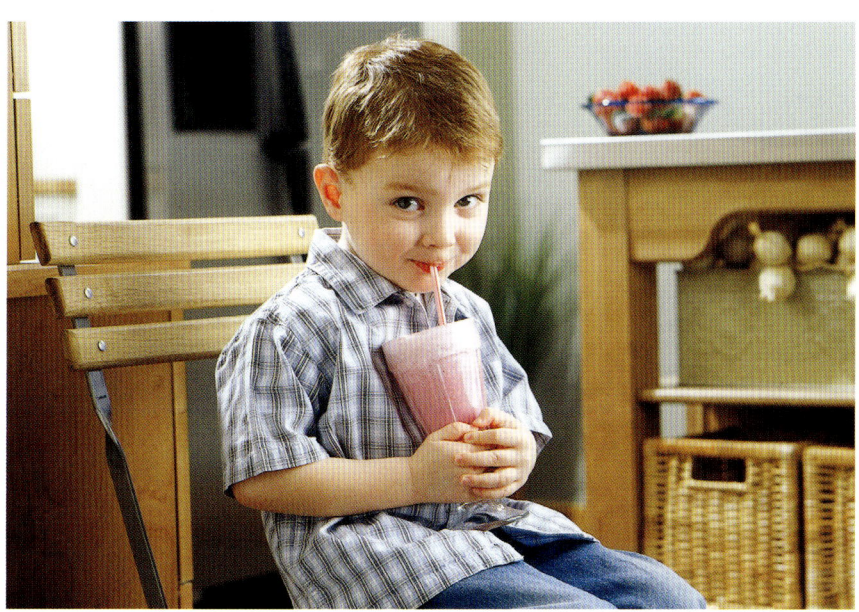

YOUR DINNER MENU	Large Meal (730 calories)	Total Carbs	NET CARBS	Small Meal (550 calories)	Total Carbs	NET CARBS
Fish with lemon slice	6 oz (175 g), cooked	0	0	6 oz (175 g), cooked	0	0
Margarine or oil (to cook fish or put on veggies)	2 tsp (10 mL)	0	0	2 tsp (10 mL)	0	0
Brown rice, cooked	1 cup (250 mL)	44	41	½ cup (125 mL)	22	20
Green peas	½ cup (125 mL)	11	7	½ cup (125 mL)	11	7
Yellow beans	1 cup (250 mL)	10	7	1 cup (250 mL)	10	7
Fruit milkshake	1 cup (250 mL)	15	8	1 cup (250 mL)	15	8
Kiwi	1 medium	10	8	1 medium	10	8
	TOTAL CARBS	90 g	71 g	TOTAL CARBS	68 g	50 g
	Total carbs minus fiber = NET CARBS ↑			NET CARBS ↑		
CARB CHOICES (1 carb choice = 15 g net carbs)			5	CARB CHOICES		3

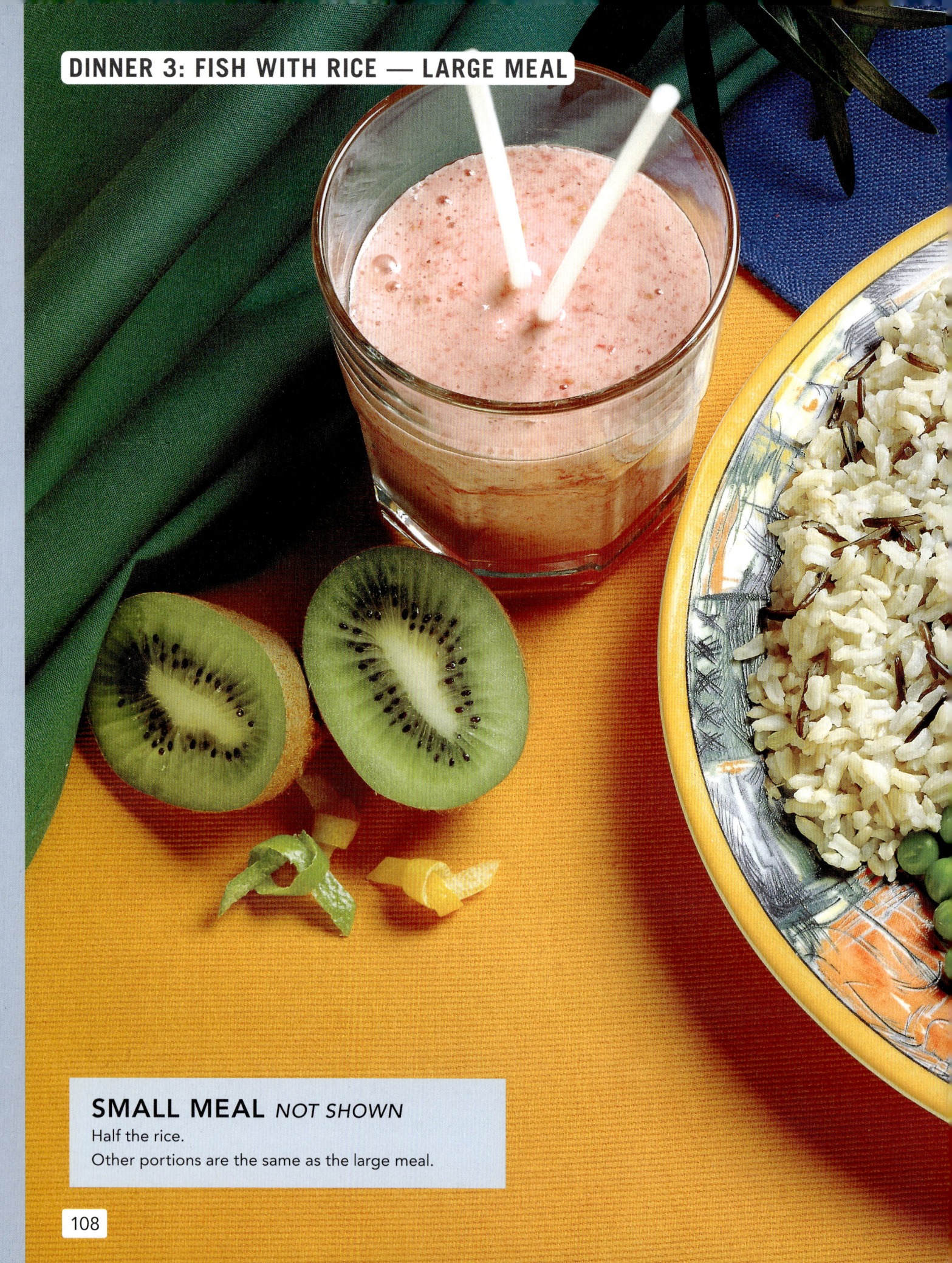

DINNER 3: FISH WITH RICE — LARGE MEAL

SMALL MEAL *NOT SHOWN*
Half the rice.
Other portions are the same as the large meal.

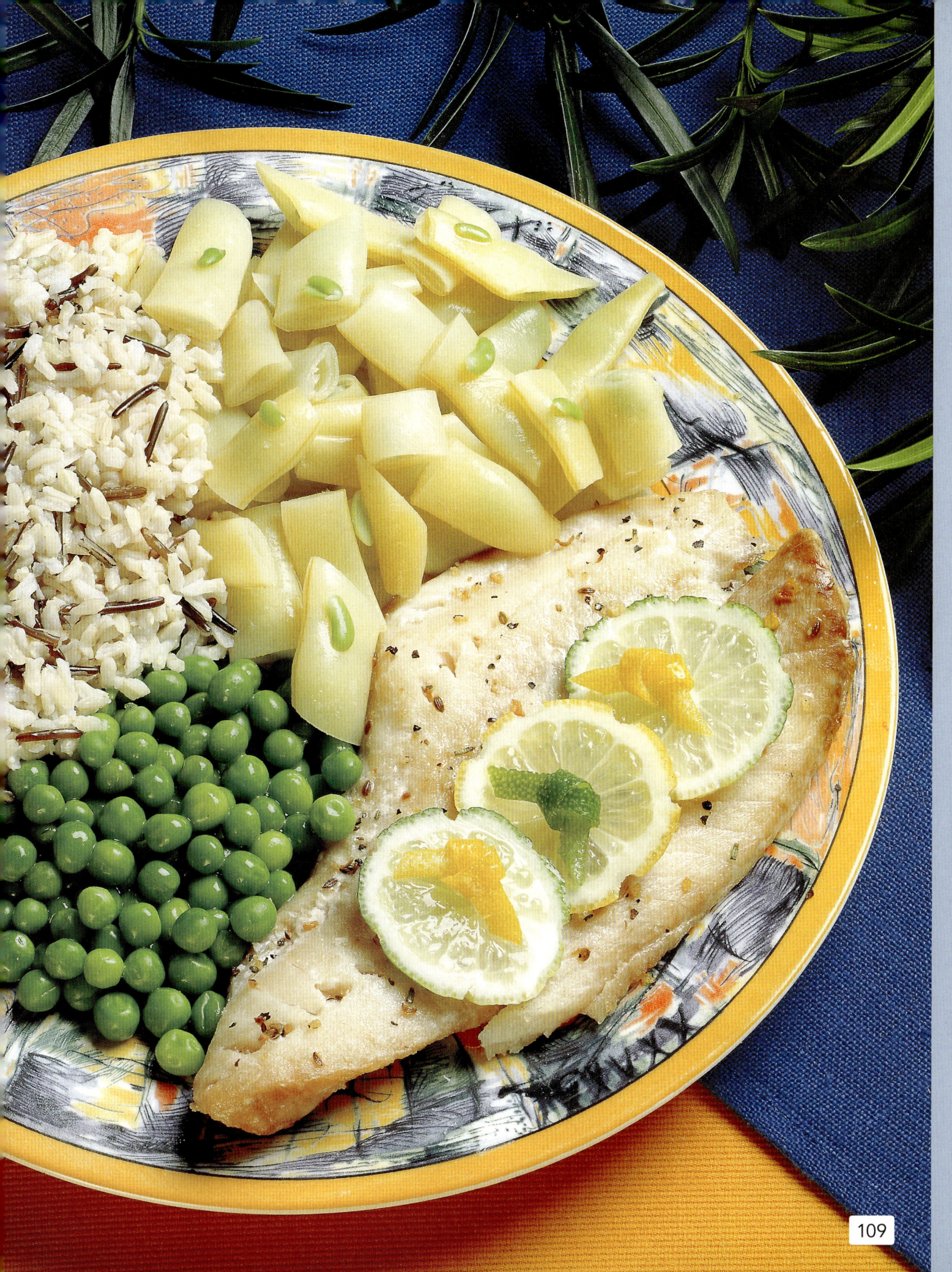

DINNER MEALS

DINNER 4

RECIPE TIP

Tender cuts of roast
- Ribeye roast marbled with fat, excellent cut
- Tenderloin
- Sirloin tip
- Top round
- Top sirloin

Talk with your supermarket butcher; they will help you choose the right cut for you.

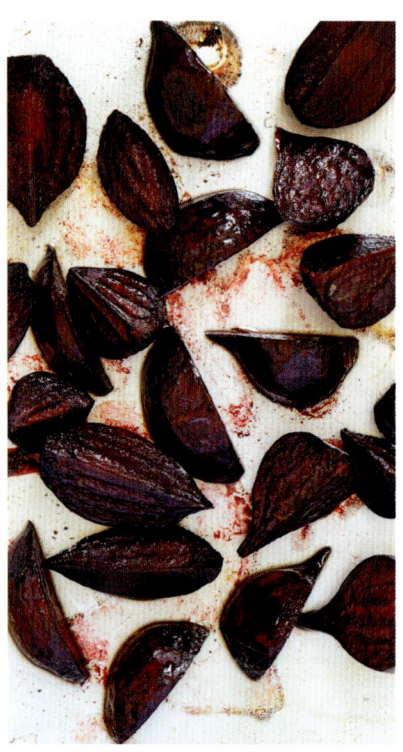

Roast Beef

A Common Way to Cook Roast Beef

- Prepare a paste of vegetable or olive oil, 2 or 3 crushed garlic cloves, and ½ tsp (2 mL) each of salt and pepper, rosemary and thyme. Rub it on all sides of the raw roast beef.

- Lay the roast on a rack in a roasting pan, with no lid. Place in a preheated hot oven of 500°F (260°C) and cook for 15 minutes. Turn the oven temperature down to 275°F (140°C) and cook another 1½ hours until the internal temperature reads 145°F (62°C).

- Once it is cooked to medium doneness, remove from the oven, cover and let it rest for at least 20 minutes before carving. Resting the roast allows the juices to flow away from the centre and back to the outer edges, ensuring the whole roast is juicy throughout.

Once your roast is ready, make your gravy using the brown gravy mix.

The oven-roasted potatoes are peeled and cooked for an hour in a similar method to the Oven-Roasted Beets below.

Oven-Roasted Beets – An Alternative to Boiled Beets

Preheat oven to 400°F (200°C)

4 medium (3-inch/7.5 cm) beets

1 tbsp (15 mL) olive or vegetable oil

Salt and pepper, to taste

1. Scrub the beets to remove any dirt. Trim off the tops and bottoms.
2. Cut into chunks and place in a large bowl with the oil and toss.
3. Sprinkle with salt and pepper.
4. Place on an oiled baking sheet, or use parchment paper, and bake for 45 minutes to an hour, until the beets are tender. Turn the beets once or twice during cooking.

DINNER MEALS

For dessert, enjoy stewed rhubarb with ice cream. Stewed rhubarb is also nice served warm on a piece of toast or on its own as a low-carb snack.

Stewed Rhubarb

Makes 1¾ cups (425 mL)

4 cups (1 L) rhubarb (fresh or frozen), cut into 1-inch (2.5 cm) pieces
2 tbsp (30 mL) water
½ tsp (2 mL) sugar-free drink mix (strawberry or raspberry)
Dash of cinnamon

PER 1 CUP (250 ML)	
Calories	62
Carbohydrate	15 g
Fiber	7 g
Net carbs	8 g
Protein	3 g
Fat, total	1 g
Fat, saturated	0 g
Cholesterol	0 mg
Sodium	23 mg

> **LOW-CARB SWAP**
>
> **LARGE AND SMALL MEAL**
>
> Swap ice cream:
> 2 tbsp (30 mL)
> **4 g net carbs**
>
> → For plain Greek yogurt:
> 2 tbsp (30 mL)
> **2 g net carbs**
>
> → For keto frozen dessert:
> 2 tbsp (30 mL)
> **0 g net carbs**
>
> See Ice Cream Swaps, page 278.

1. Add rhubarb and water to a heavy pot and simmer at a low temperature for about 15 minutes, until rhubarb is soft. Add more water as needed.
2. While still warm, add sugar-free drink mix and cinnamon.
3. Store in the fridge.

YOUR DINNER MENU	Large Meal (730 calories)	Total Carbs	NET CARBS	Small Meal (550 calories)	Total Carbs	NET CARBS
Roast beef	5 oz (150 g), cooked	0	0	5 oz (150 g), cooked	0	0
Horseradish	1 tbsp (15 mL)	2	1	1 tbsp (15 mL)	2	1
Baked onions	3 small or 1 medium	3	2	3 small or 1 medium	3	2
Roasted potatoes (no skin)	1½ medium	47	42	½ medium	16	14
Brown gravy mix (regular or 25% less salt)	¼ cup (60 mL)	4	4	¼ cup (60 mL)	4	4
Boiled beets	½ cup (125 mL)	8	6	½ cup (125 mL)	8	6
Salad	Small	2	1	Small	2	1
Salad dressing	1 tbsp (15 mL) oil and vinegar	0	0	1 tbsp (15 mL) fat-free Italian	2	2
Stewed Rhubarb	1 cup (250 mL)	15	8	1 cup (250 mL)	15	8
Ice cream	2 tbsp (30 mL)	4	4	2 tbsp (30 mL)	4	4
	TOTAL CARBS	85 g	68 g	TOTAL CARBS	56 g	42 g
	Total carbs minus fiber = NET CARBS ↑				NET CARBS ↑	
	CARB CHOICES (1 carb choice = 15 g net carbs)		4	CARB CHOICES		3

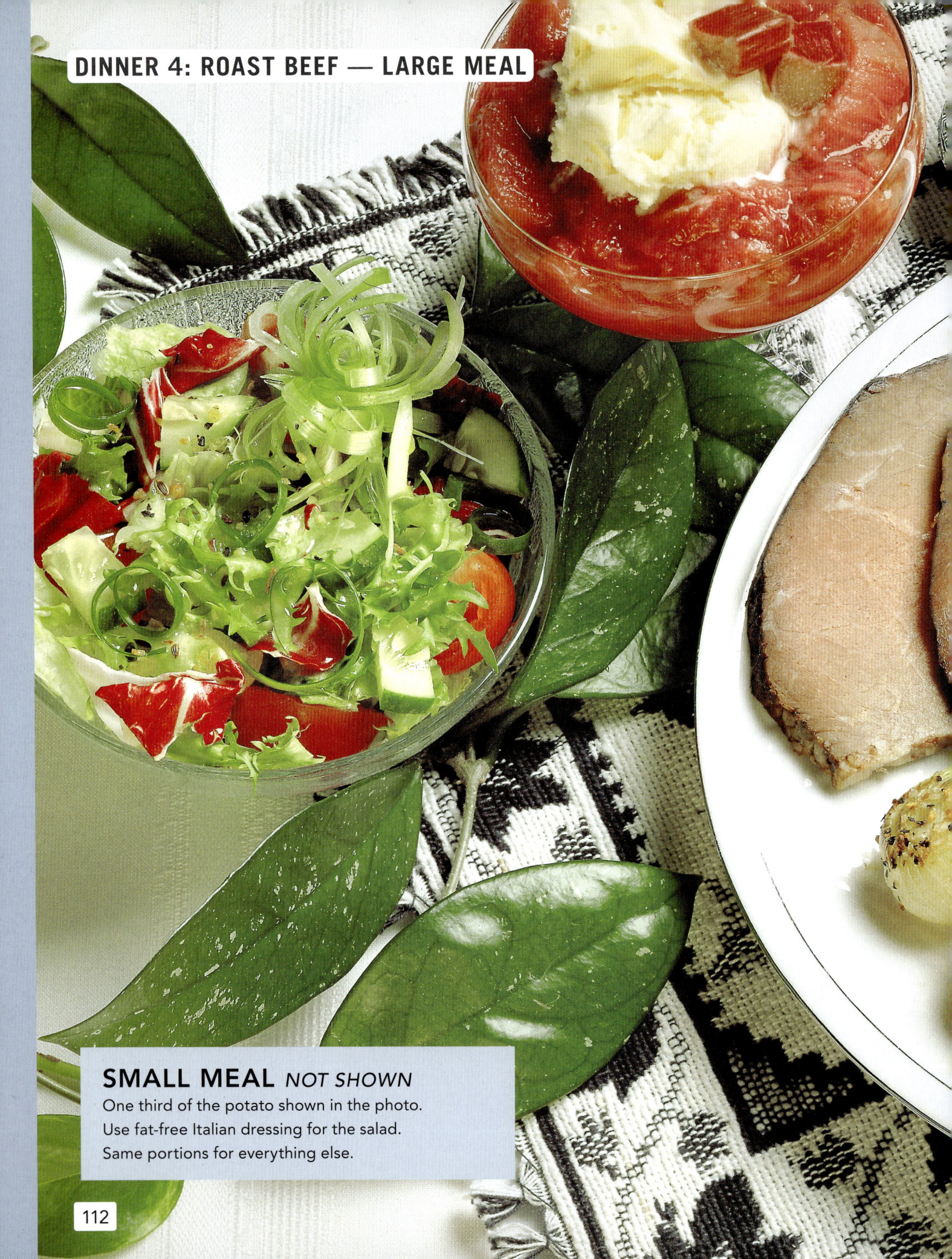

DINNER 4: ROAST BEEF — LARGE MEAL

SMALL MEAL *NOT SHOWN*
One third of the potato shown in the photo.
Use fat-free Italian dressing for the salad.
Same portions for everything else.

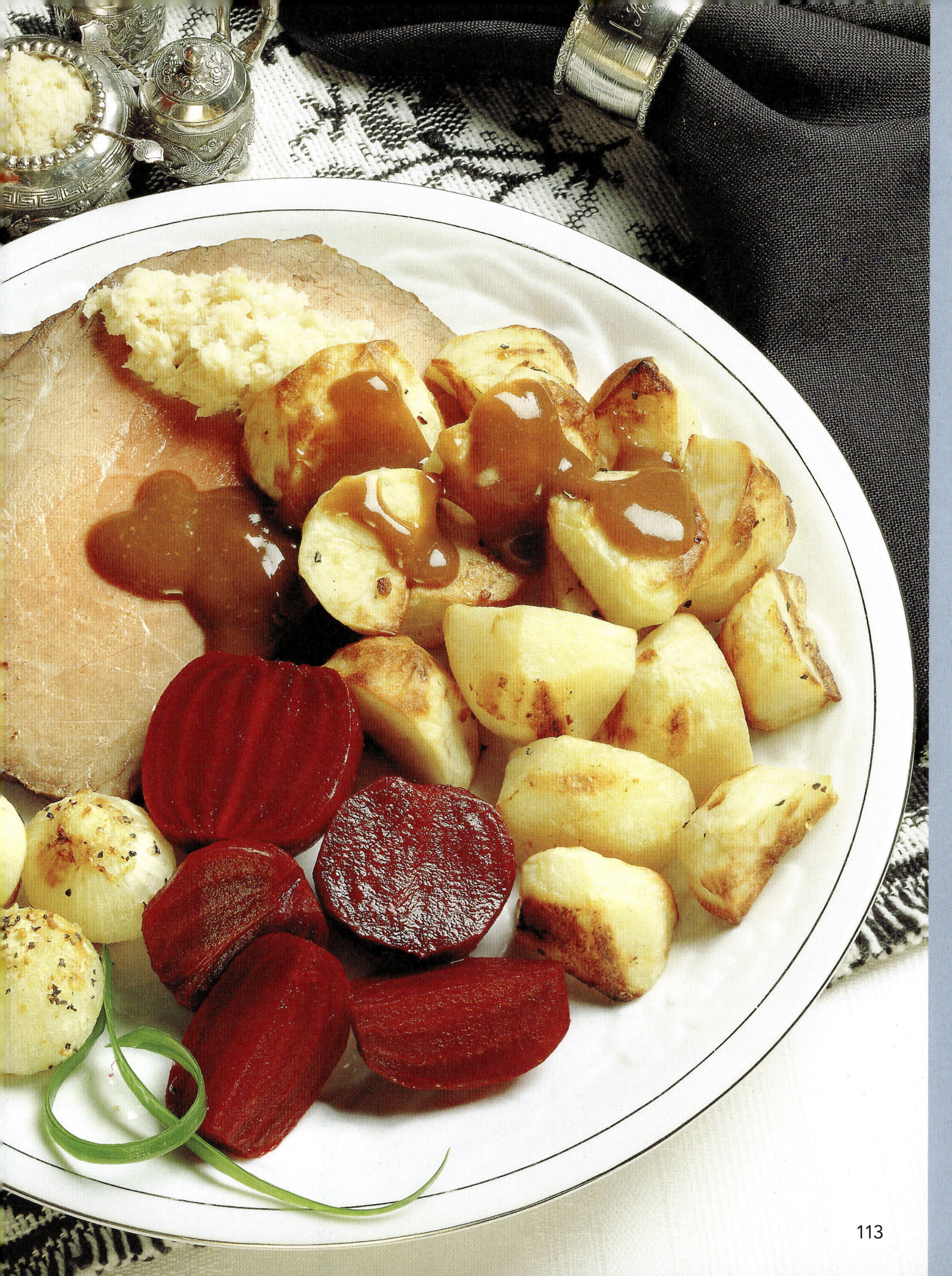

DINNER MEALS

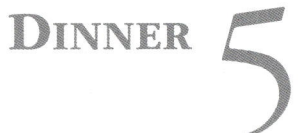

Cold Plate Dinner

This is a quick and easy meal to prepare. It's different every time depending on the vegetables and the choice of fish and cheese.

Fish choices include canned (or leftover cooked and chilled) salmon, tuna, sardines, shrimp, crab or lobster. If you don't like fish, replace it with two large hard-boiled eggs, or 2 oz (60 g) of cold cooked meat.

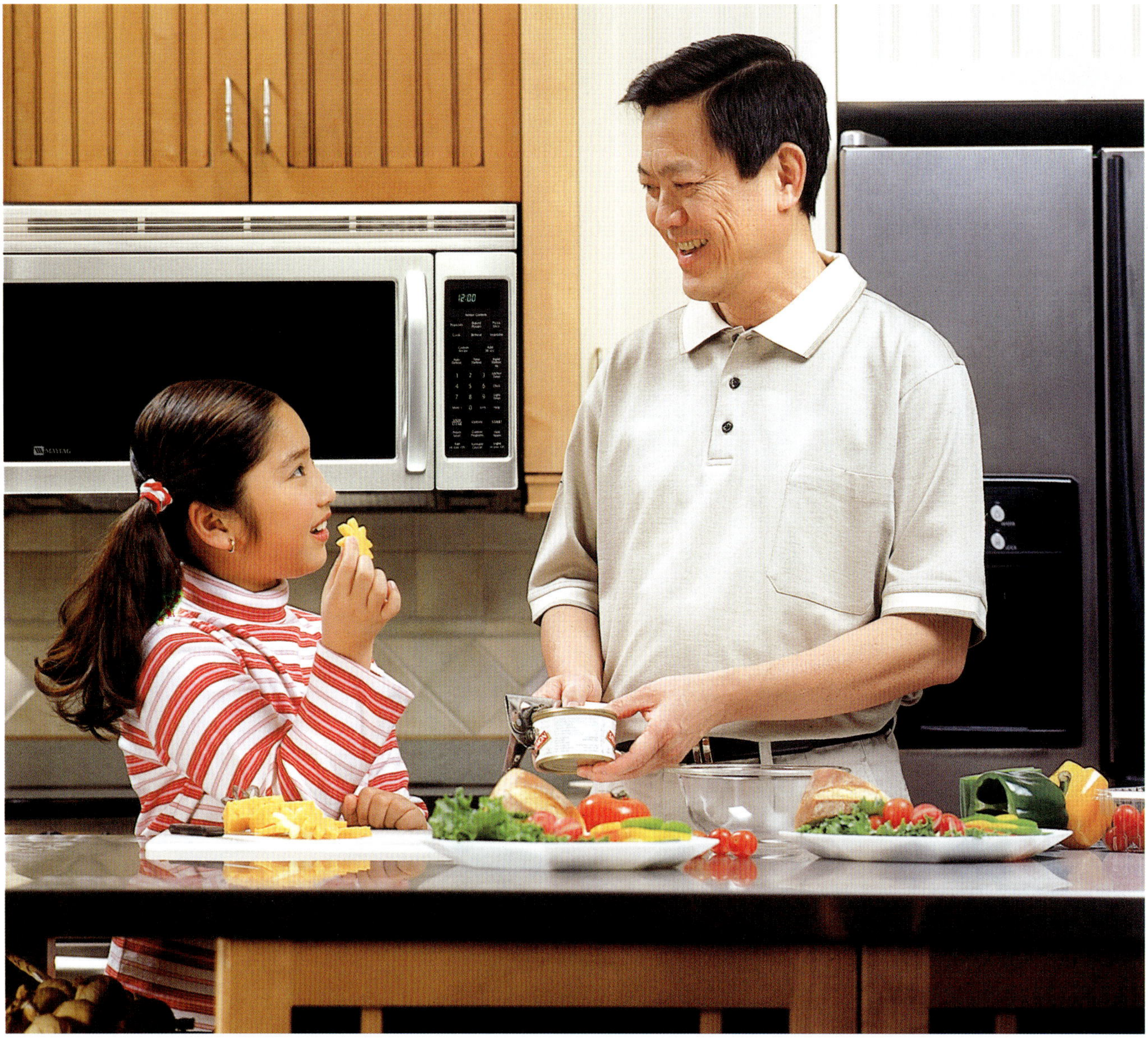

DINNER MEALS

Rice pudding is a great way to use up day-old rice. This pudding is delicious when warm. It is a heavier dessert and goes best with a light dinner. It also makes a great large snack or a breakfast!

Rice Pudding

Makes four 1-cup (250 mL) servings

Preheat oven to 350°F (180°C)

1 large egg
1½ cups (375 mL) 2% milk
2 tbsp (30 mL) sugar
½ tsp (2 mL) ground cinnamon
½ tsp (2 mL) vanilla
2 cups (500 mL) cooked rice (long-grain brown or white or converted)
¼ cup (60 mL) raisins

1. In a large bowl, beat egg, milk, sugar or sweetener, cinnamon and vanilla. Use a whisk or spoon.
2. Stir in rice and raisins.
3. Pour into a greased casserole dish, about 6 to 8 inches (15 to 20 cm) across.
4. Bake for 45 minutes, or until the center is set.

PER 1 CUP (250 ML)	
Calories	231
Carbohydrate	41 g
Fiber	2 g
Net Carbs	39 g
Protein	6 g
Fat, total	3 g
Fat, saturated	1 g
Cholesterol	41 mg
Sodium	50 mg

⟳ LOW-CARB SWAP

LARGE MEAL
Swap Rice Pudding made with sugar:
1 cup (250 mL)
39 g net carbs
→ For Rice Pudding made with zero-calorie sweetener:
1 cup (250 mL)
33 g net carbs

SMALL MEAL
Swap Rice Pudding made with sugar:
¾ cup (175 mL)
30 g net carbs
→ For Rice Pudding made with zero-calorie sweetener:
25 g net carbs

See Sugar Swaps, page 29.

YOUR DINNER MENU	Large Meal (730 calories)	Total Carbs	NET CARBS	Small Meal (550 calories)	Total Carbs	NET CARBS
COLD PLATE DINNER						
• lettuce or spinach	A plateful	0	0	A plateful	0	0
• tomato	½ medium	2	1	½ medium	2	1
• green & red pepper	5 rings	3	2	5 rings	3	2
• cucumber	4 thick slices	1	1	4 thick slices	1	1
• radishes	2 large	1	0	2 large	1	0
• salmon	½ cup (125 mL)	0	0	½ cup (125 mL)	0	0
• Cheddar cheese	2 oz (60 g)	1	1	2 oz (60 g)	1	1
• bun, whole wheat	1 small	23	20	4 whole-wheat soda crackers	9	8
• margarine	1 tsp (5 mL)	0	0	—	—	—
Rice Pudding	1 cup (250 mL)	41	39	¾ cup (175 mL)	31	30
	TOTAL CARBS	**72 g**	**64 g**	TOTAL CARBS	**48 g**	**43 g**
	Total carbs minus fiber = NET CARBS ↑			NET CARBS ↑		
	CARB CHOICES (1 carb choice = 15 g net carbs)	4		CARB CHOICES	3	

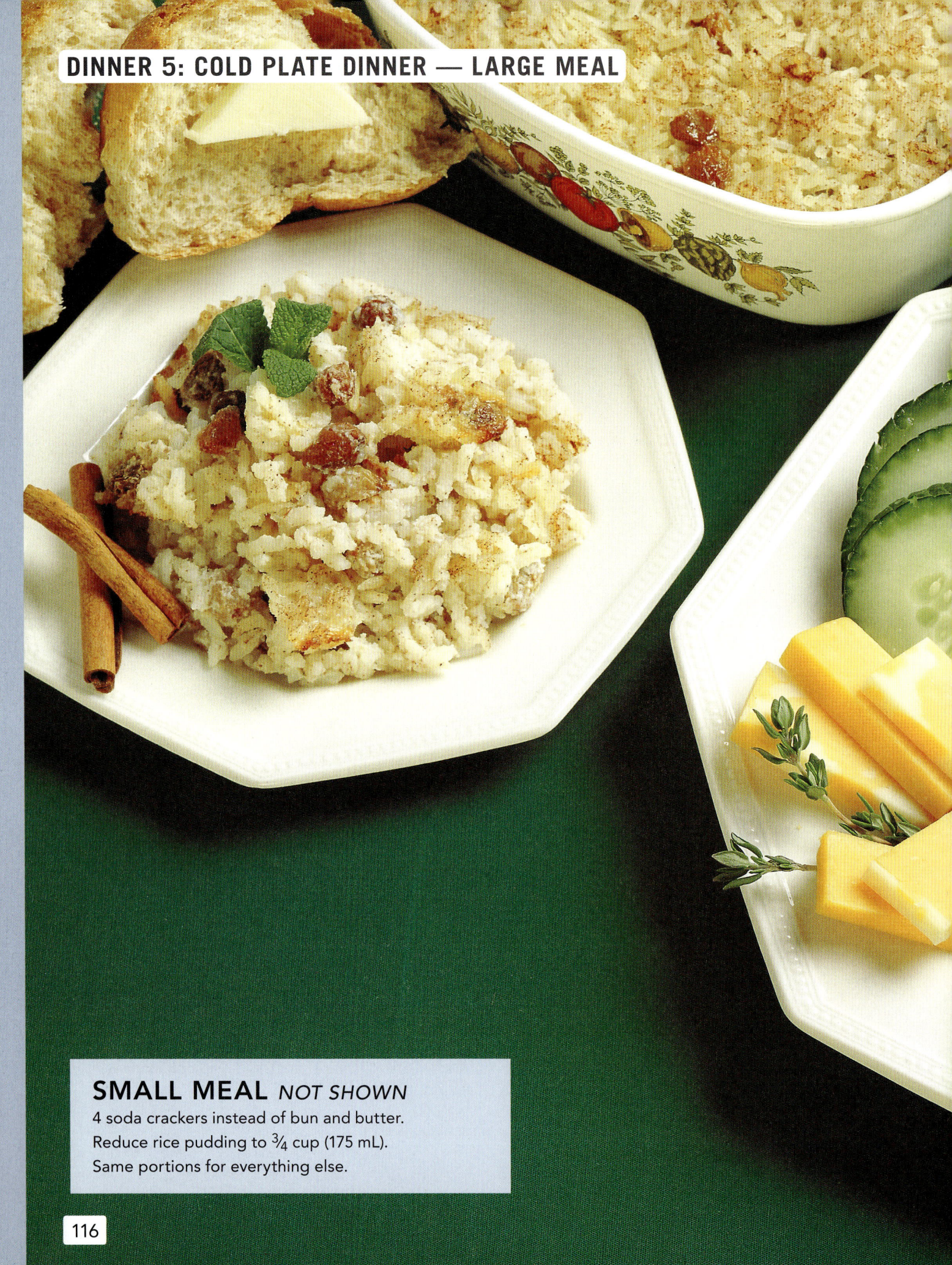

DINNER 5: COLD PLATE DINNER — LARGE MEAL

SMALL MEAL *NOT SHOWN*
4 soda crackers instead of bun and butter. Reduce rice pudding to ¾ cup (175 mL). Same portions for everything else.

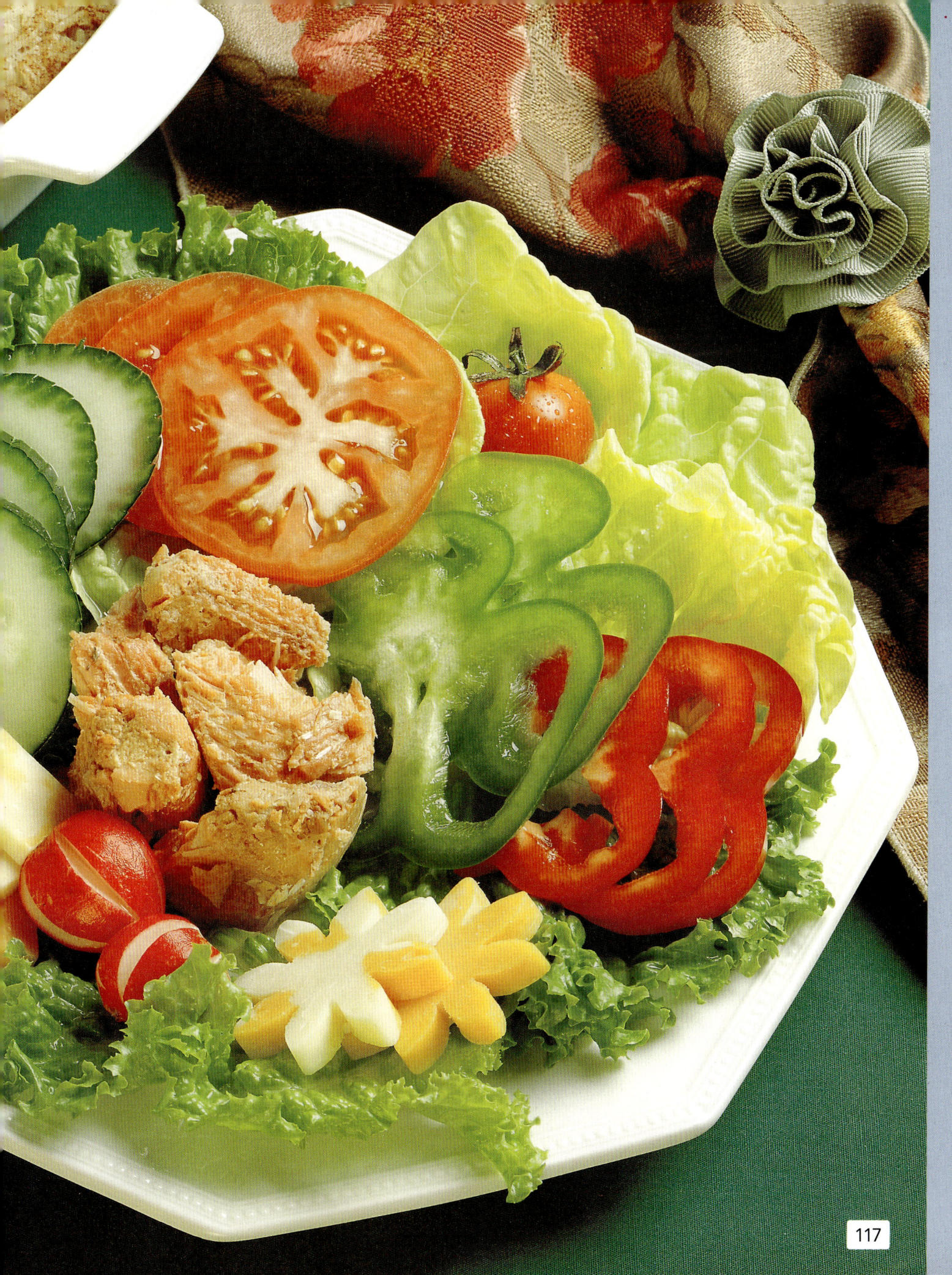

DINNER MEALS

DINNER 6

HEALTH TIP

You don't need to add salt to recipes that use canned soup or canned vegetables.

Look for the low-sodium canned varieties. Frozen vegetables are your best choice for low salt, plus they are handy and ready in your freezer when you want them.

◯ LOW-CARB SWAP

HAMBURGER SOUP RECIPE

Swap 1½ cups (375 mL) of soup made with 1½ cups (375 mL) corn
24 g net carbs

→ For 1½ cups (375 mL) of soup made with an additional 2 cups (500 mL) of chopped low-carb vegetables and no corn
20 g net carbs

See page 134 for a list of low-carb vegetables.

Hamburger Soup & Bannock

This hearty soup is nutritious and a favorite when served with bannock. Leftovers freeze well.

Hamburger Soup

Makes 10 cups (2.5 L)

1 lb (500 g) lean ground beef
  (or chopped or ground wild meat)
1 medium onion, chopped
4 cloves garlic, finely chopped, or
  1 tsp (5 mL) garlic powder
19 oz (540 mL) can tomatoes
10 oz (284 mL) can tomato soup
1 tsp (5 mL) Worcestershire sauce
¼ tsp (1 mL) black pepper
4 cups (1 L) water
½ to 1 packet (2.25 to 4.5 g) reduced-salt beef bouillon mix
3 medium carrots, peeled and sliced
1 cup (250 mL) chopped cabbage
1½ cups (375 mL) frozen corn or 12 oz (341 mL) can
  corn kernels
¼ cup (60 mL) dry macaroni

PER 1½ CUPS (375 ML)	
Calories	232
Carbohydrate	27 g
Fiber	3 g
Net carbs	24 g
Protein	16 g
Fat, total	7 g
Fat, saturated	3 g
Cholesterol	36 mg
Sodium	453 mg

1. In a large, heavy pot on the stove, brown ground beef. Drain off fat.
2. Add onions and garlic, and cook at low heat until onions are soft.
3. Add tomatoes, tomato soup, Worcestershire sauce, pepper, water and bouillon mix.
4. Bring to a boil, cover and simmer for 30 minutes.
5. Add vegetables and macaroni. Cover and simmer for another 30 minutes.

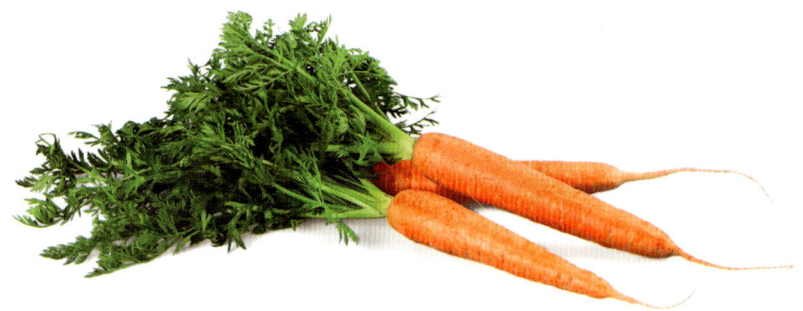

DINNER MEALS

Low-Carb Bannock

Makes one 9-inch (23 cm) bannock (or 10 pieces)

Preheat oven to 375°F (190°C)

1½ cups (375 mL) flour

1½ cups (375 mL) almond flour

1½ tsp (7 mL) baking powder

½ tsp (2 mL) salt

1 tbsp (15 mL) sugar

2 tbsp (30 mL) vegetable oil, or other fat, melted

1 cup (250 mL) skim milk

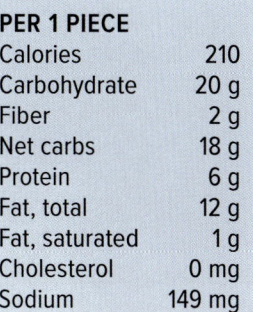

PER 1 PIECE	
Calories	210
Carbohydrate	20 g
Fiber	2 g
Net carbs	18 g
Protein	6 g
Fat, total	12 g
Fat, saturated	1 g
Cholesterol	0 mg
Sodium	149 mg

RECIPE TIP

When you use milk instead of water in this bannock recipe, the milk adds flavor and nutrition and helps with rising.

1. In a large bowl, mix together the two flours, baking powder, salt and sugar.
2. Mix vegetable oil with milk and add to flour. Mix with a large spoon to make a soft dough. Add a bit of flour if too wet or a bit of liquid if too dry.
3. With your hands, flatten the dough on a floured surface and shape it into one 9-inch (23 cm) piece.
4. Place on a greased baking sheet. Bake in the oven for 25 minutes, or until lightly browned.
5. Cut into 10 pieces.

To cook bannock on a campfire:

This is a half recipe without added oil in the dough. You'll need a cast iron pan.

- Without preheating, spread the 1 tbsp (15 mL) oil, or other fat, evenly on the bottom of the cast iron pan.
- Once the dough is mixed in your bowl, place it directly into the greased cast iron pan and form the shape with your floured hands.
- Fry the bannock on low-medium embers on the fire for 8 minutes on the first side and 5 minutes on the flip side, or until cooked through. This is a thinner version with a crunchy crust.

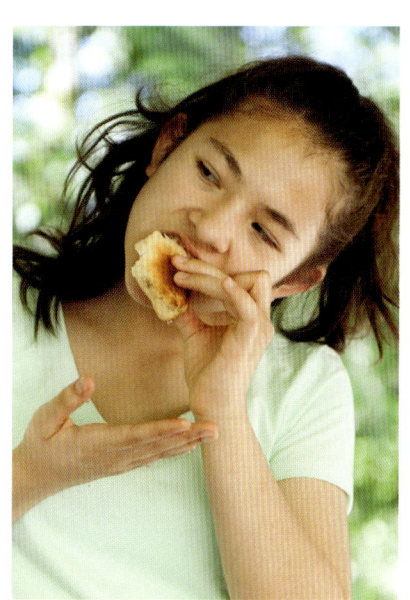

YOUR DINNER MENU	Large Meal (730 calories)	Total Carbs	NET CARBS	Small Meal (550 calories)	Total Carbs	NET CARBS
Hamburger Soup	1½ cups (375 mL)	27	24	1½ cups (375 mL)	27	24
Bannock	2 pieces	40	35	1 piece	20	18
Margarine	1 tsp (5 mL)	0	0	1 tsp (5 mL)	0	0
Orange	1 medium	15	13	1 medium	15	13
	TOTAL CARBS	82 g	72 g	TOTAL CARBS	62 g	55 g
	Total carbs minus fiber = NET CARBS ↑			NET CARBS ↑		
	CARB CHOICES (1 carb choice = 15 g net carbs)		5	CARB CHOICES		4

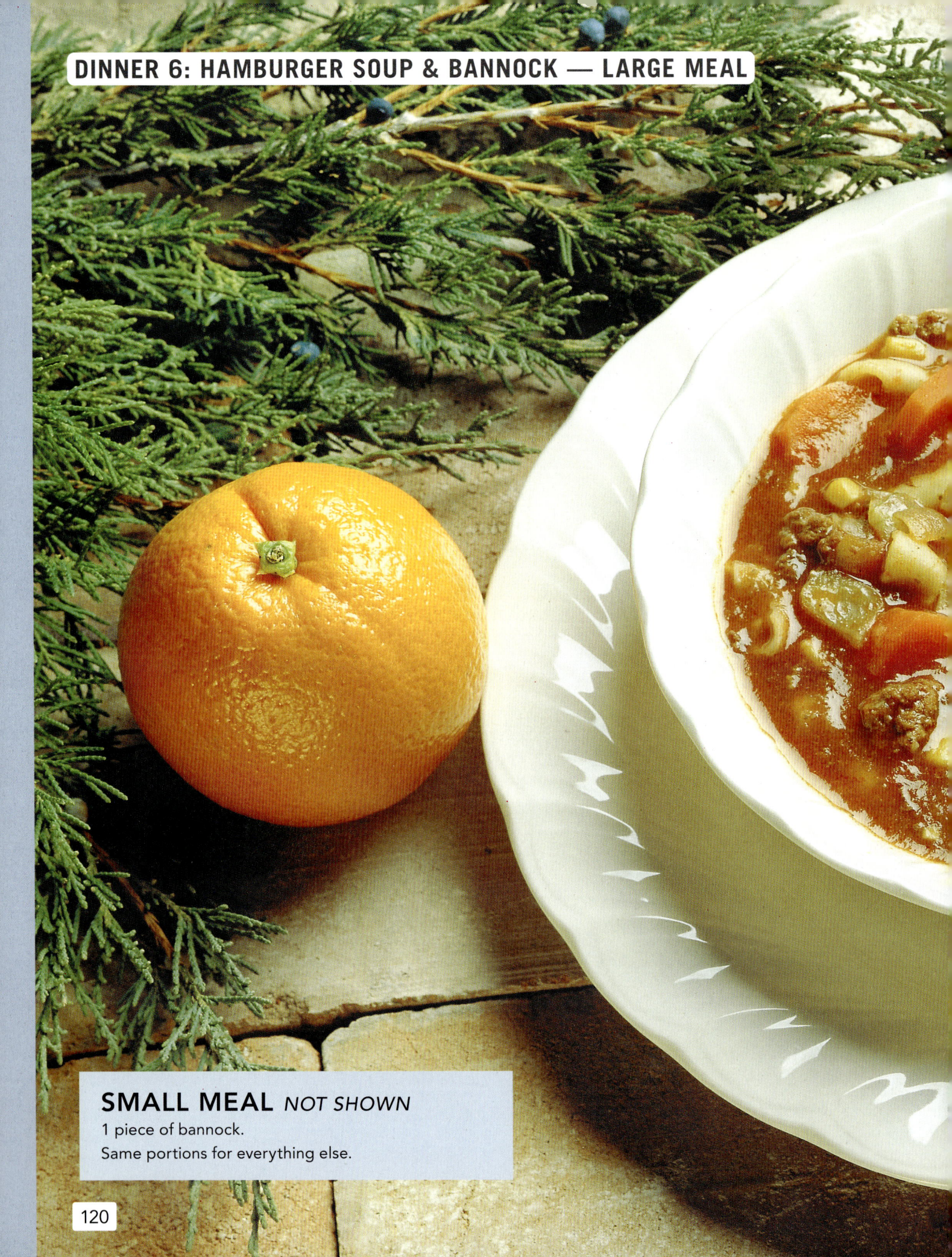

DINNER 6: HAMBURGER SOUP & BANNOCK — LARGE MEAL

SMALL MEAL *NOT SHOWN*
1 piece of bannock.
Same portions for everything else.

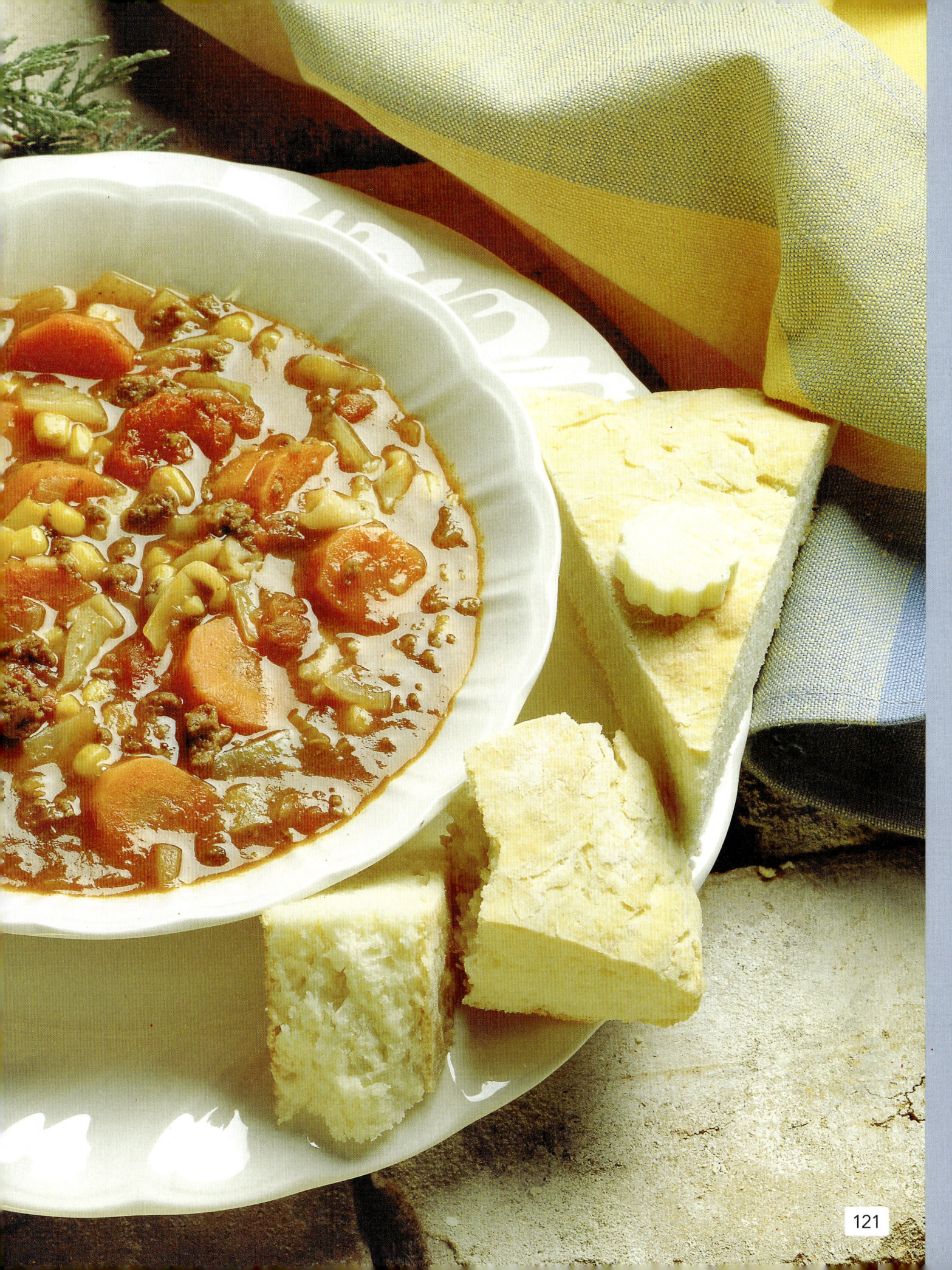

DINNER MEALS

DINNER 7

Beans & Wieners

This meal has low-fat home-baked beans that are high in fiber and protein. Wieners are a popular combination with beans. As they are high in fat and salt, just four wieners are included in the full recipe.

Beans & Wieners

Makes 5 cups (1.25 L)

3 cups (750 mL) Home-Baked Beans or a 14 oz (398 mL) can of brown beans

4 regular wieners (each wiener weighs 1½ oz/45 g)

1. Place the beans in a pot or casserole dish.
2. Cut the wieners in slices and add to the beans.
3. Heat on the stove or in a microwave oven.

PER 1 CUP (250 ML)	
Calories	342
Carbohydrate	42 g
Fiber	9 g
Net carbs	33 g
Protein	17 g
Fat, total	12 g
Fat, saturated	5 g
Cholesterol	22 mg
Sodium	393 mg

Low-Salt Home-Baked Beans

Makes 4½ cups (1.125 L)

Preheat oven to 275°F (140°C)

2 cups (500 mL) dry white beans (navy, small white or Great Northern)

1 medium onion, chopped

2 cloves garlic, finely chopped

1 tbsp (15 mL) dry mustard

¼ tsp (1 mL) black pepper

2 cups (500 mL) water

3 tbsp (45 mL) ketchup

2 tbsp (30 mL) molasses

Dash of hot pepper sauce

PER 1 CUP (250 ML)	
Calories	364
Carbohydrate	68 g
Fiber	15 g
Net carbs	53 g
Protein	21 g
Fat, total	2 g
Fat, saturated	0 g
Cholesterol	0 mg
Sodium	109 mg

1. Rinse beans in cold water, removing any discolored beans. Place in a pot with enough cold water to cover.
2. Cover and bring to a boil over high heat; boil for 5 minutes. Remove from heat and let stand, covered, for 1 hour.
3. Drain the water from the beans and transfer beans to a casserole dish or bean pot. Add other ingredients.
4. Cover and bake in oven, or in a slow cooker on low, for 6 to 8 hours, or until beans are tender. Stir periodically and add extra water if beans are drying out.

RECIPE TIP

These Home-Baked Beans have just 157 mg of sodium per cup.

Store-bought canned baked beans have 850 mg of sodium per cup.

DINNER MEALS

This dessert recipe is so easy, thick and delectable.

Chocolate Mousse

Makes six ½-cup (125 mL) servings

1½ cups (375 mL) skim milk

1 package (4-serving size) of light, fat-free, chocolate instant pudding mix

1 cup (250 mL) frozen light whipped topping, thawed until soft

PER ½ CUP (125 ML)	
Calories	76
Carbohydrate	12 g
Fiber	1 g
Net carbs	11 g
Protein	2 g
Fat, total	2 g
Fat, saturated	2 g
Cholesterol	1 mg
Sodium	245 mg

1. In a medium bowl, pour the skim milk and then add pudding mix. Beat with an electric mixer until thickened (about 2 minutes).
2. Fold in the thawed whipped topping until well blended (or if you want a marbled look, fold in the topping gently and don't fully mix).
3. Pour into six dessert dishes and serve.

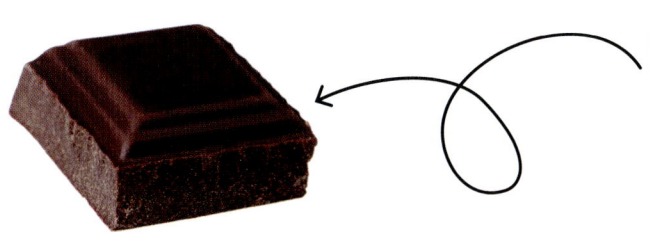

⟲ LOW-CARB SWAP

LARGE AND SMALL MEAL

Swap Chocolate Mousse: ½ cup (125 mL)

11 g net carbs

→ For 80% dark chocolate: 10 g (about 1 piece)
2 g net carbs

See Candy Swaps, page 281.

YOUR DINNER MENU	Large Meal (730 calories)	Total Carbs	NET CARBS	Small Meal (550 calories)	Total Carbs	NET CARBS
Beans & Wieners	1⅓ cups (325 mL)	56	**44**	1 cup (250 mL)	42	**33**
Toast, light rye	1 slice	15	**13**	½ slice	7	**6**
Margarine	1 tsp (5 mL)	0	**0**	1 tsp (5 mL)	0	**0**
Tossed salad	Medium	3	**2**	Medium	3	**2**
Salad dressing	1 tbsp (15 mL), oil and vinegar, or French	0	**0**	1 tbsp (15 mL), fat-free Italian	2	**2**
Chocolate Mousse	½ cup (125 mL)	12	**11**	½ cup (125 mL)	12	**11**
	TOTAL CARBS	**86 g**	**70 g**	TOTAL CARBS	**66 g**	**54 g**
	Total carbs minus fiber = NET CARBS ↑				NET CARBS ↑	
	CARB CHOICES (1 carb choice = 15 g net carbs)		**5**	CARB CHOICES		**4**

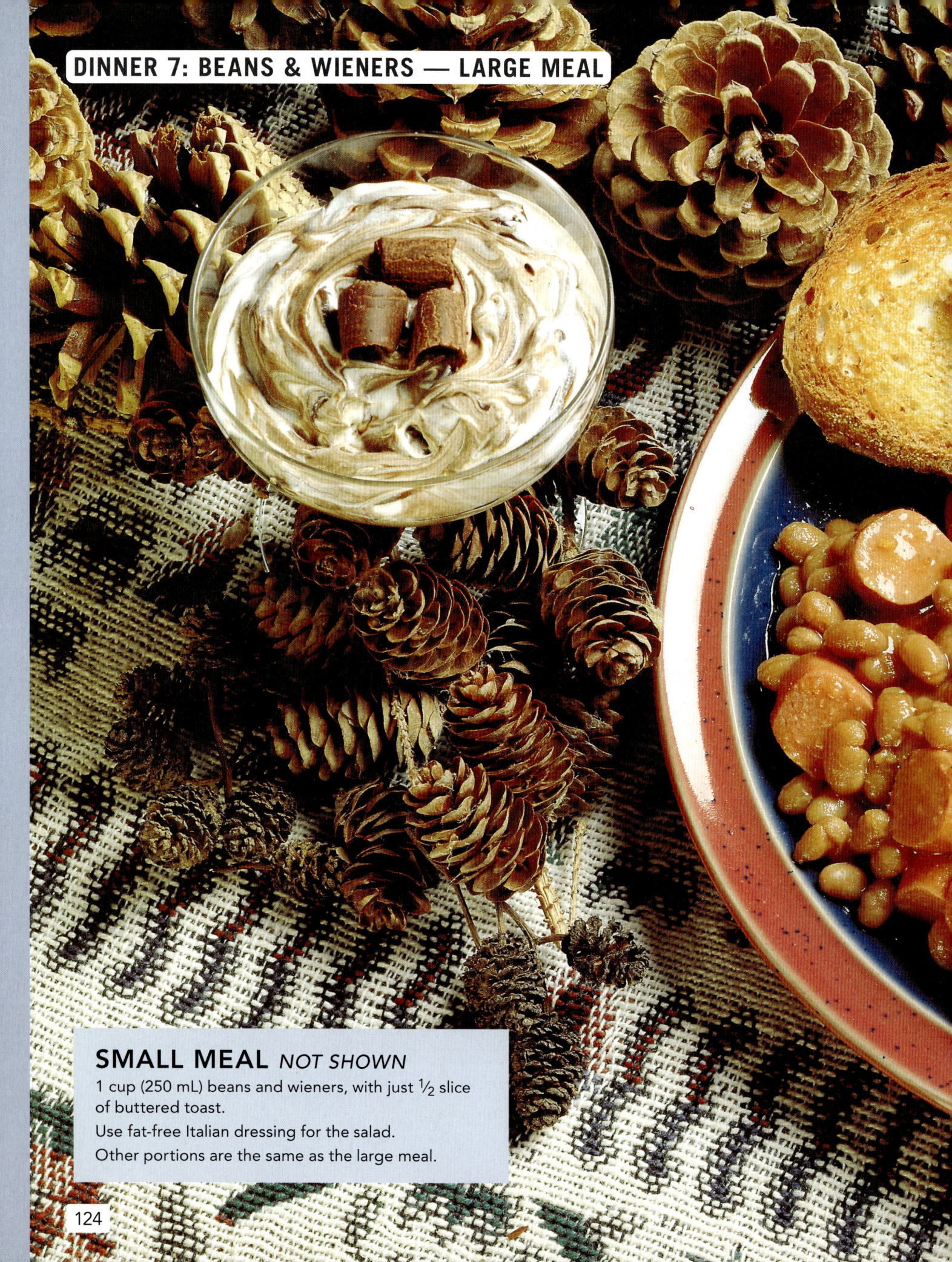

DINNER 7: BEANS & WIENERS — LARGE MEAL

SMALL MEAL *NOT SHOWN*
1 cup (250 mL) beans and wieners, with just ½ slice of buttered toast.
Use fat-free Italian dressing for the salad.
Other portions are the same as the large meal.

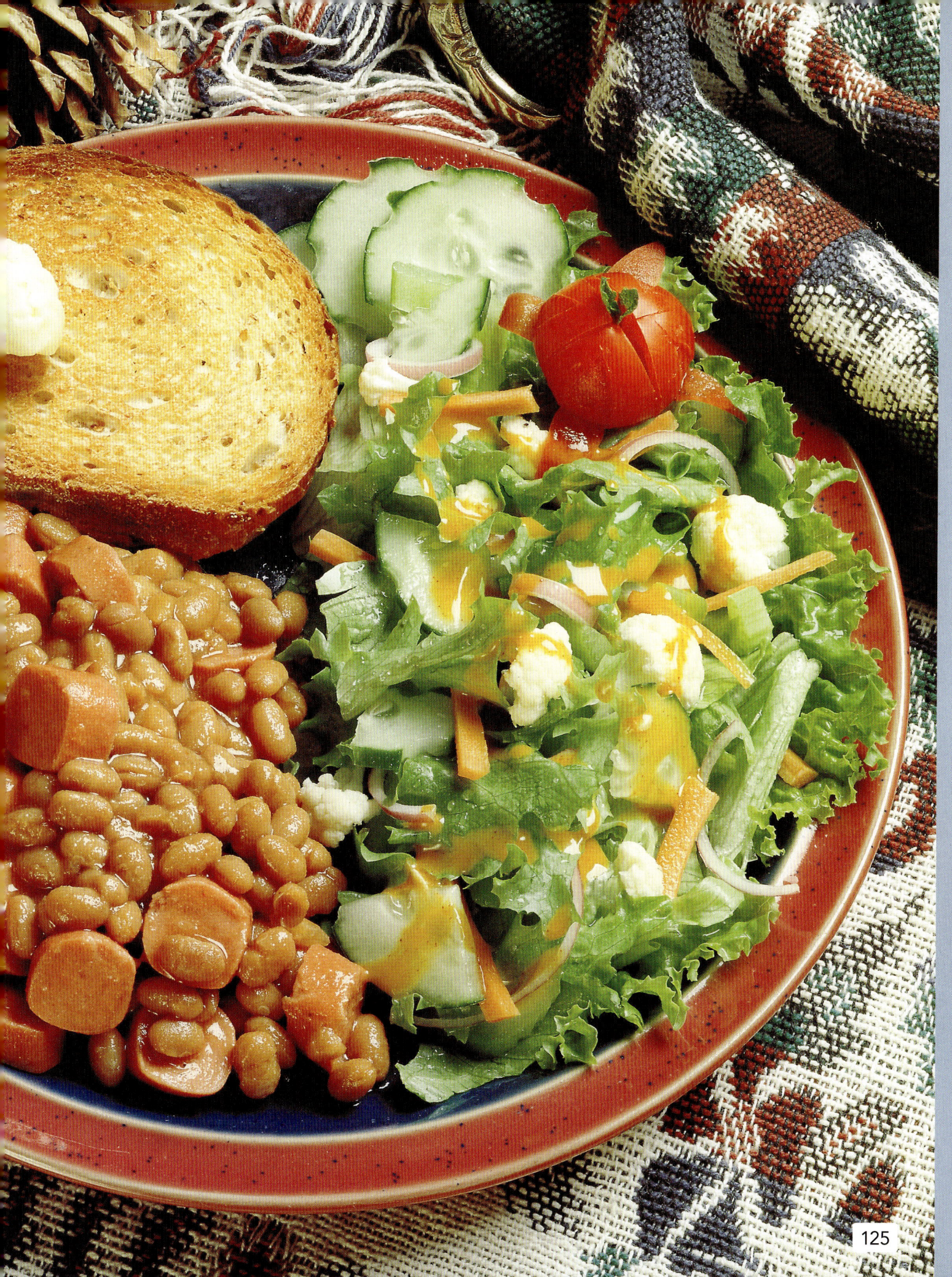

DINNER MEALS

DINNER 8

Steak & Potato

When we think of steak, we think of barbecue. But steaks can also be broiled in the oven or pan-fried on the stove.

20 minutes before cooking, take the steaks out of the fridge. Cold steaks will not cook evenly. Season to your liking. The seasoning recipe below is salt-free.

If you are frying steaks, use a nonstick pan or an oiled cast iron pan. On high heat, sear the outside of the steak for about 2 to 3 minutes on each side. This keeps the meat juicy and tender inside. Then let the steak rest, covered, for several minutes after cooking, which gives time for the juices to distribute evenly through the steak.

RECIPE TIP
Cuts of steak

As a rule, the more expensive the steak, the more tender it will be. Tender steaks are sometimes labeled as "grilling steaks." They are: rib eye, T-bone, tenderloin, filet and top sirloin.

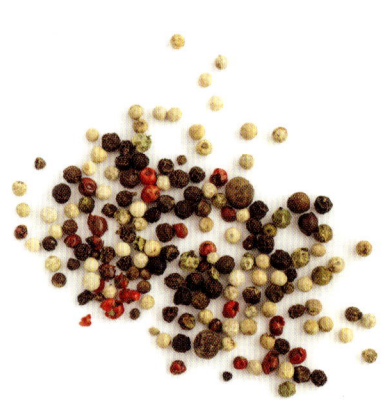

Steak Seasoning

Makes 6 tbsp (90 mL)

- 1 tbsp (15 mL) cayenne or chili powder
- 2 tbsp (30 mL) regular or smoked paprika
- 1 tbsp (15 mL) garlic powder
- 1 tbsp (15 mL) ground black pepper
- 1 tbsp (15 mL) dry mustard

PER ½ TSP (2 ML)	
Calories	4
Carbohydrate	1 g
Fiber	0 g
Net carbs	1 g
Protein	0 g
Fat, total	0 g
Fat, saturated	0 g
Cholesterol	0 mg
Sodium	2 mg

1. Put spices in a jar and shake. Sprinkle on meat, potato or vegetables.

Mashed Potatoes

Makes 4 cups (1 L)

- 6 medium potatoes (a medium potato is about 2–3 inches/5–7.5 cm)
- ⅔ cup (150 mL) skim or 2% milk
- 2 tbsp (30 mL) butter or margarine

PER ½ CUP (125 ML)	
Calories	113
Carbohydrate	20 g
Fiber	2 g
Net carbs	18 g
Protein	2 g
Fat, total	3 g
Fat, saturated	2 g
Cholesterol	8 mg
Sodium	48 mg

1. Wash and peel potatoes and cut into quarters.
2. Place potatoes in a large pot with enough water to cover. Bring to a boil, then reduce heat, cover and boil gently for about 20 minutes or until fork-tender.
3. Remove from heat, add milk and butter, and mash.

If you have leftover Mashed Potatoes, you can use them to make Salmon Potato Dish: see page 190.

DINNER MEALS

🔴 LOW-CARB SWAP RECIPE: Mashed Potatoes with Cauliflower

LARGE MEAL
Swap Mashed Potatoes:
1 cup (250 mL)
36 g net carbs

→ For Mashed Potatoes with Cauliflower:
1 cup (250 mL)
13 g net carbs

→ For mashed cauliflower:
1 cup (250 mL)
7 g net carbs

SMALL MEAL
Swap Mashed Potatoes:
½ cup (125 mL)
18 g net carbs

→ For Mashed Potatoes with Cauliflower:
½ cup (125 mL)
6 g net carbs

→ For mashed cauliflower:
½ cup (125 mL)
4 g net carbs

See Potato Swaps, page 275.

This recipe adds cauliflower to the potatoes, which reduces calories and carbs in your serving but keeps the potato flavor.

1 CUP	
Calories	86
Total carbs	15 g
Net carbs	13 g

Makes five 1-cup (250 mL) servings

2 medium potatoes, peeled and diced
½ head of cauliflower, diced
2 tbsp (30 mL) skim or 2% milk
1 tbsp (15 mL) butter or margarine
Parsley for topping, optional

1. Add potatoes and cauliflower to a pot and cover with water. Bring to a boil and put the lid on. Reduce the heat but continue boiling for 10 minutes or until tender.
2. Drain off water from cooked potatoes and cauliflower.
3. Add the milk and butter, and mash together until smooth.

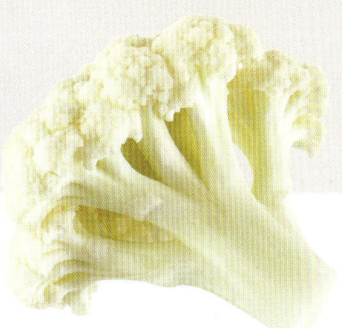

YOUR DINNER MENU	Large Meal (730 calories)	Total Carbs	NET CARBS	Small Meal (550 calories)	Total Carbs	NET CARBS
Steak	5 oz (150 g), cooked	0	0	4 oz (120 g), cooked	0	0
Mashed Potatoes	1 cup (250 mL)	39	36	½ cup (125 mL)	20	18
Mushrooms	½ cup (125 mL)	4	2	½ cup (125 mL)	4	2
Brussels sprouts	¾ cup (175 mL)	8	4	¾ cup (175 mL)	8	4
Salad	Small	2	1	Small	2	1
Salad dressing, creamy	1 tbsp (15 mL)	2	2	1 tbsp (15 mL)	2	2
Sherbert	½ cup (125 mL)	23	21	⅓ cup (75 mL)	15	14
	TOTAL CARBS	78 g	66 g	TOTAL CARBS	51 g	41 g
	Total carbs minus fiber = NET CARBS ↑			NET CARBS ↑		
	CARB CHOICES (1 carb choice = 15 g net carbs)		4	CARB CHOICES		3

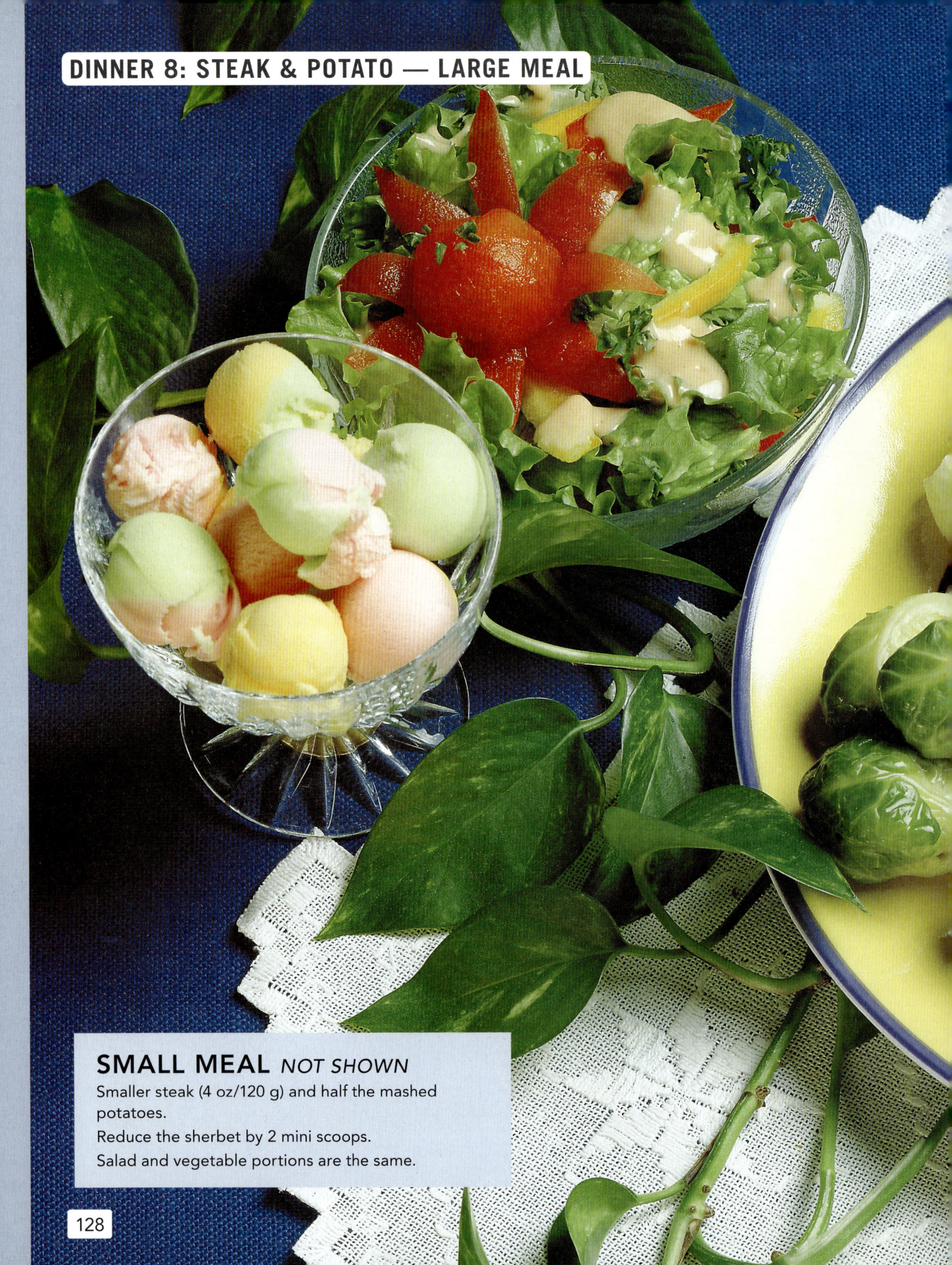

DINNER 8: STEAK & POTATO — LARGE MEAL

SMALL MEAL *NOT SHOWN*

Smaller steak (4 oz/120 g) and half the mashed potatoes.
Reduce the sherbet by 2 mini scoops.
Salad and vegetable portions are the same.

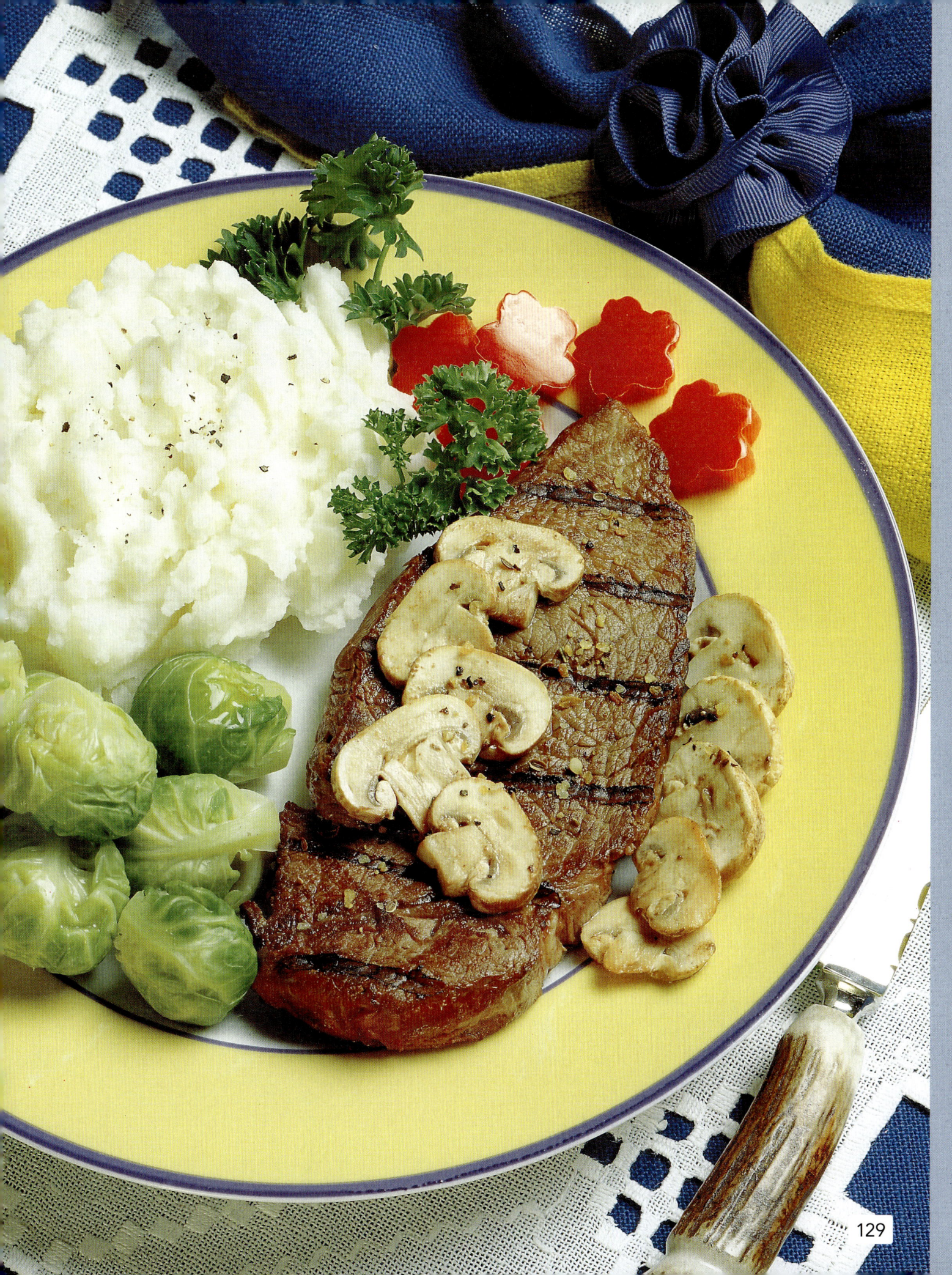

DINNER MEALS

DINNER 9

Cheese Omelet

An omelet or scrambled eggs makes a fast-and-easy nutritious dinner.

RECIPE TIP

Veg up your omelet

Before you cook the omelet, fry in butter until soft some veggies, such as: chopped onion, celery and bell peppers. Set aside. Cook the omelet in the same pan. After you cook the eggs with the cheese, add the cooked veggies and fold the omelet in half.

Cheese Omelet

2 large eggs

1 oz (30 g) cheese, grated or sliced

1. In a small bowl, whisk the eggs. Pour into a greased nonstick pan.
2. Place the cheese on top.
3. Put a lid on and cook at low heat for about 5 minutes.
4. Fold in half.

PER OMELET	
Calories	260
Carbohydrate	1 g
Fiber	0 g
Net carbs	1 g
Protein	19 g
Fat, total	19 g
Fat, saturated	9 g
Cholesterol	402 mg
Sodium	297 mg

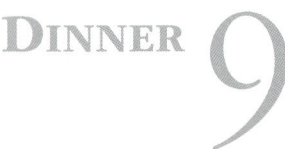

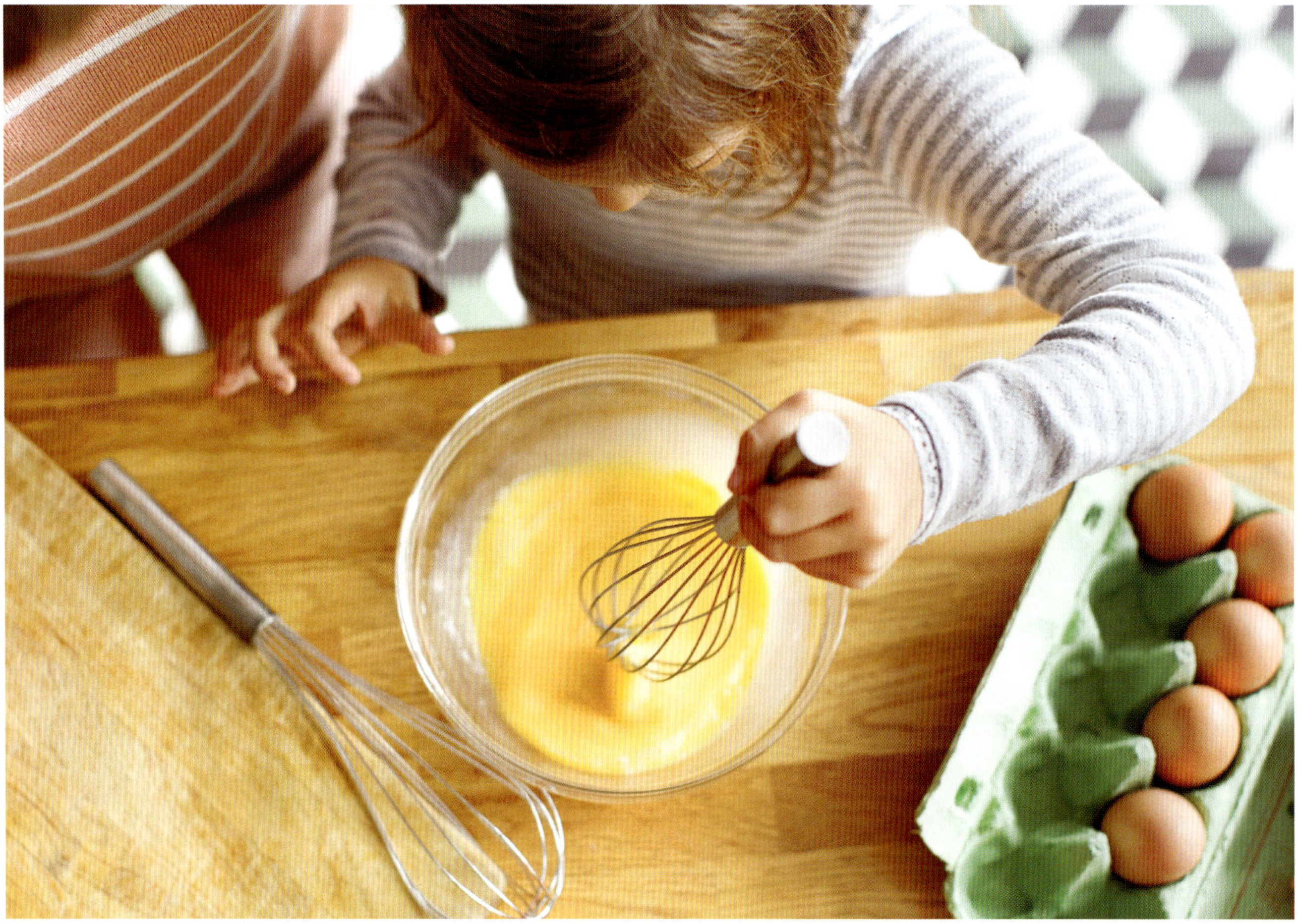

DINNER MEALS

Oatmeal Cookies

Makes 36 cookies

Preheat oven to 375°F (190°C)

⅓ cup (75 mL) butter
¾ cup (175 mL) sugar
1 large egg
1 tsp (5 mL) vanilla
½ cup (125 mL) flour
½ cup (125 mL) almond flour
1 tsp (5 mL) baking powder
1 tsp (5 mL) baking soda
1 tsp (5 mL) ground cinnamon
1½ cups (375 mL) quick-cooking oats
½ cup (125 mL) raisins
½ cup (125 mL) walnuts, chopped

PER COOKIE	
Calories	82
Carbohydrate	11 g
Fiber	1 g
Net carbs	10 g
Protein	2 g
Fat, total	4 g
Fat, saturated	1 g
Cholesterol	11 mg
Sodium	50 mg

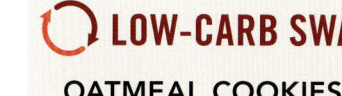

LOW-CARB SWAP

OATMEAL COOKIES RECIPE

Swap 1 cookie made with ¾ cup (175 mL) sugar
10 g net carbs

→ For 1 cookie made with ½ cup (125 mL) sugar and ⅓ cup (75 mL) zero-calorie sweetener
8 g net carbs

See Sugar Swaps, page 29.

1. In a large mixing bowl, add butter, sugar, egg and vanilla. Beat with a wooden spoon until smooth.
2. In a medium bowl, mix together all-purpose flour and almond flour, baking powder, baking soda, cinnamon and quick-cooking oats.
3. Add the flour mixture to the butter mixture. Stir well. Add raisins and nuts and stir again.
4. Shape dough into 1-inch (2.5 cm) balls. Place on an ungreased baking sheet. You'll need two baking sheets: three rows of six cookies on each sheet.
5. Bake for 10 minutes, or until light golden.

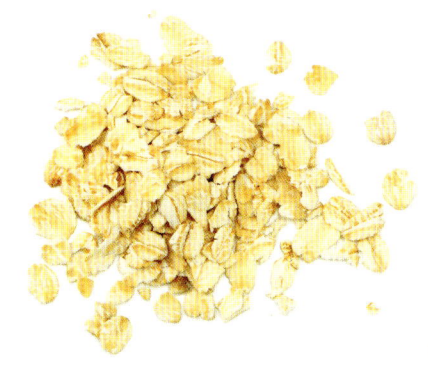

YOUR DINNER MENU	Large Meal (730 calories)	Total Carbs	NET CARBS	Small Meal (550 calories)	Total Carbs	NET CARBS
Cheese Omelet	1	1	1	1	1	1
Toast, whole wheat	2 slices	32	27	1 slice	16	14
Margarine	2 tsp (10 mL)	0	0	½ tsp (2 mL)	0	0
Broccoli pieces	2 cups (500 mL)	10	7	2 cups (500 mL)	10	7
Light cheese spread	1 tbsp (15 mL)	1	1	1 tbsp (15 mL)	1	1
Oatmeal Cookies	2	22	20	1	11	10
Strawberries, fresh	½ cup (125 mL)	6	4	1 cup (250 mL)	12	8
	TOTAL CARBS	**72 g**	**60 g**	TOTAL CARBS	**51 g**	**41 g**
	Total carbs minus fiber = NET CARBS ↑			NET CARBS ↑		
	CARB CHOICES (1 carb choice = 15 g net carbs)		4	CARB CHOICES		3

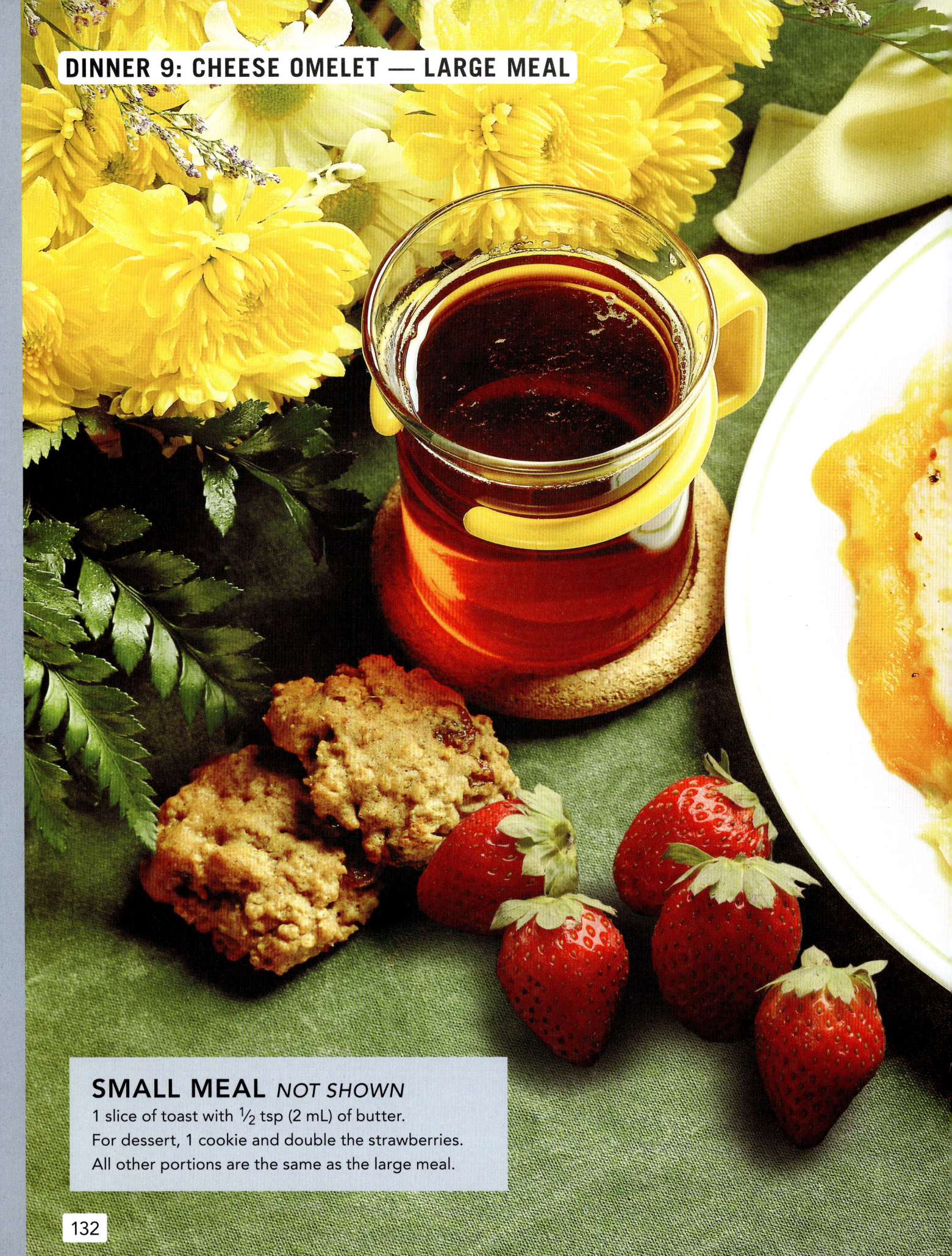

DINNER 9: CHEESE OMELET — LARGE MEAL

SMALL MEAL *NOT SHOWN*
1 slice of toast with ½ tsp (2 mL) of butter. For dessert, 1 cookie and double the strawberries. All other portions are the same as the large meal.

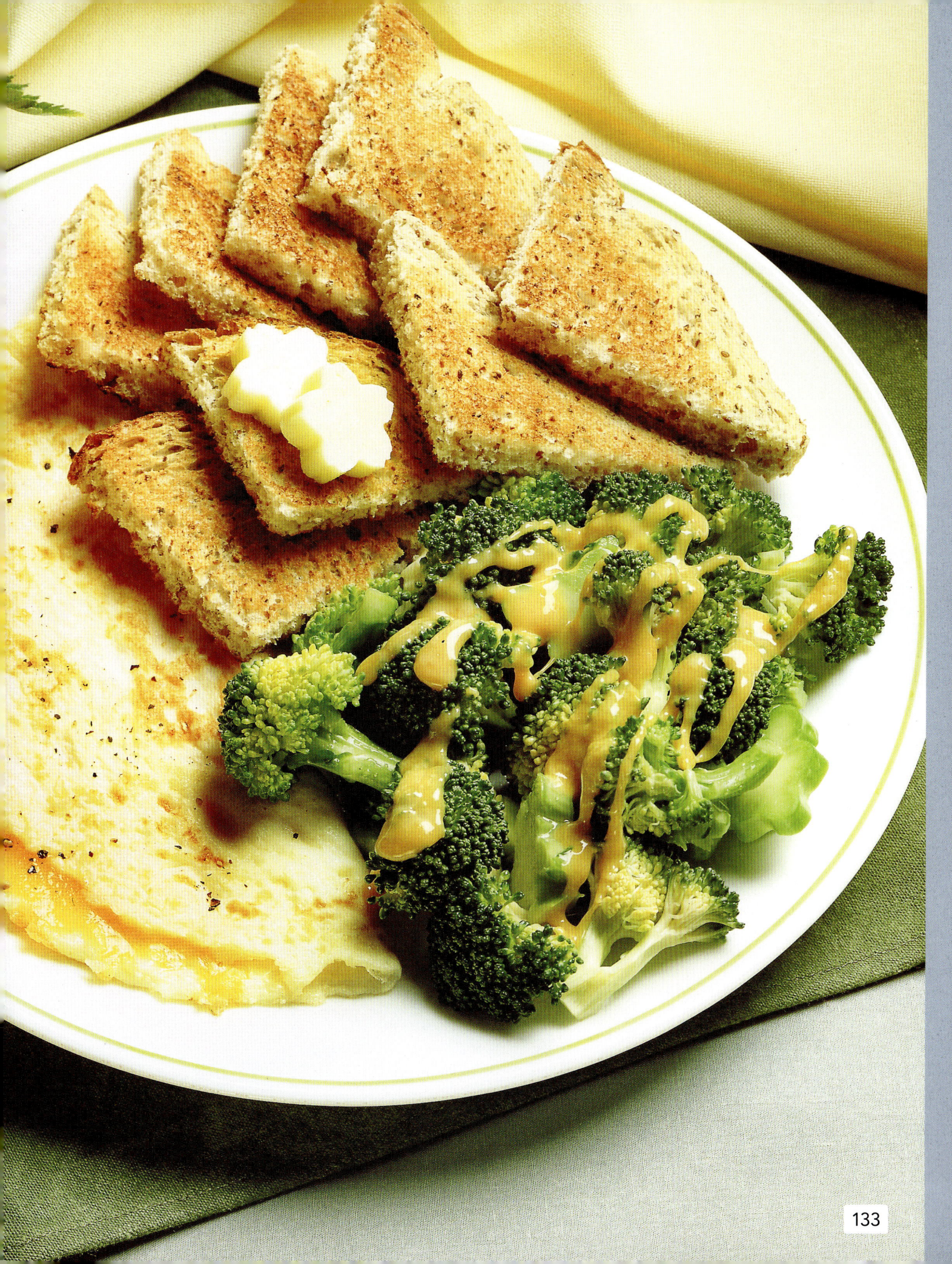

DINNER MEALS

Dinner 10

🔴 LOW-CARB SWAP

LARGE MEAL

Swap sweet potato:
1 large
43 g net carbs

➔ For butternut squash, cubed and cooked:
1½ cups (375 mL)
28 g net carbs

SMALL MEAL

Swap sweet potato:
½ large
21 g net carbs

➔ For butternut squash, cubed and cooked:
¾ cup (175 mL)
14 g net carbs

See Potato Swaps, page 275.

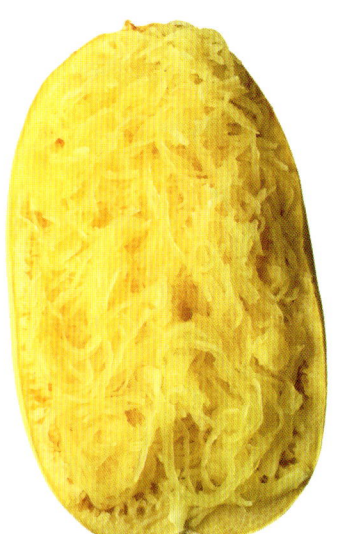

Ham & Sweet Potato

Ham

Place your cooking ham on a rack in a roasting pan. Bake for about 25 minutes per pound (1½ hours per kg) at 325°F (160°C), or to an internal temperature of 160°F (71°C). Add slices of pineapple on top of the ham for the last 30 minutes of the cooking.

Sweet Potato

A sweet potato has different vitamins and minerals than a regular potato. Variety in your food makes for a healthy diet. Like orange squash and carrots, sweet potato is rich in vitamin A, which is important for healthy eyes.

To bake sweet potato in the oven, poke the skin with a fork and place on the oven rack beside the ham until tender (about 1 hour). To microwave, poke the skin and cook on high for 6 to 10 minutes. Or try the Roasted Herbed Sweet Potatoes recipe below.

Roasted Herbed Sweet Potatoes

Wash sweet potato and cut into chunks. You don't have to remove the skin. In a bowl, toss the sweet potato with a small amount of olive oil. Sprinkle with Italian seasoning or thyme leaves, or your own favorite herbs. Spread out evenly on a baking sheet and bake in a 425°F (220°C) oven for 30 minutes, or until tender and golden brown. Once cooked, drizzle lightly with balsamic vinegar before serving.

Low-carb vegetables

- asparagus
- bean sprouts
- beans (green or yellow)
- bok choy
- broccoli
- Brussels sprouts
- cabbage
- cauliflower
- celery
- cucumber
- edamame beans
- eggplant
- fiddleheads
- leafy greens, such as lettuce, arugula, kale and spinach
- mushrooms
- okra
- onions
- peppers (red, green, yellow, orange)
- radishes
- spaghetti squash
- spinach
- tomato
- zucchini

DINNER MEALS

Whipped Gelatin

Makes 4 cups (1 L)

1 package (4-serving size) light gelatin of your favorite flavor

1. Make the gelatin according to the directions on the box.
2. Remove the gelatin from the fridge after about 45 minutes. It should be as thick as an unbeaten egg white. Beat the gelatin with a beater until it is foamy and has doubled in size.
3. Put it back in the fridge until firm.

PER 1 CUP (250 ML)	
Calories	5
Carbohydrate	2 g
Fiber	0 g
Net carbs	2 g
Protein	0 g
Fat, total	0 g
Fat, saturated	0 g
Cholesterol	0 mg
Sodium	25 mg

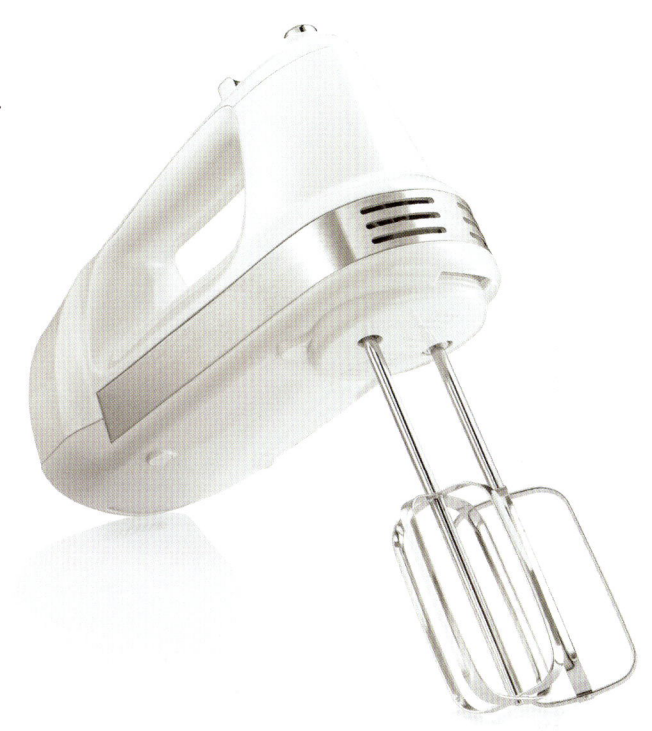

YOUR DINNER MENU	Large Meal (730 calories)	Total Carbs	NET CARBS	Small Meal (550 calories)	Total Carbs	NET CARBS
Baked ham	1 thick slice (5 oz/150 g, cooked)	1	1	1 thick slice (5 oz/150 g, cooked)	1	1
Pineapple, packed in juice	2 rings, no juice	13	12	2 rings, no juice	13	12
Sweet potato	1 large	46	43	½ large	23	21
Margarine or butter	3 tsp (15 mL)	0	0	1 tsp (5 mL)	0	0
Cauliflower	2 cups (500 mL)	8	5	2 cups (500 mL)	8	5
Dried Parmesan cheese	Sprinkle	0	0	Sprinkle	0	0
Skim or 1% milk	1 cup (250 mL)	12	12	1 cup (250 mL)	12	12
Whipped Gelatin	1 cup (250 mL)	2	2	1 cup (250 mL)	2	2
	TOTAL CARBS	82 g	75 g	TOTAL CARBS	59 g	53 g
	Total carbs minus fiber = NET CARBS ↑			NET CARBS ↑		
	CARB CHOICES (1 carb choice = 15 g net carbs)		5	CARB CHOICES		4

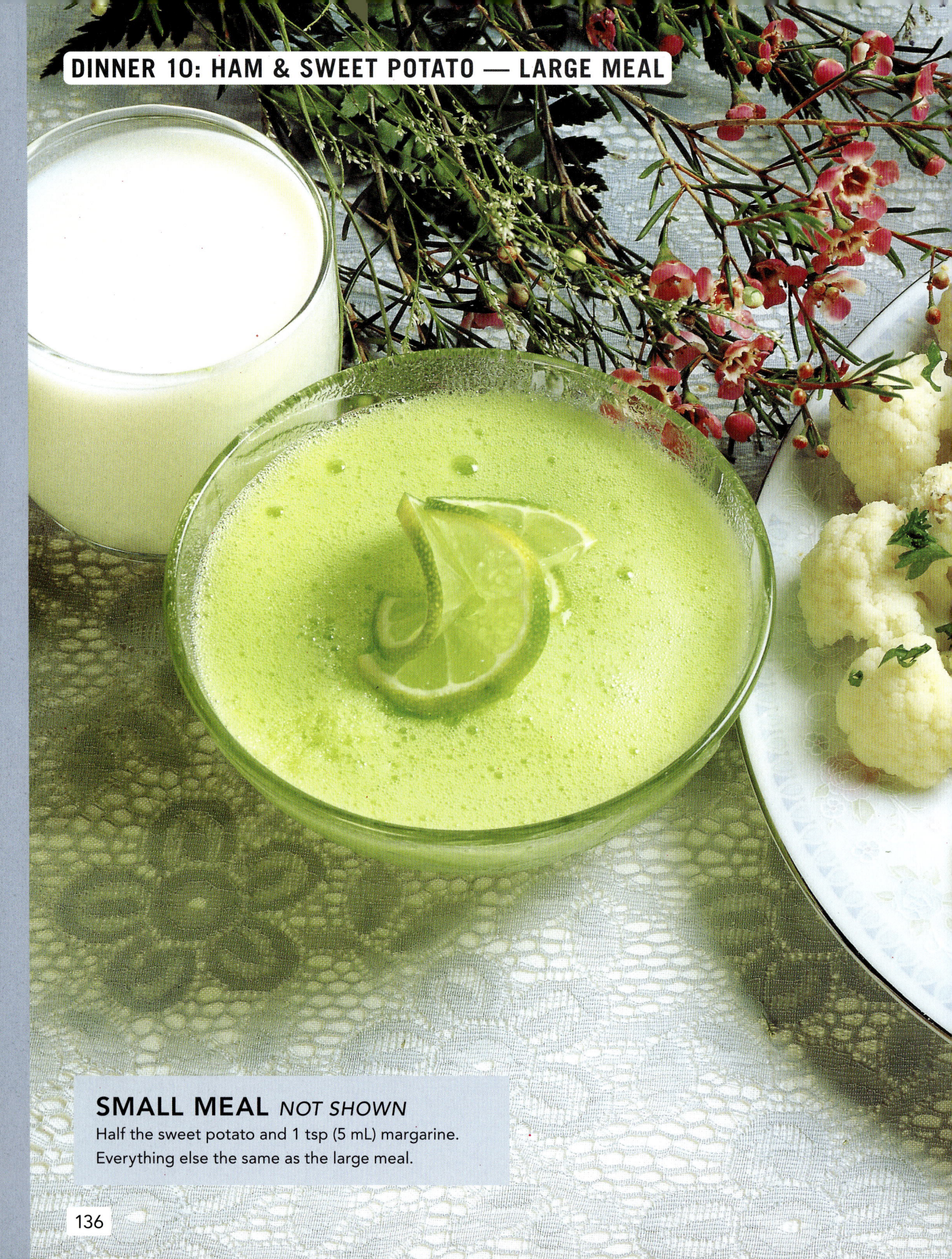

DINNER 10: HAM & SWEET POTATO — LARGE MEAL

SMALL MEAL *NOT SHOWN*
Half the sweet potato and 1 tsp (5 mL) margarine. Everything else the same as the large meal.

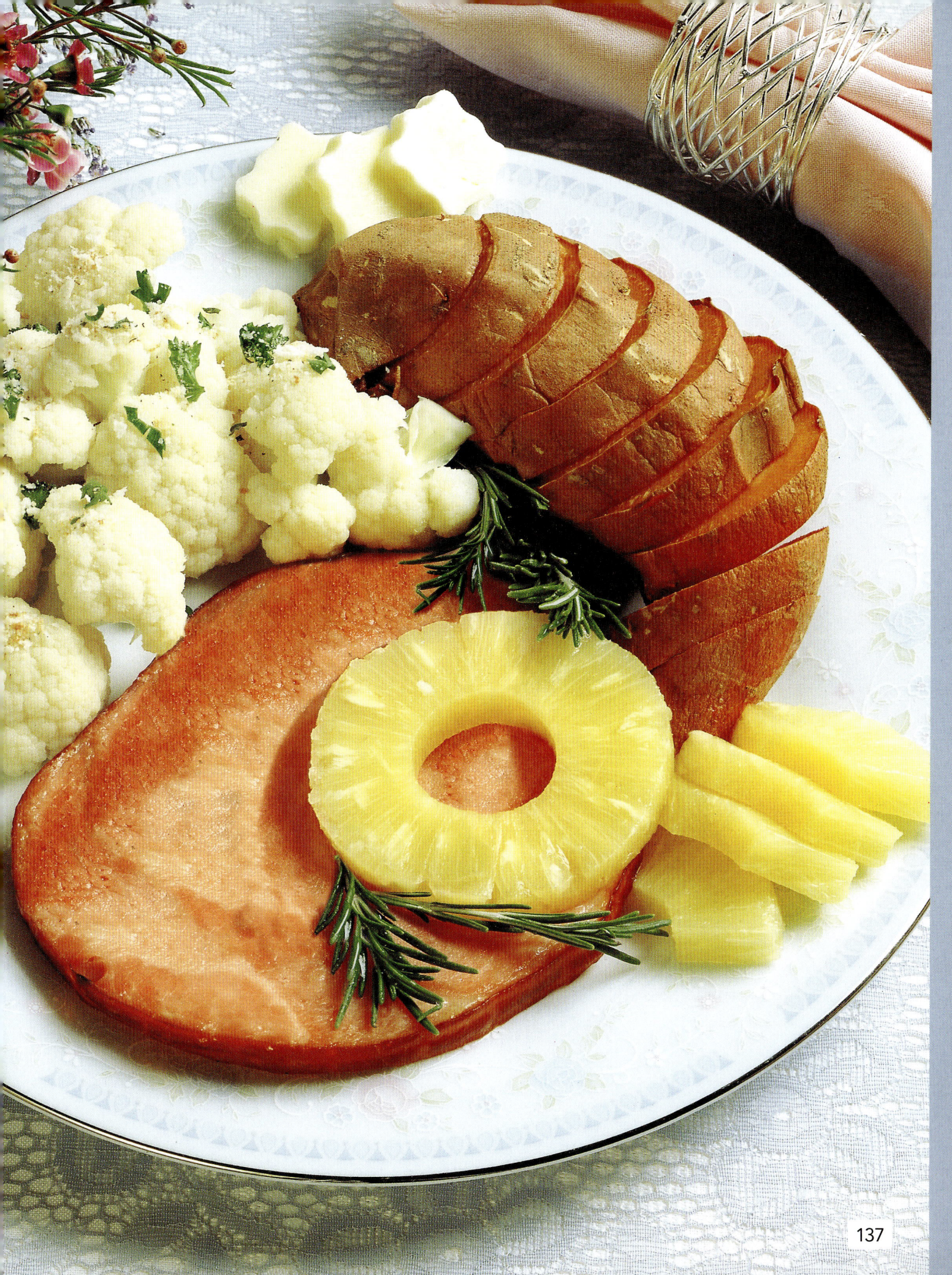

DINNER MEALS

DINNER 11

Beef Stew

Beef stew is an old favorite. With this meal, it is served with potatoes, a slice of bread to soak up the stew, and sliced cucumbers. For dessert, enjoy a serving of melon or other fruit.

⟳ LOW-CARB SWAP

Swap the slice of bread:
13 g net carbs
→ For cheese (serve with the melon or other fruit):
1 oz (30 g)
0 g net carbs

Beef Stew

Makes 8 cups (2 L)

- 2 tbsp (30 mL) margarine or oil
- 2 medium onions, chopped
- 2 cloves garlic, finely chopped (or ½ tsp/2 mL garlic powder)
- 1½ lb (750 g) stewing beef, fat removed, chopped into bite-size pieces
- 2 tbsp (30 mL) flour
- 1 to 2 packets (4.5 g each) reduced-salt beef bouillon, mixed in 2 cups (500 mL) hot water
- 2 bay leaves (remove before serving) or 2 tsp (10 mL) dried basil
- 2 large stalks of celery, sliced
- 3 medium carrots, sliced
- 2 cups (500 mL) other fresh vegetables (or frozen mixed vegetables)
- ⅛ tsp (0.5 mL) black pepper
- ¼ cup (60 mL) dry wine (or wine vinegar)

PER 1 CUP (250 ML)	
Calories	195
Carbohydrate	12 g
Fiber	2 g
Net carbs	10 g
Protein	18 g
Fat, total	8 g
Fat, saturated	2 g
Cholesterol	35 mg
Sodium	188 mg

1. In a heavy pot, add margarine, onions and garlic and stir often on medium heat until onions become clear.
2. Add meat and stir until cooked on the outside (about 5 minutes). Sprinkle flour over onion and meat mixture, and stir until flour disappears.
3. Take pot off the heat and stir in the rest of the ingredients. Return to heat, and bring to a boil. Then turn heat down to low. Cover and simmer for about an hour. Stir occasionally.
4. If you are using frozen mixed vegetables instead of fresh vegetables, add them just at the end and simmer for 10 minutes.

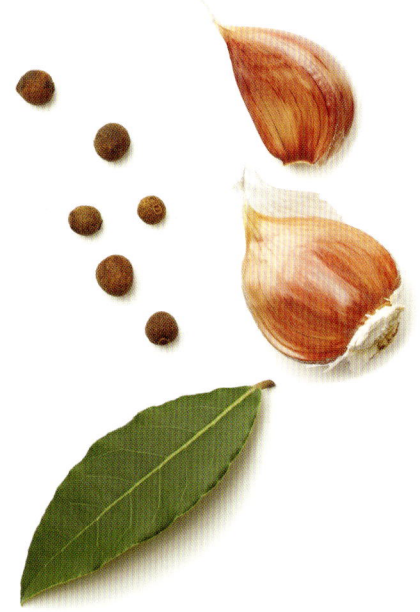

DINNER MEALS

Moroccan Beef Stew (Tagine) and Couscous

Here is an interesting spicy variation of the Beef Stew, a traditional Moroccan stew called Tagine. It is lovely served with couscous and mint tea.

Tagine refers to both the cone-shaped, clay-fired pot with lid (see photo) as well as the stew that's cooked inside it. Traditionally, it was cooked over a charcoal fire.

Moroccan Beef Stew

Follow the Beef Stew ingredients, and adjust as below:

- Omit bay leaves.
- Add the following spices: 1 tsp (5 mL) each of turmeric, coriander, ginger, cumin and cinnamon.
- Instead of celery and carrots, use diced pumpkin or orange squash such as acorn or butternut.
- Omit the wine.

Cook according to the Beef Stew directions. This stew can be cooked in a casserole in the oven at 325°F (160°C) for 2 hours or until meat and vegetables are tender.

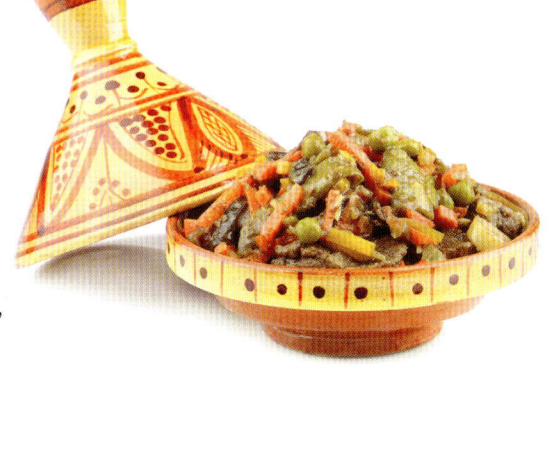

How Moroccan Stew Fits into Your Dinner Menu

Have 2 cups of the Moroccan Beef Stew. Couscous replaces the potato and bread. With the large meal have 1⅓ cup (300 mL) of cooked couscous, and for the small meal, ⅔ cup (150 mL). Follow the cooking directions on the couscous package. For both the large and small meals, enjoy the cucumbers and melon as shown in the menu box below.

See page 276 for carbohydrate information on couscous. Couscous is made from wheat, so it is like a type of pasta, but because it looks more like rice, it is in the Rice Swaps chart.

YOUR BREAKFAST MENU	Large Meal (730 calories)	Total Carbs	NET CARBS	Small Meal (550 calories)	Total Carbs	NET CARBS
Beef Stew	2 cups (500 mL)	24	**19**	2 cups (500 mL)	24	**19**
Boiled potatoes	1 medium	32	**29**	½ medium	16	**15**
Bread, rye	1 slice	15	**13**	1 slice	15	**13**
Margarine	1 tsp (5 mL)	0	**0**	½ tsp (2 mL)	0	**0**
Sliced cucumbers	½ medium cucumber	1	**1**	½ medium cucumber	1	**1**
Melon	2 slices (1 cup/250 mL diced)	15	**13**	1 slice (½ cup/125 mL diced)	7	**6**
	TOTAL CARBS	**87 g**	**75 g**	TOTAL CARBS	**63 g**	**54 g**
	Total carbs minus fiber = NET CARBS ↑			NET CARBS ↑		
	CARB CHOICES (1 carb choice = 15 g net carbs)		5	CARB CHOICES		4

139

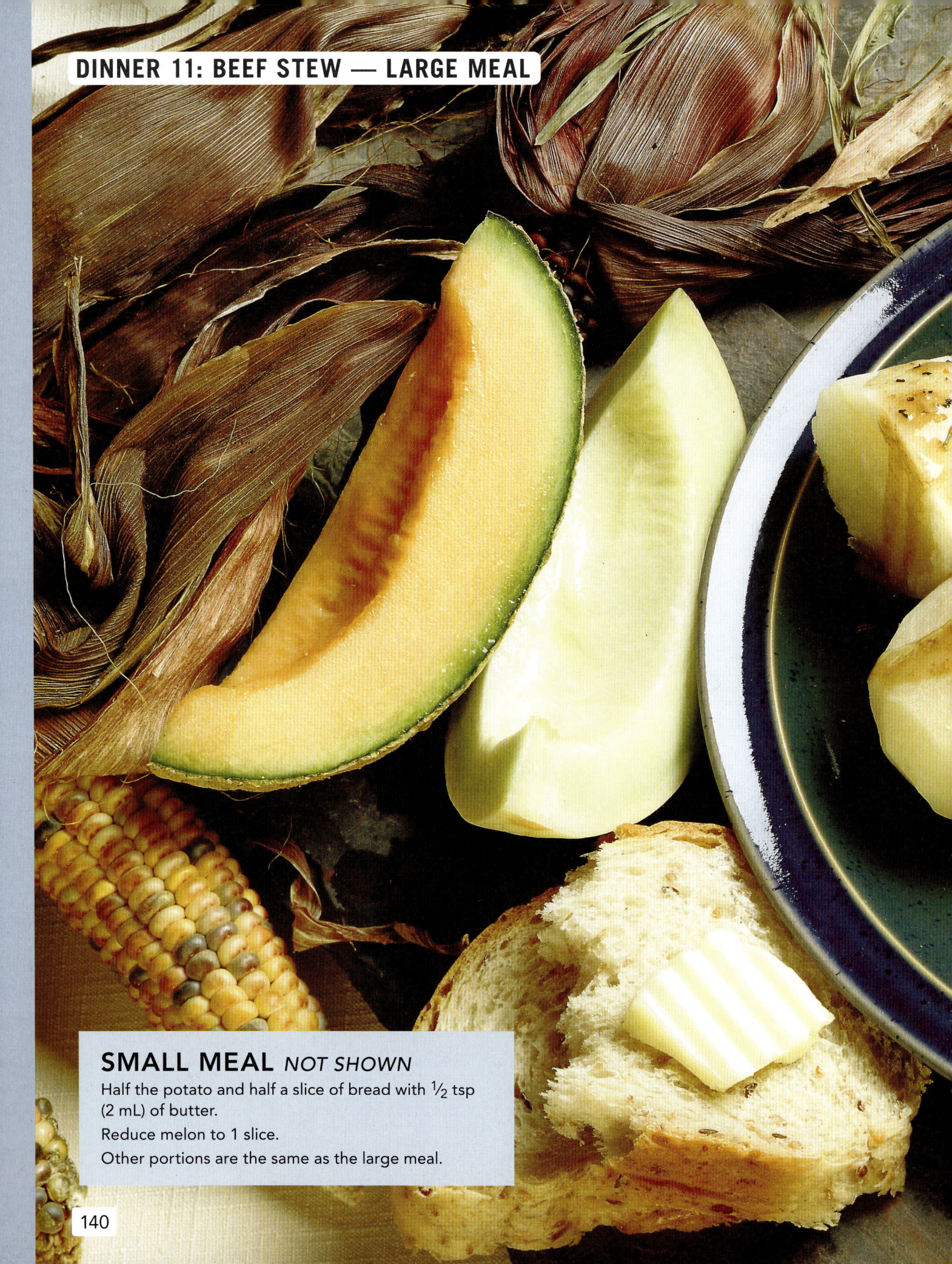

DINNER 11: BEEF STEW — LARGE MEAL

SMALL MEAL *NOT SHOWN*

Half the potato and half a slice of bread with ½ tsp (2 mL) of butter.

Reduce melon to 1 slice.

Other portions are the same as the large meal.

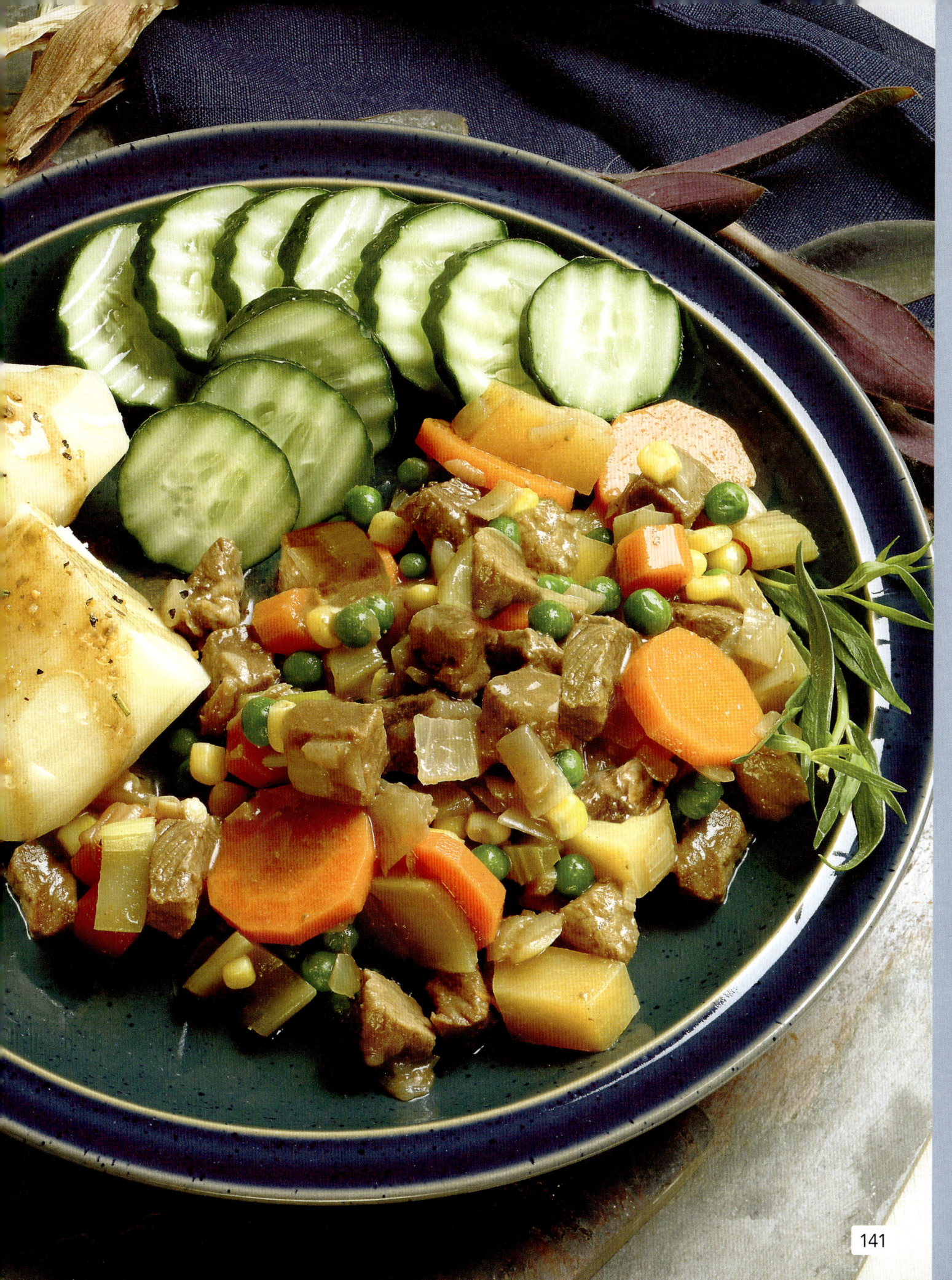

DINNER MEALS

DINNER 12

Fish & Chips

Fish Fillets

Look for "lightly breaded" fish fillets. These have fewer carbohydrates and less sodium than the standard heavily breaded fish sticks. Simply fry in a pan from frozen or bake in the oven along with the frozen French fries, according to the package instructions.

Homemade French Fries

Cut potato into wedges, toss in a small amount of oil, place on a baking sheet, and bake at 450°F (230°C) for 15 minutes.

Roasted Acorn Squash

Peel and cut the squash into chunks. In a bowl, toss the squash with a small amount of olive oil. Sprinkle with salt and pepper or herbs, optional. Spread out evenly on a greased or parchment-covered baking sheet, and cook with the fish and chips for 15 minutes, or until tender.

Microwaved Squash

Here's a quick way to cook squash. Poke holes with a fork all over the outside of the squash. Microwave on high for 7 minutes. It will be very hot; let it cool slightly. Slice in half, remove seeds and scoop out the squash. You can also quickly cook yams and potatoes in the microwave.

HEALTH TIP

Compare the calories of 10 French fries:

- 160 calories: fried in oil from a restaurant
- 90 calories: frozen fries baked in the oven

LOW-CARB SWAP

LARGE OR SMALL MEAL

Swap acorn squash:
½ cup (125 mL)
13 g net carbs

→ For spaghetti squash:
½ cup (125 mL)
4 g net carbs

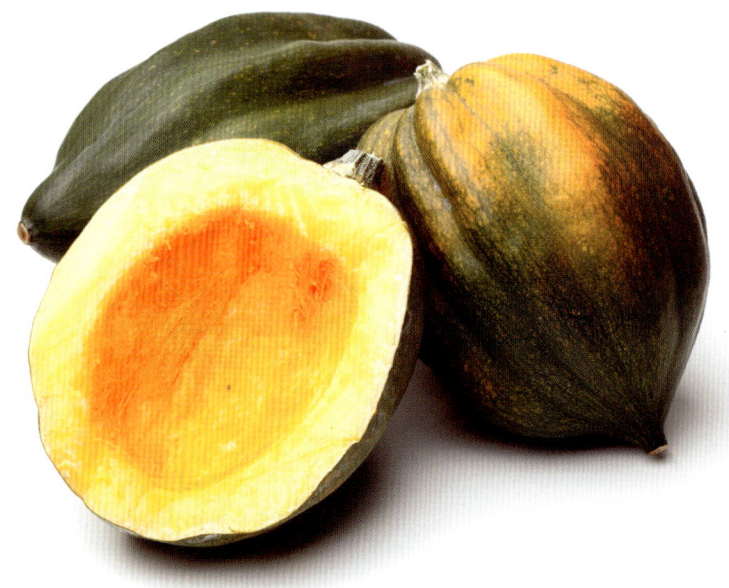

DINNER MEALS

Try this Light Jellied Vegetable Salad. It is colorful and tasty and low in carbs and calories. The flavor is refreshing with the fish and chips.

Light Jellied Vegetable Salad

Makes 2½ cups (625 mL) (5 servings)

1 package (4-serving size) light lime gelatin

1½ cups (375 mL) boiling water

2 tbsp (30 mL) lime or lemon juice

½ cup (125 mL) radish, finely chopped

½ cup (125 mL) celery, finely chopped

½ cup (125 mL) cabbage, finely chopped

1 tbsp (15 mL) fresh parsley, chopped, or 1 tsp (5 mL) dried parsley

PER ½ CUP (125 ML)	
Calories	18
Carbohydrate	4 g
Fiber	1 g
Net carbs	3 g
Protein	1 g
Fat, total	0 g
Fat, saturated	0 g
Cholesterol	0 mg
Sodium	41 mg

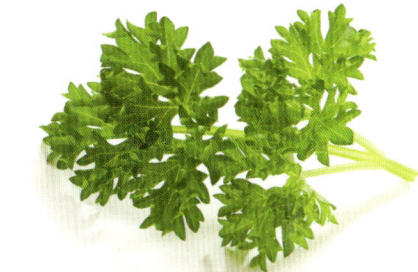

1. In a medium bowl, place the gelatin powder. Add boiling water and stir until gelatin is mixed in. Add the lime or lemon juice. Put this mixture in the fridge.
2. Once the gelatin is slightly thickened (about 45 minutes), stir in all the chopped vegetables.
3. Chill until set (about another hour).

Jellied Vegetable Salad can be a low-carb vegetable choice with any lunch or dinner meal: ½ cup (125 mL) has only 3 g net carbs.

YOUR DINNER MENU	Large Meal (730 calories)	Total Carbs	NET CARBS	Small Meal (550 calories)	Total Carbs	NET CARBS
Lightly breaded fish fillets	1½ fillets (210 g or 3 wedges)	20	18	1½ fillets (210 g or 3 wedges)	20	18
Oven-baked frozen French fries	20	31	28	12	18	16
Ketchup	1 tbsp (15 mL)	4	4	1 tbsp (15 mL)	4	4
Roasted Acorn Squash	¾ cup (175 mL)	22	19	½ cup (125 mL)	15	13
Oil (for the squash)	1 tsp (5 mL)	0	0	½ tsp (2 mL)	0	0
Light Jellied Vegetable Salad	½ cup (125 mL)	4	3	½ cup (125 mL)	4	3
	TOTAL CARBS	81 g	72 g	TOTAL CARBS	61 g	54 g
	Total carbs minus fiber = NET CARBS ↑			NET CARBS ↑		
	CARB CHOICES (1 carb choice = 15 g net carbs)		5	CARB CHOICES		4

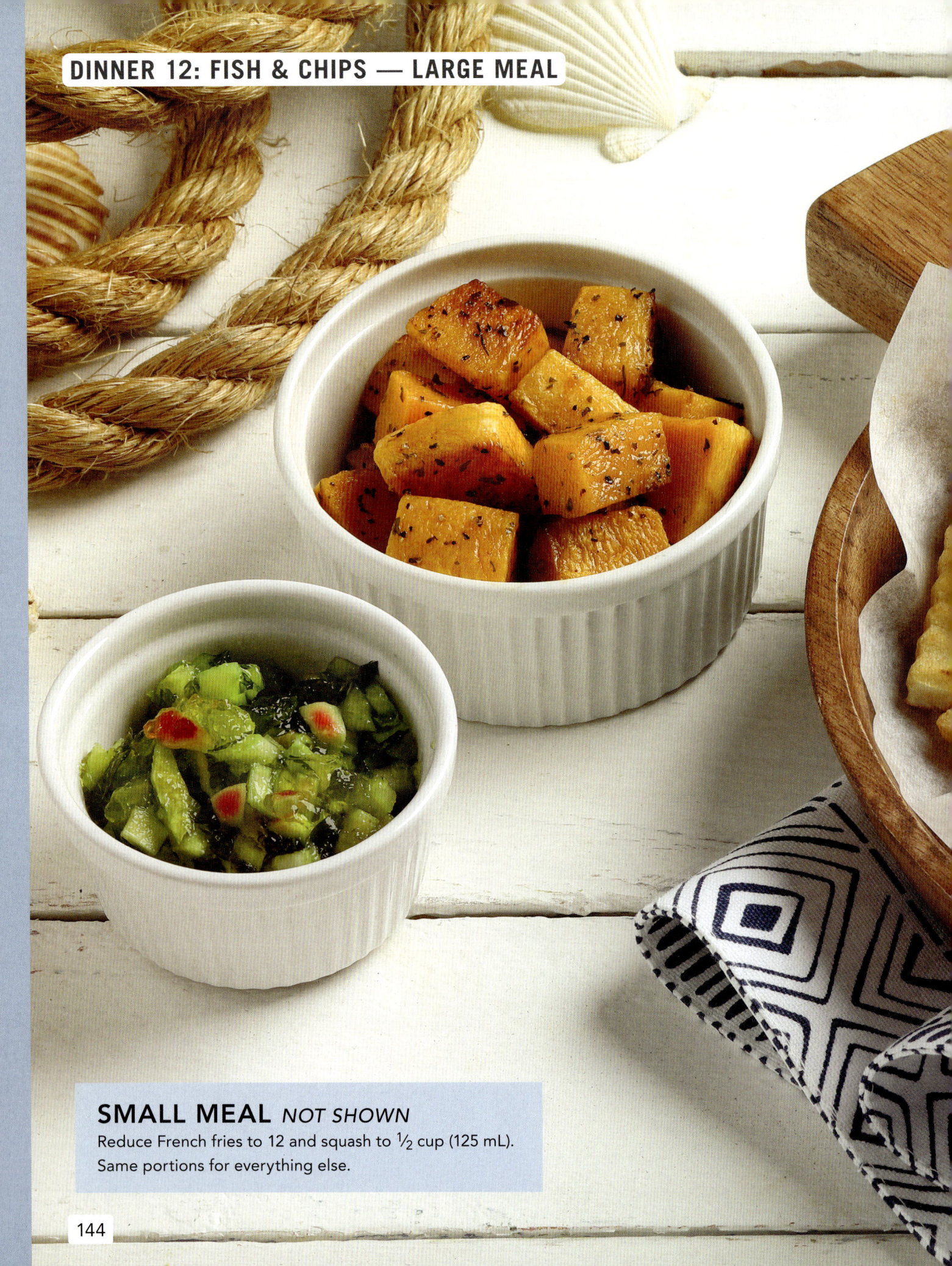

DINNER 12: FISH & CHIPS — LARGE MEAL

SMALL MEAL *NOT SHOWN*
Reduce French fries to 12 and squash to ½ cup (125 mL).
Same portions for everything else.

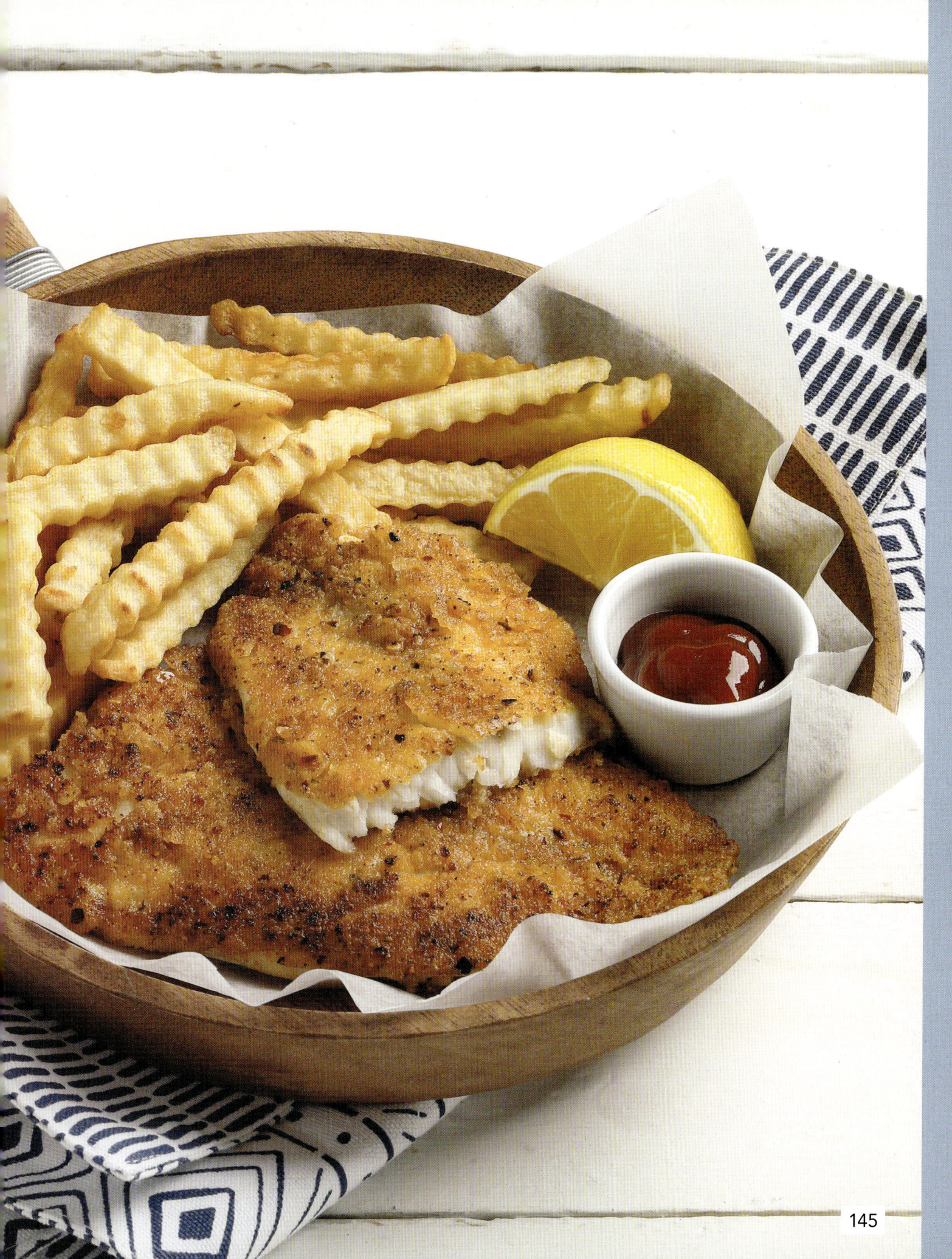

DINNER MEALS

Dinner 13

Sausages & Cornbread

Here is a favorite meal! Sausages are high in saturated fat and salt, so only choose them once in a while in the portions shown. This reduced-carb cornbread recipe can be enjoyed for dinner, lunch or a snack.

Cornbread or Corn Muffins

Makes an 8-inch (2 L) square pan (12 pieces) or 12 muffins

Preheat oven to 400°F (200°C)

- ¾ cup (175 mL) cornmeal
- 1¼ cups (300 mL) skim milk
- 1 large egg
- 2 tbsp (30 mL) oil or melted margarine, butter or shortening
- ½ cup (125 mL) flour
- ½ cup (125 mL) almond flour
- 1 tbsp (15 mL) baking powder
- ½ tsp (2 mL) salt
- ¼ cup (60 mL) sugar

PER PIECE (1/12 OF RECIPE)	
Calories	136
Carbohydrate	18 g
Fiber	1 g
Net carbs	17 g
Protein	4 g
Fat, total	6 g
Fat, saturated	1 g
Cholesterol	16 mg
Sodium	163 mg

RECIPE TIP

Jalapeno Corn Cornbread

For this variation of the cornbread recipe, use the recipe below: after you combine the cornmeal mixture and the flour mixture (step 3), add ½ cup (125 mL) of kernel corn and 1 finely chopped jalapeno pepper. Remove the seeds of the pepper unless you want it hot! This variation adds only an extra 1 g of net carb per muffin.

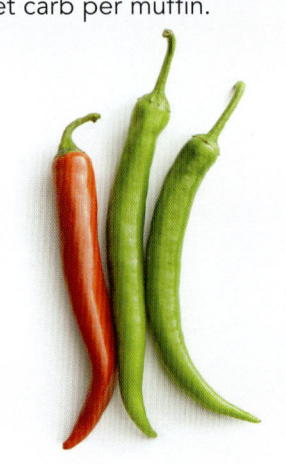

1. In a medium bowl, mix together cornmeal, milk, egg and oil (or melted fat).
2. In a large bowl, mix together the two kinds of flour, baking powder, salt and sugar.
3. Add cornmeal mixture to the flour mixture. Stir until combined. Pour into a greased 8-inch (2 L) square pan or muffin tin.
4. Bake for about 20 minutes (15 minutes for muffins), or until lightly browned.
5. Cut into 12 pieces (about 3 inches by 2 inches/8 cm by 5 cm).

Serve the meal with lightly steamed zucchini and Coleslaw (see recipe on page 72).

RECIPE TIP

Ratatouille

Another way to prepare sliced zucchini is to sauté it in a small amount of oil with additional vegetables: chopped onion, garlic and eggplant, fresh or canned chopped tomatoes and chopped bell pepper. Sprinkle with dried Parmesan. It's delicious!

DINNER MEALS

Dessert

Choose a light fudge ice cream bar, or swap with a keto ice cream bar.

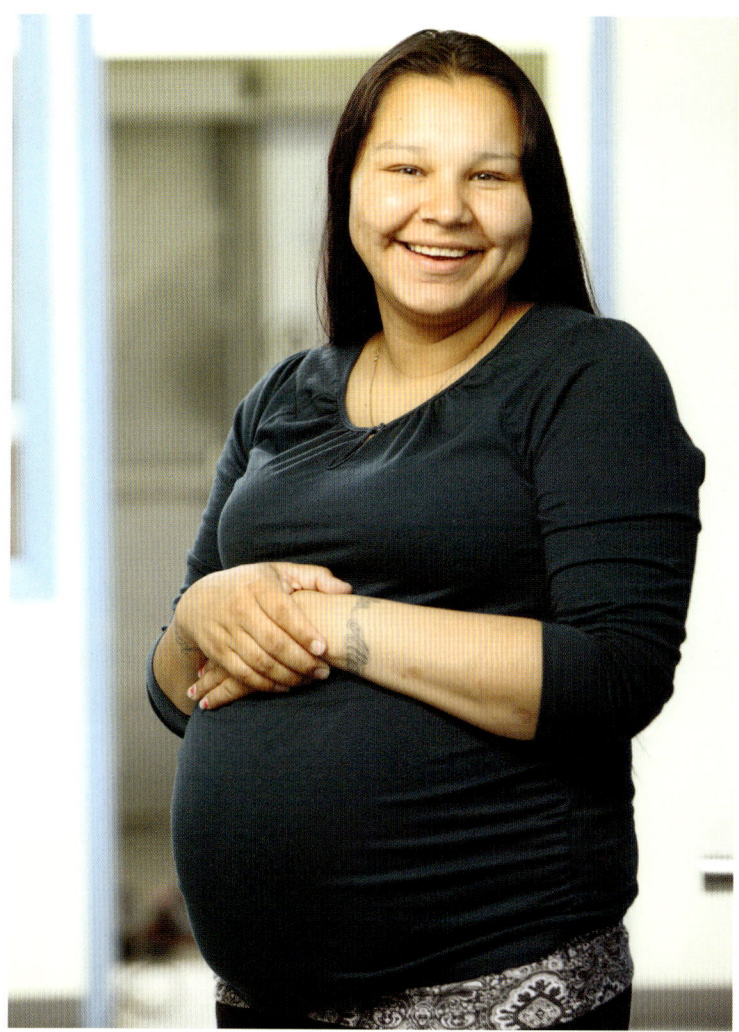

Craving ice cream? Enjoy the light fudge ice cream bar with this meal or try the Low-Carb Swap below.

⟲ LOW-CARB SWAP

Swap light fudge ice cream bar:
9 g net carbs
→ For keto frozen dessert bar (labeled as 0 gram sugar):
2 g net carbs

Note: While carbs are lower in keto frozen dessert bars, the fat and calories are a lot higher.

See Ice Cream Swaps, page 278.

YOUR DINNER MENU	Large Meal (730 calories)	Total Carbs	NET CARBS	Small Meal (550 calories)	Total Carbs	NET CARBS
Sausages	4 small links	1	1	4 small links	1	1
Cornbread	2½ pieces	45	42	1½ pieces	27	25
Margarine or butter	2 tsp (10 mL)	0	0	—	—	—
Steamed zucchini	2 cups (500 mL)	14	8	2 cups (500 mL)	14	8
Dried Parmesan cheese	Sprinkle	0	0	Sprinkle	0	0
Coleslaw (page 72)	½ cup (125 mL)	5	4	½ cup (125 mL)	5	4
Light fudge ice cream bar	1 bar	10	9	1 bar	10	9
	TOTAL CARBS	75 g	64 g	**TOTAL CARBS**	57 g	47 g
	Total carbs minus fiber = NET CARBS ↑			NET CARBS ↑		
	CARB CHOICES (1 carb choice = 15 g net carbs)		4	CARB CHOICES		3

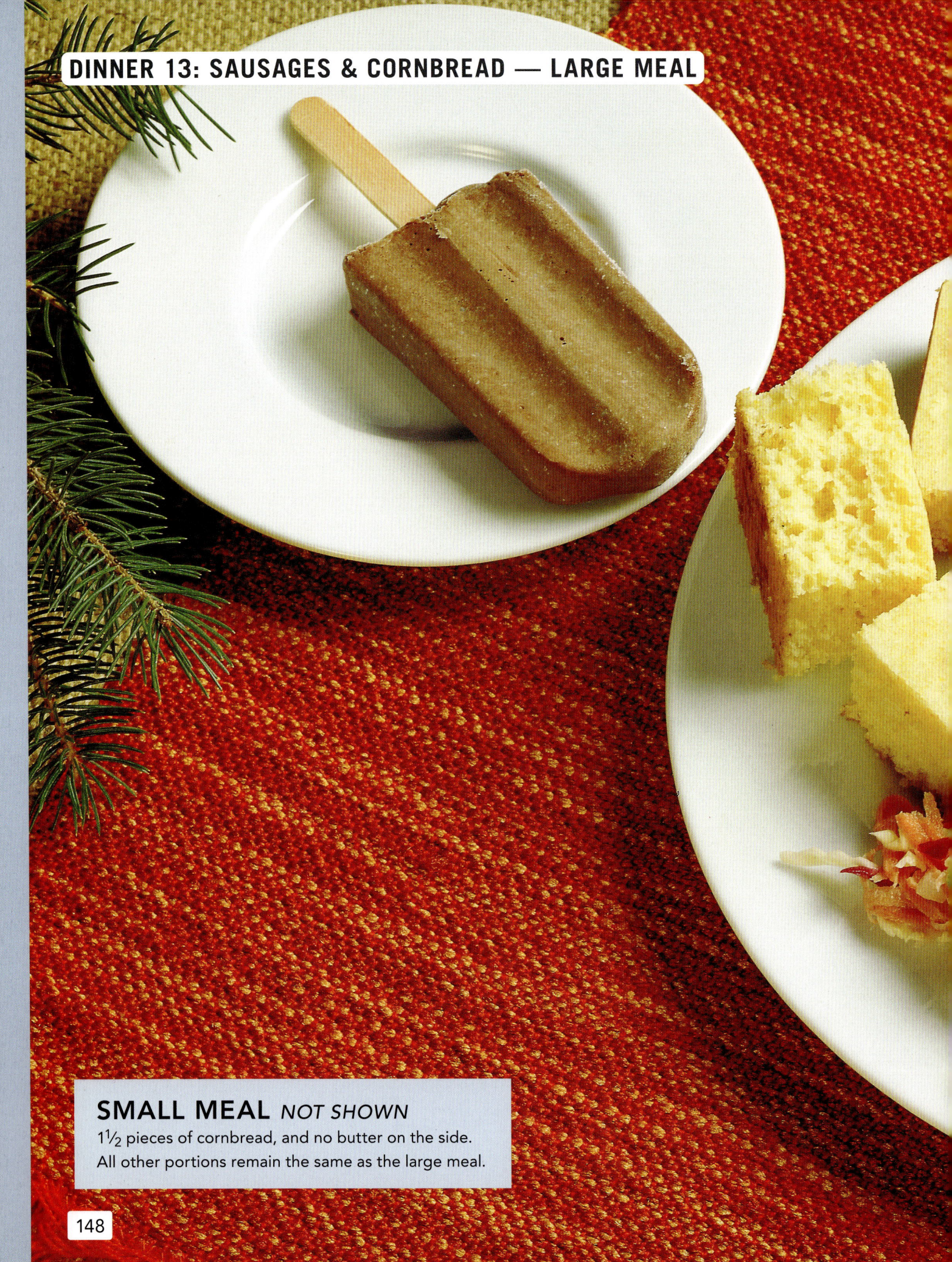

DINNER 13: SAUSAGES & CORNBREAD — LARGE MEAL

SMALL MEAL *NOT SHOWN*
1½ pieces of cornbread, and no butter on the side. All other portions remain the same as the large meal.

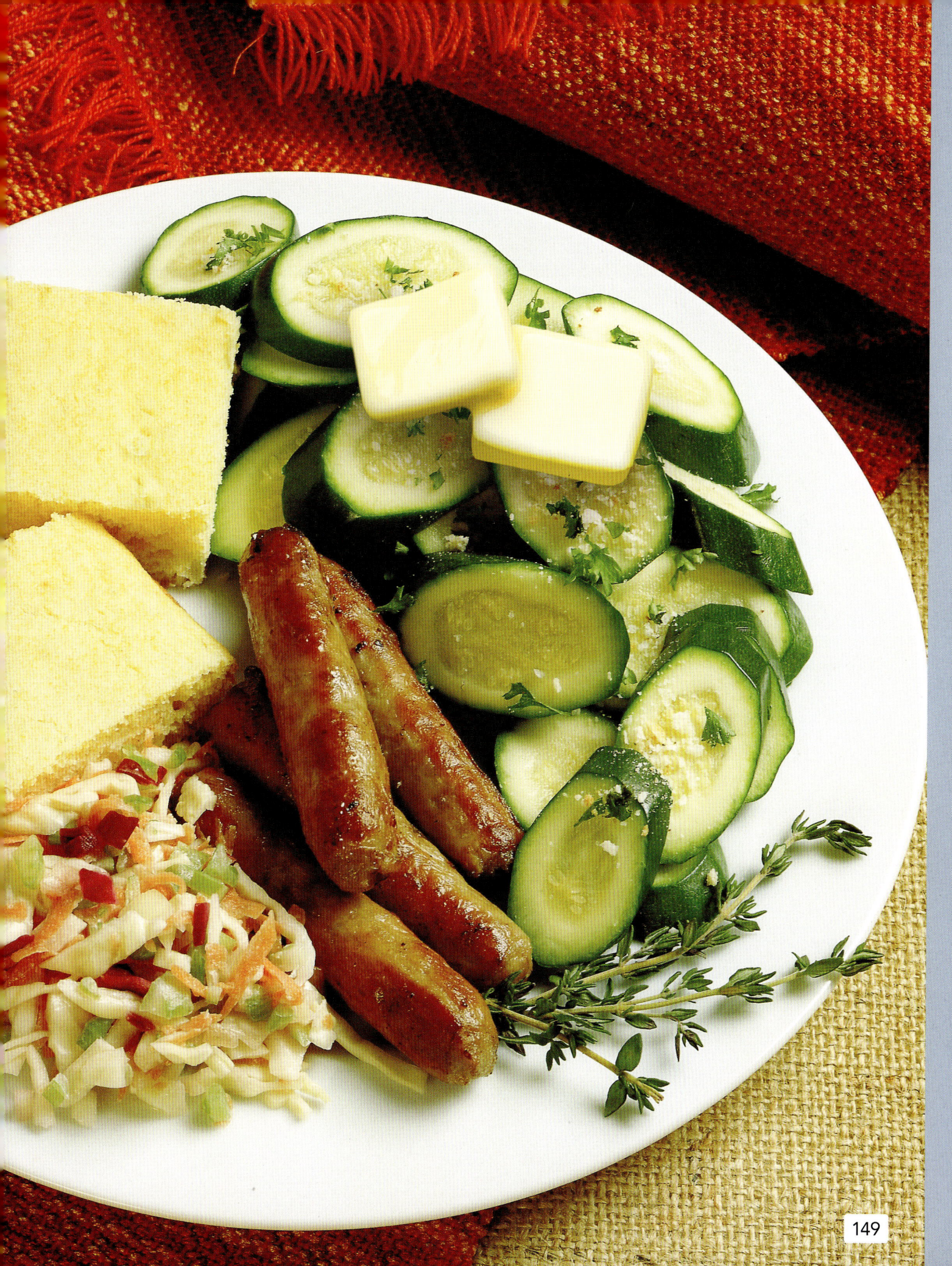

DINNER MEALS

DINNER 14

Chili Con Carne

Chili Con Carne

Makes 6¼ cups (1.55 L)

- 1 lb (500 g) lean ground beef
- 2 medium onions, chopped
- 28 oz (796 mL) can kidney beans, drained and rinsed
- 10 oz (284 mL) can tomato soup
- 1 cup (250 mL) water
- ¼ tsp (1 mL) black pepper
- 1 tsp (5 mL) chili powder
- 1 tbsp (15 mL) vinegar
- 1 tsp (5 mL) Worcestershire sauce
- 1 cup (250 mL) chopped vegetables, such as celery or green pepper

PER 1 CUP (250 ML)	
Calories	270
Carbohydrate	29 g
Fiber	7 g
Net carbs	22 g
Protein	21 g
Fat, total	8 g
Fat, saturated	3 g
Cholesterol	38 mg
Sodium	601 mg

1. In a large, heavy pot, brown ground beef. Drain off extra fat.
2. Add all the other ingredients to the pot.
3. Cover with a lid and cook for 2 to 3 hours on low heat. Stir every now and then so the chili doesn't stick. Add extra water if it gets too thick.

Your meal includes carrots and green beans with the Chili. For the large meal, brown or white rice is also included.

HEALTH TIP

Canned beans

Kidney beans are a good source of protein and fiber. Be sure to pick up the large size of can for this recipe.

Rinse canned beans to remove about 30% of the salt.

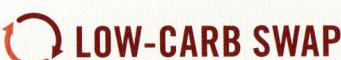

LOW-CARB SWAP

LARGE MEAL

Swap cooked rice:
⅓ cup (75 mL)
14 g net carbs

→ For riced cauliflower:
⅓ cup (75 mL)
1 g net carbs

See Rice Swaps, page 276.

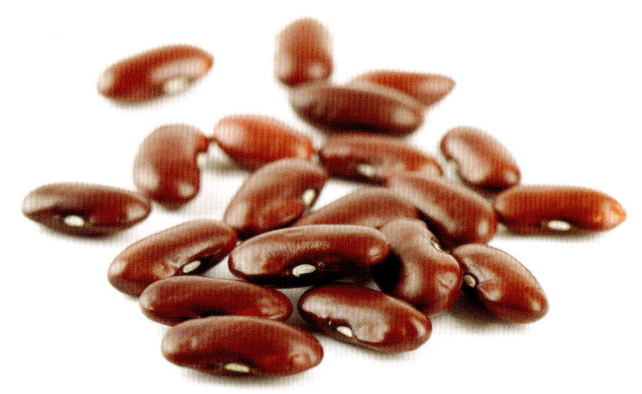

DINNER MEALS

For a dessert treat, try these baked apples. They have a lovely glaze from the combination of brown sugar and butter. Margarine can be used, but butter makes the syrup thicker. Regular sugar is used because zero-calorie sweeteners tend to make the syrup thin.

Baked Apples

Makes 2 baked apples

Preheat oven to 350°F (180°C)

2 small apples
1 tbsp (15 mL) butter or margarine
2 tsp (10 mL) brown sugar
¼ tsp (1 mL) ground cinnamon
¼ tsp (1 mL) lemon juice
Dash of nutmeg
1 tbsp (15 mL) raisins

PER APPLE	
Calories	147
Carbohydrate	25 g
Fiber	2 g
Net carbs	23 g
Protein	0 g
Fat, total	6 g
Fat, saturated	4 g
Cholesterol	15 mg
Sodium	46 mg

RECIPE TIP

Here's a quick microwave option. Core the two apples, then chop or slice them. Mix them with the other ingredients in a microwaveable bowl. Microwave for about 3 minutes, or until the apples are soft.

1. Remove apple core, cutting from the top of the apple. Don't cut right through to the bottom. Prick apples with a fork.
2. In a small bowl, mix together other ingredients and spoon into the apples.
3. Place the apples in a pan with 2 tbsp (30 mL) of water and bake for 30 minutes.
4. Enjoy with a piece of cheese.

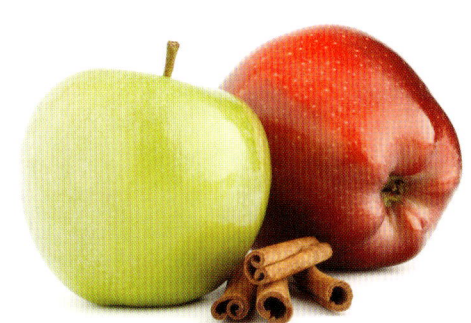

YOUR DINNER MENU	Large Meal (730 calories)	Total Carbs	NET CARBS	Small Meal (550 calories)	Total Carbs	NET CARBS
Chili Con Carne	1¼ cups (310 mL)	35	**28**	¾ cup (175 mL)	22	**17**
Rice, long-grain, converted	⅓ cup (75 mL)	14	**14**	—	—	—
Green beans	1 cup (250 mL)	10	**6**	1 cup (250 mL)	10	**6**
Carrot sticks	1 medium carrot	6	**4**	1 medium carrot	6	**4**
Baked Apple	1	25	**23**	1	25	**23**
Cheddar cheese	1 oz (30 g)	0	**0**	1 oz (30 g)	0	**0**
	TOTAL CARBS	90 g	**75 g**	**TOTAL CARBS**	63 g	**50 g**
Total carbs minus fiber = NET CARBS ↑				NET CARBS ↑		
CARB CHOICES (1 carb choice = 15 g net carbs)			5	CARB CHOICES		3

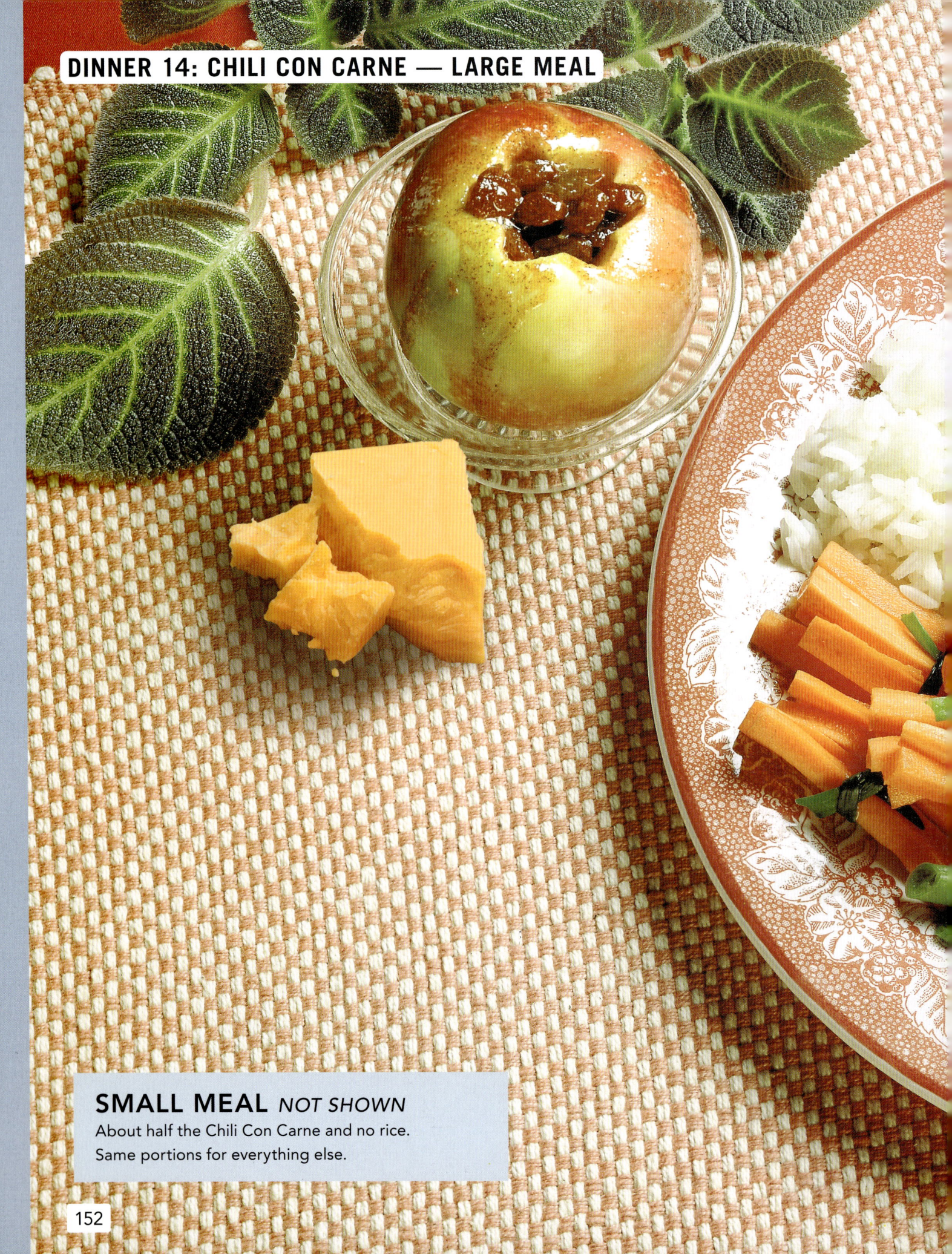

DINNER 14: CHILI CON CARNE — LARGE MEAL

SMALL MEAL *NOT SHOWN*
About half the Chili Con Carne and no rice. Same portions for everything else.

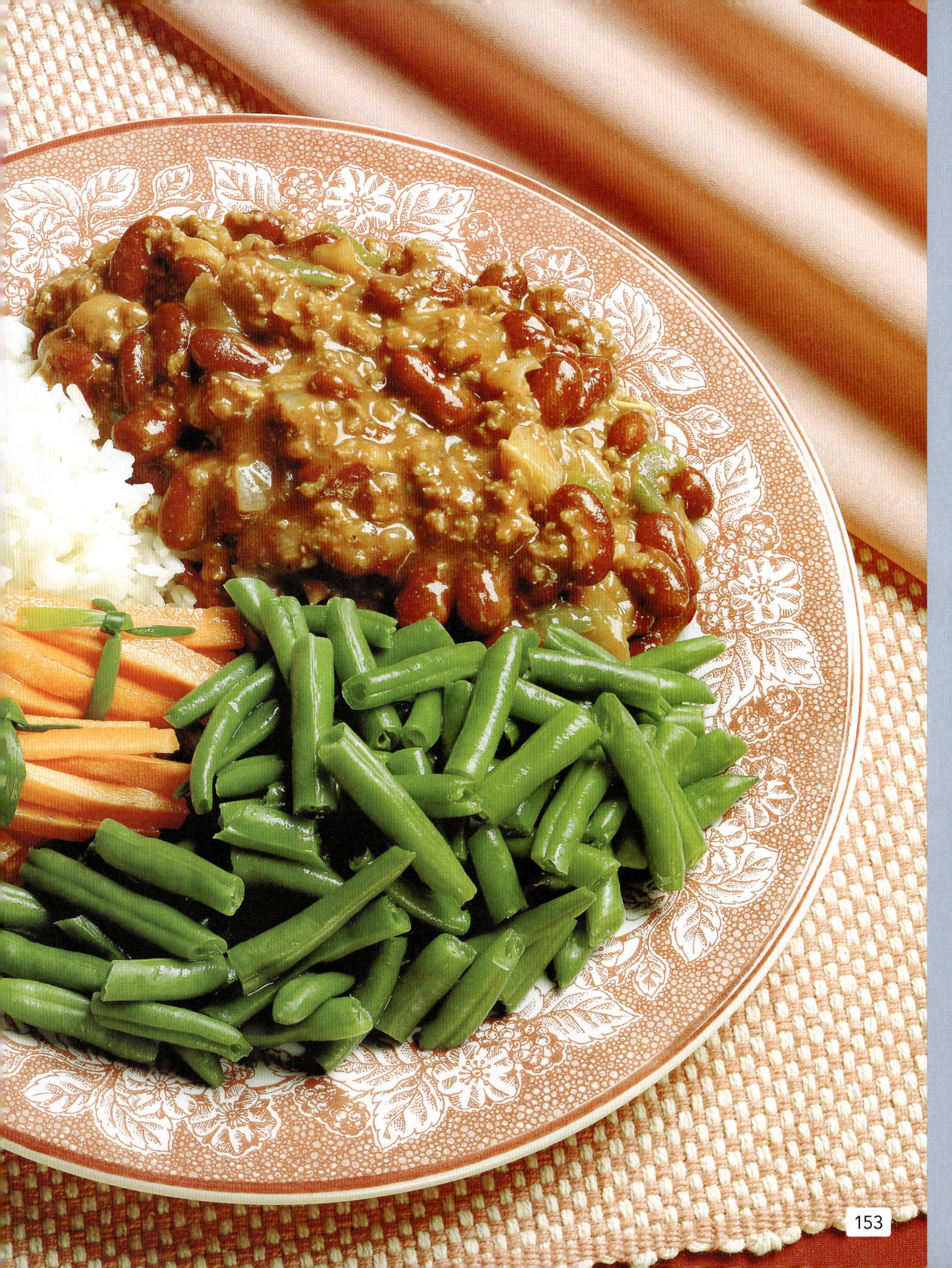

DINNER MEALS

Dinner 15

Perogies

Perogies come with many fillings, such as cheese, potato and cottage cheese. The carbs in perogies can add up quickly, so be careful not to eat more than the number shown in the menu.

First, fry a sliced half small onion on low heat in 2 tsp (10 mL) of butter or margarine. Once the onion is soft, remove and set aside. Fry the perogies in the same pan.

If using frozen perogies, boil them for 5 to 10 minutes until they float to the top. Then remove them with a slotted spoon and add to the frying pan. Fresh perogies can go directly into the pan. Fry the perogies until lightly browned.

Instead of having a 2 oz (60 g) piece of garlic sausage (kielbasa) with the large meal, you could have:

- ½ cup (125 mL) 2% cottage cheese
- 1 small fast-fry pork chop (3 oz/85 g)
- 2 slices bologna, broiled, or fried without added fat

Sauerkraut is a low-carb vegetable that has healthy bacteria.

A low-salt alternative to sauerkraut would be a small salad or coleslaw.

LOW-CARB SWAP

LARGE OR SMALL MEAL

Swap 1 perogy:
9 g net carbs

→ For 2 tbsp (30 mL) extra shredded cheese:
0 g net carbs

HEALTH TIP

Sauerkraut and Diabetes

Sauerkraut is salted, fermented (pickled) cabbage. During the fermenting process, healthy bacteria grow. These are called probiotic bacteria. While helping to digest food, probiotic bacteria slow down the rise in blood sugar after a meal.

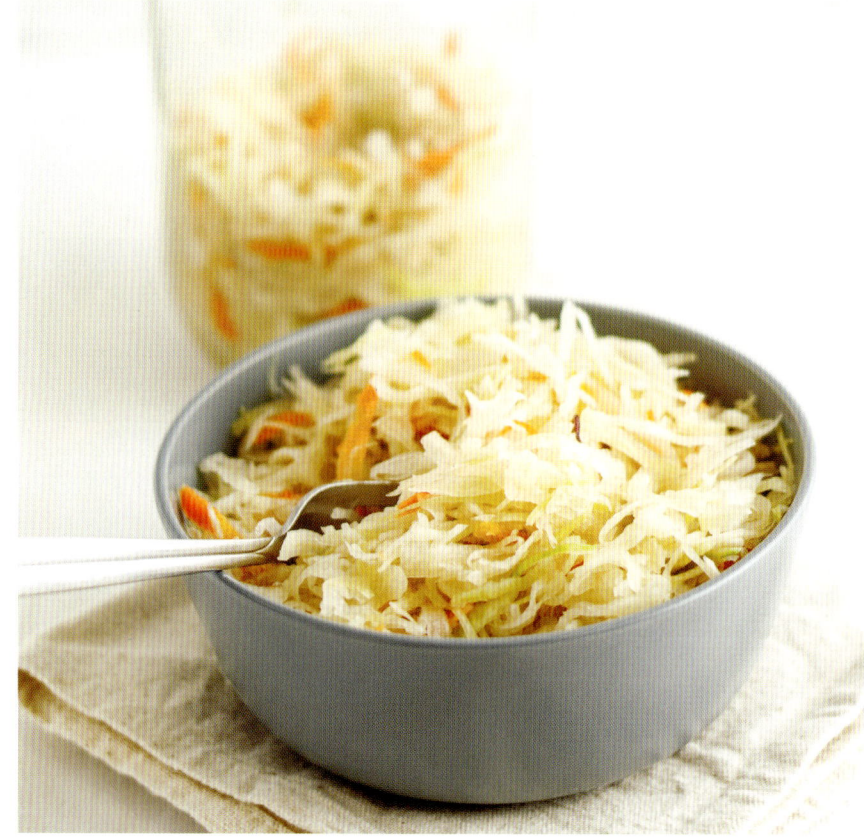

Dinner Meals

Easy Beet Soup

Makes 3½ cups (875 mL)

10 oz (284 mL) can diced beets (unsweetened), drained and rinsed

1½ cups (375 mL) vegetable juice (such as V8)

½ cup (125 mL) water

2 cups (500 mL) chopped cabbage

¼ tsp (1 mL) dried dill

PER 1 CUP (250 ML)	
Calories	46
Carbohydrate	10 g
Fiber	2 g
Net carbs	8 g
Protein	2 g
Fat, total	0 g
Fat, saturated	0 g
Cholesterol	0 mg
Sodium	363 mg

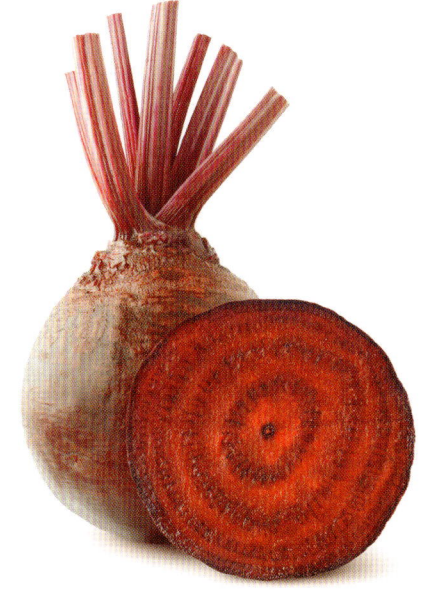

1. Place all ingredients in a pot.
2. Cover and simmer; stir regularly. It will take about 15 minutes to cook.

Beet Soup Options

Instead of the 1 cup (250 mL) of beet soup, have:

- 1 cup (250 mL) boiled or roasted beets (see page 110), or
- ½ cup (125 mL) of jarred pickled beets; these have added sugar so are a smaller portion

Dessert

For the large meal, enjoy one fresh peach when in season. Canned peaches are just as delicious: two halves with 2 tbsp (30 mL) of juice is equal to one fresh. Choose fruit canned in water or juice.

YOUR DINNER MENU	Large Meal (730 calories)	Total Carbs	NET CARBS	Small Meal (550 calories)	Total Carbs	NET CARBS
Perogies	5	50	**45**	4	40	36
Sour cream, 2–5%	2 tbsp (30 mL)	4	4	1 tbsp (15 mL)	2	2
Cheddar cheese, shredded	2 tbsp (30 mL)	0	0	2 tbsp (30 mL)	0	0
Cooked sliced onion in butter or margarine	½ small onion 2 tsp (10 mL)	3 0	2 0	½ small onion 2 tsp (10 mL)	3 0	2 0
Garlic sausage (kielbasa)	2 oz (60 g)	2	2	2 oz (60 g)	2	2
Easy Beet Soup	1 cup (250 mL)	10	8	1 cup (250 mL)	10	8
Cherry tomatoes	2, or 2 slices of tomato	1	1	2, or 2 slices of tomato	1	1
Sauerkraut	½ cup (125 mL)	3	1	½ cup (125 mL)	3	1
Peach	1 medium	13	11	—	—	—
	TOTAL CARBS	86 g	74 g	**TOTAL CARBS**	61 g	52 g
	Total carbs minus fiber = NET CARBS ↑			NET CARBS ↑		
	CARB CHOICES (1 carb choice = 15 g net carbs)		5	CARB CHOICES		3

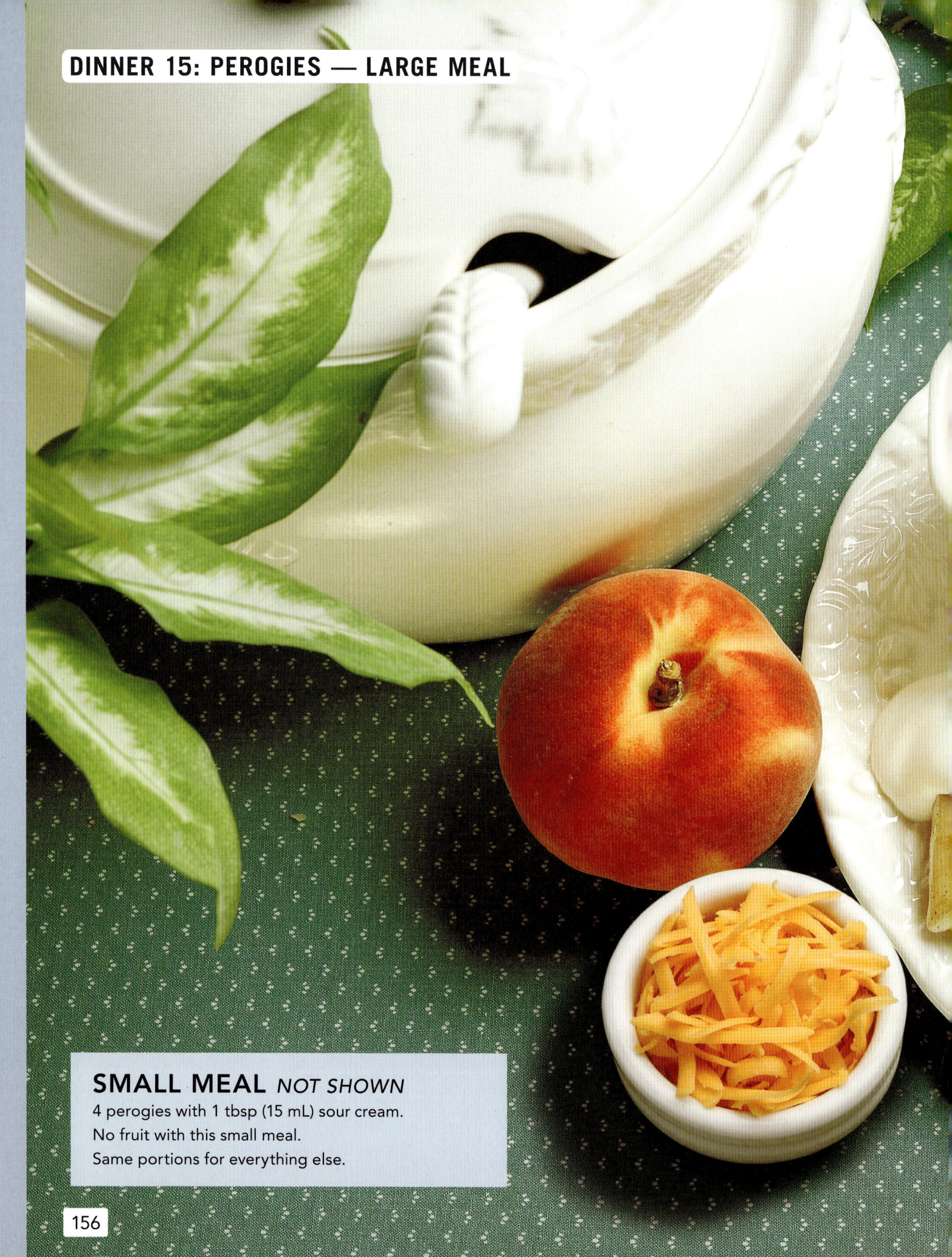

DINNER 15: PEROGIES — LARGE MEAL

SMALL MEAL *NOT SHOWN*
4 perogies with 1 tbsp (15 mL) sour cream.
No fruit with this small meal.
Same portions for everything else.

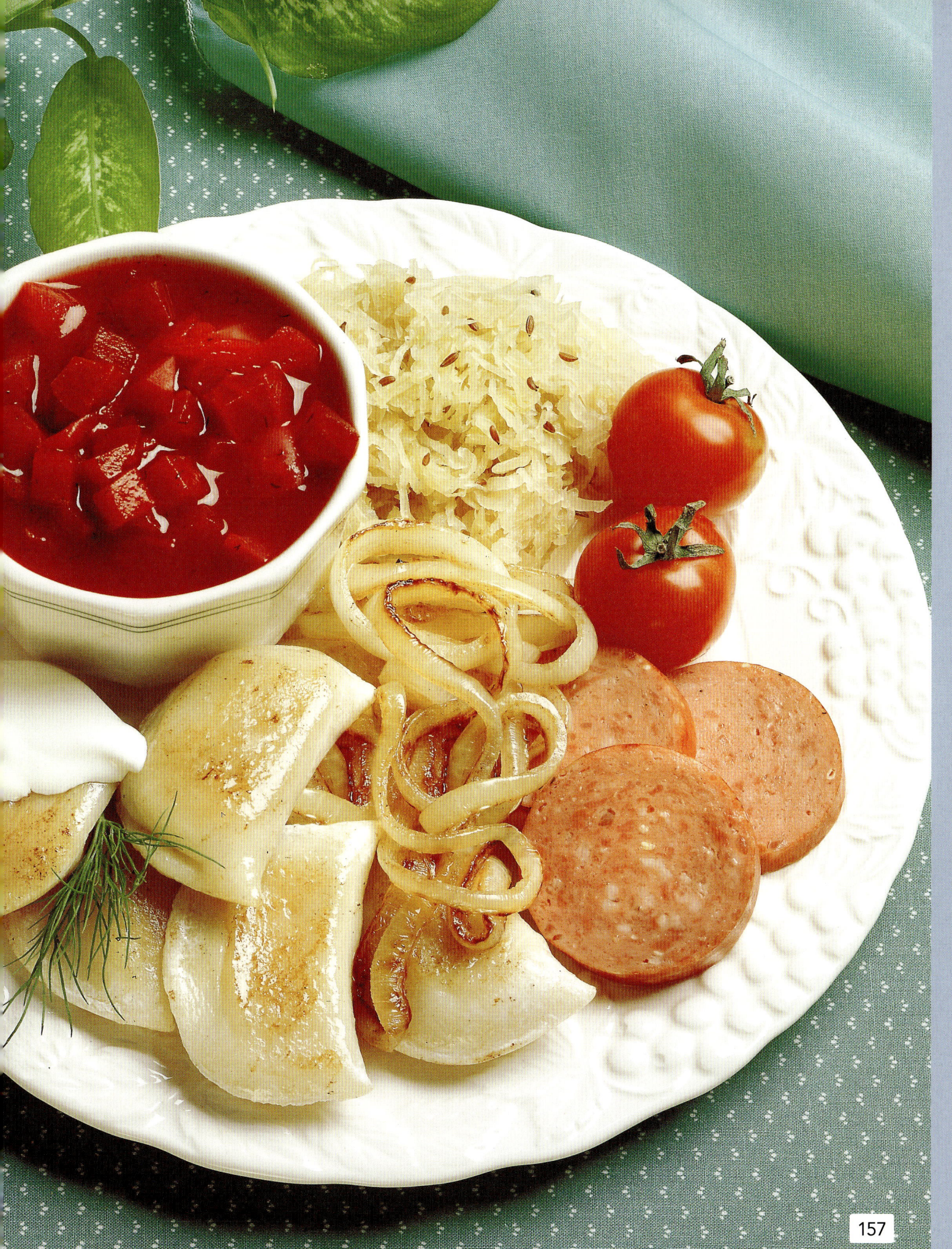

DINNER MEALS

DINNER 16

Hamburger with Potato Salad

HEALTH TIP

Hamburger and Potato Salad Safety

Cook hamburgers until well done with no pink showing. Then they are safe to eat.

The mayonnaise in the potato salad can quickly become unsafe to eat if left in the sun at an outdoor barbecue.

Refrigerate all hamburger and potato salad leftovers right away.

Use lean or extra-lean ground beef when you make hamburgers. One pound (500 g) of lean ground beef will make about 4 beef patties.

For extra flavor, you can mix into the pound of raw meat 2 tsp (10 mL) of Five Spice Blend (page 98) or Mrs. Dash type of salt-free blend. Options that would lightly salt your hamburger include ¼ to ½ tsp (1 to 2 mL) of your favorite seasoning salt.

There are several ways to cook your hamburgers:

- Grill on a barbecue.
- Place them on a rack and broil in the oven.
- Fry them in a nonstick pan, then place on a paper towel to soak up the extra fat.

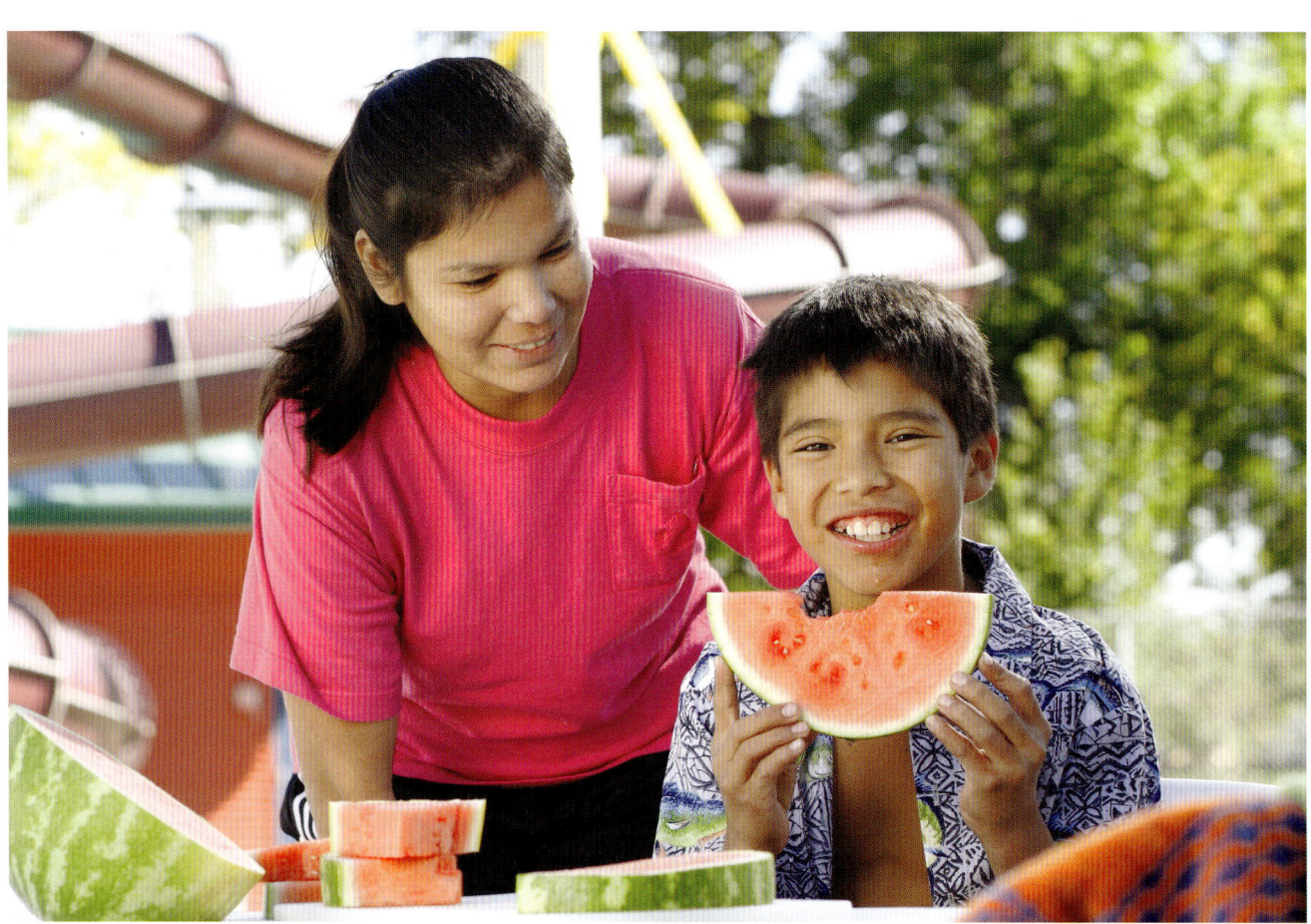

Potato Salad

Makes 4 cups (1 L)

2 medium (2 cups/500 mL cubed) cooked potatoes, chopped

½ green pepper, finely chopped

2 stalks celery, finely chopped

2 to 3 green onions, chopped (or 1 small onion, finely chopped)

5 radishes, sliced

2 tbsp (30 mL) vinegar

2 tbsp (30 mL) mayonnaise

½ tsp (2 mL) prepared mustard

Salt and pepper, to taste

2 large hard-boiled eggs, sliced or chopped

Sprinkle of paprika

1. In a large bowl, mix together potatoes, green pepper, celery, green onions and radishes.
2. In a small bowl, mix together vinegar, mayonnaise, mustard, salt and pepper, and add to the potatoes. Gently add egg pieces or place on top of salad. Sprinkle with paprika.
3. Keep refrigerated until ready to eat.

PER ½ CUP (125 ML)	
Calories	82
Carbohydrate	9 g
Fiber	1 g
Net carbs	8 g
Protein	3 g
Fat, total	4 g
Fat, saturated	1 g
Cholesterol	48 mg
Sodium	54 mg

LOW-CARB SWAP

FOR POTATO SALAD RECIPE

Substitute cooked rutabagas for the cooked potatoes. Half of a 5-inch (12.5 cm) rutabaga (300 g peeled weight) is equal to two medium potatoes.

LARGE MEAL

Swap Potato Salad: ¾ cup (175 mL)

12 g net carbs

→ For salad made with rutabaga: **6 g net carbs**

SMALL MEAL

Swap Potato Salad: ½ cup (125 mL)

8 g net carbs

→ For salad made with rutabaga: **4 g net carbs**

See Potato Swaps, page 275.

Light Iced Tea

Check the label of the light iced tea package to be sure it has fewer than 20 calories in a serving. The label will probably say "diet," "calorie-reduced," "light" or "lite."

Make your own light iced tea by mixing leftover cold tea with lemon juice and a zero-calorie sweetener to suit your taste.

YOUR DINNER MENU	Large Meal (730 calories)	Total Carbs	NET CARBS	Small Meal (550 calories)	Total Carbs	NET CARBS
Cheeseburger with bun and toppings as shown	4 oz (120 g) burger	26	24	3 oz (90 g) burger	26	24
Potato Salad	¾ cup (175 mL)	14	12	½ cup (125 mL)	9	8
Celery sticks	2 stalks	4	2	2 stalks	4	2
Dill pickles	2 small or 1 medium	1	1	2 small or 1 medium	1	1
Light iced tea	12 oz (375 mL)	1	1	12 oz (375 mL)	1	1
Watermelon	3 small slices	21	20	1 small slice	7	7
	TOTAL CARBS	**67 g**	**60 g**	**TOTAL CARBS**	**48 g**	**43 g**
	Total carbs minus fiber = NET CARBS ↑			NET CARBS ↑		
	CARB CHOICES (1 carb choice = 15 g net carbs)		4	CARB CHOICES		3

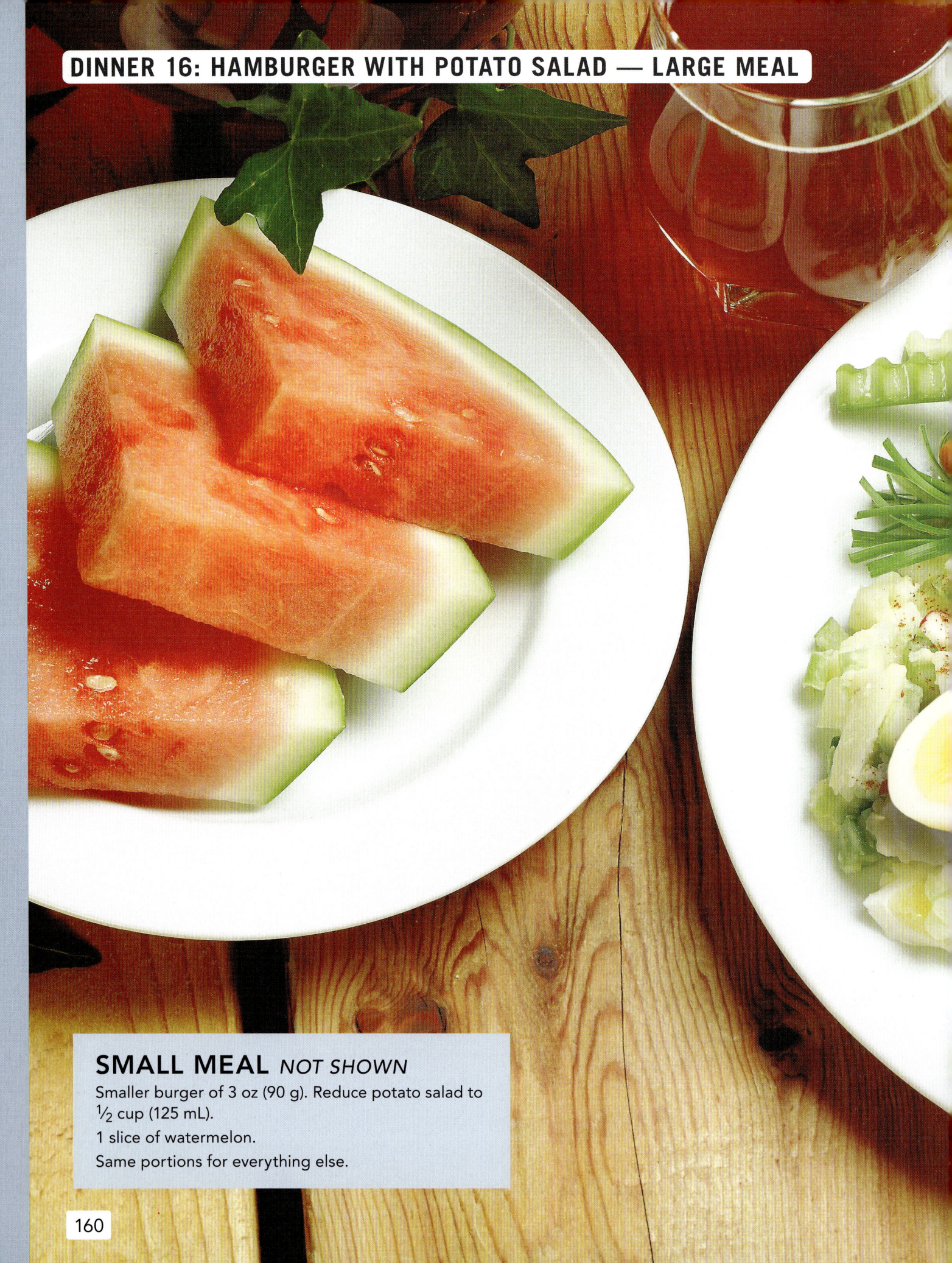

DINNER 16: HAMBURGER WITH POTATO SALAD — LARGE MEAL

SMALL MEAL *NOT SHOWN*

Smaller burger of 3 oz (90 g). Reduce potato salad to ½ cup (125 mL).

1 slice of watermelon.

Same portions for everything else.

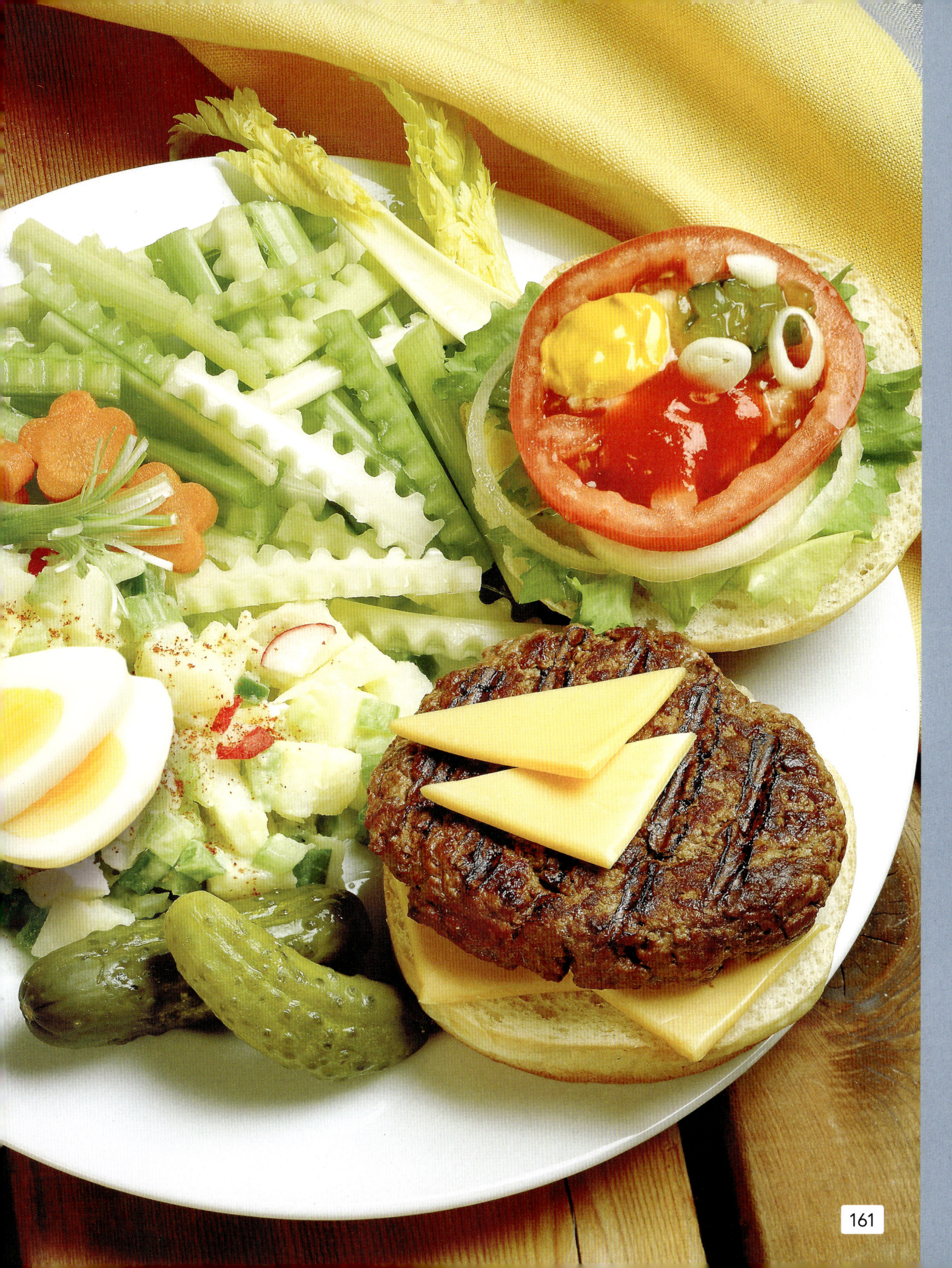

DINNER MEALS

DINNER 17

Roast Turkey Dinner

Roast turkey is a great meal to have at Thanksgiving – or any time of the year! The leftovers come in so handy for sandwiches, soups and other meals. There is a fabulous Turkey Noodle Soup recipe in our companion book, *Diabetes Essentials* (see the back cover of this book).

LOW-CARB SWAP

LARGE MEAL
Swap Mashed Potatoes:
¾ cup (175 mL)
27 g net carbs

→ For Mashed Potatoes with Cauliflower (see recipe on page 127):
¾ cup (175 mL)
10 g net carbs

→ For mashed cauliflower:
1 cup (250 mL)
5 g net carbs

SMALL MEAL
Swap Mashed Potatoes:
⅓ cup (75 mL)
12 g net carbs

→ For Mashed Potatoes with Cauliflower (see recipe on page 127)
⅓ cup (75 mL)
4 g net carbs

→ For mashed cauliflower:
1 cup (250 mL)
2 g net carbs

See Potato Swaps, page 275.

Cooking the Turkey

Place the thawed unstuffed turkey breast-side-up on a rack in a roasting pan. Cover with the lid. Bake in a 350°F (180°C) oven for about 15 minutes per pound. Baste with juices every hour, using a turkey baster or a large spoon. For the last 15 to 30 minutes, uncover the pan so the turkey skin can brown nicely. Turkey is cooked when a thermometer in the inner thigh measures 170°F (77°C); when you pierce it with a fork, the juices will run clear.

Make your gravy according to the directions on the package.

Stuffing is not included in this meal because of the additional carbs. But if you have a favorite recipe, you can replace the Mashed Potatoes carb-for-carb with stuffing. Or you can measure half potatoes and half stuffing.

Prepare the Light Jellied Vegetable Salad to accompany the meal. See page 143.

Enjoy cranberry sauce on the side.

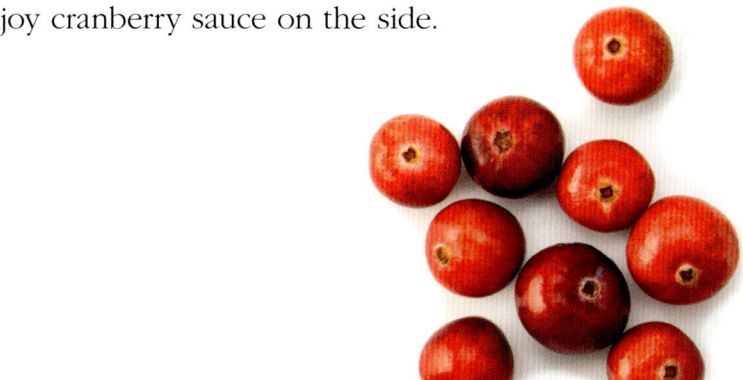

Mashed Potatoes

Use the recipe for Mashed Potatoes on page 126.

Check out the Low-Carb Swap for Mashed Potatoes on the side of this page.

Wine Spritzer

This is made with half wine and half diet ginger ale, diet 7-Up or soda water. If you prefer, you can use a dealcoholized wine.

DINNER MEALS

Crustless Pumpkin Pie

Makes 6 slices (9-inch/23 cm glass pie plate)

Preheat oven to 400°F (200°C)

14 oz (398 mL) can pure 100% pumpkin
⅓ cup (75 mL) sugar
½ tsp (2 mL) salt
½ tsp (2 mL) ground ginger
1 tsp (5 mL) ground cinnamon
¼ tsp (1 mL) ground nutmeg
¼ tsp (1 mL) ground cloves
2 large eggs, slightly beaten
13 oz (385 mL) can evaporated skim milk

PER SLICE	
Calories	147
Carbohydrate	25 g
Fiber	2 g
Net carbs	23 g
Protein	8 g
Fat, total	2 g
Fat, saturated	1 g
Cholesterol	65 mg
Sodium	259 mg

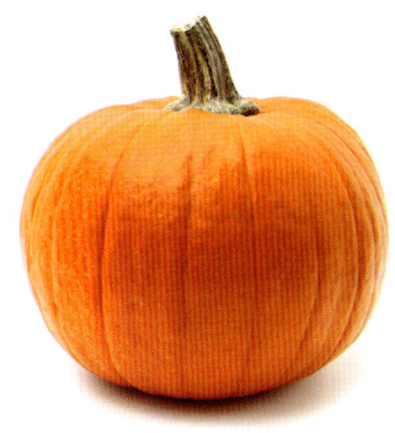

1. In a large bowl, mix pumpkin, sugar, salt and spices.
2. Stir in the 2 slightly beaten eggs and mix well.
3. Add the evaporated skim milk (shake can before opening) and stir until smooth.
4. Pour into a greased glass pie plate (not metal). Bake for about 40 minutes, or until knife inserted near the center of the pie comes out clean.

Serve cooled with whipped cream or Greek yogurt.

YOUR DINNER MENU	Large Meal (730 calories)	Total Carbs	NET CARBS	Small Meal (550 calories)	Total Carbs	NET CARBS
Turkey (white and dark meat)	5 oz (150 g)	0	0	4 oz (120 g)	0	0
Cranberry sauce	1 tbsp (15 mL)	7	7	½ tbsp (7 mL)	3	3
Mashed Potatoes (see page 126)	¾ cup (175 mL)	29	27	⅓ cup (75 mL)	13	12
Turkey gravy (from mix)	¼ cup (60 mL)	4	4	¼ cup (60 mL)	4	4
Peas and carrots	½ cup (125 mL)	8	6	½ cup (125 mL)	8	6
Asparagus	7 stalks	4	2	7 stalks	4	2
Dill pickle	1 medium	1	1	1 medium	1	1
Light Jellied Vegetable Salad (see page 143)	½ cup (125 mL)	4	3	½ cup (125 mL)	4	3
Wine spritzer (half wine, half diet soda)	6 oz (175 mL)	0	0	6 oz (175 mL)	0	0
Crustless Pumpkin Pie	1 slice	25	23	1 slice	25	23
Whipped cream	2 tbsp (30 mL)	1	1	2 tbsp (30 mL)	1	1
	TOTAL CARBS	**83 g**	**74 g**	**TOTAL CARBS**	**63 g**	**55 g**
	Total carbs minus fiber = NET CARBS ↑			NET CARBS ↑		
	CARB CHOICES (1 carb choice = 15 g net carbs)		5	CARB CHOICES		4

DINNER 17: ROAST TURKEY DINNER — LARGE MEAL

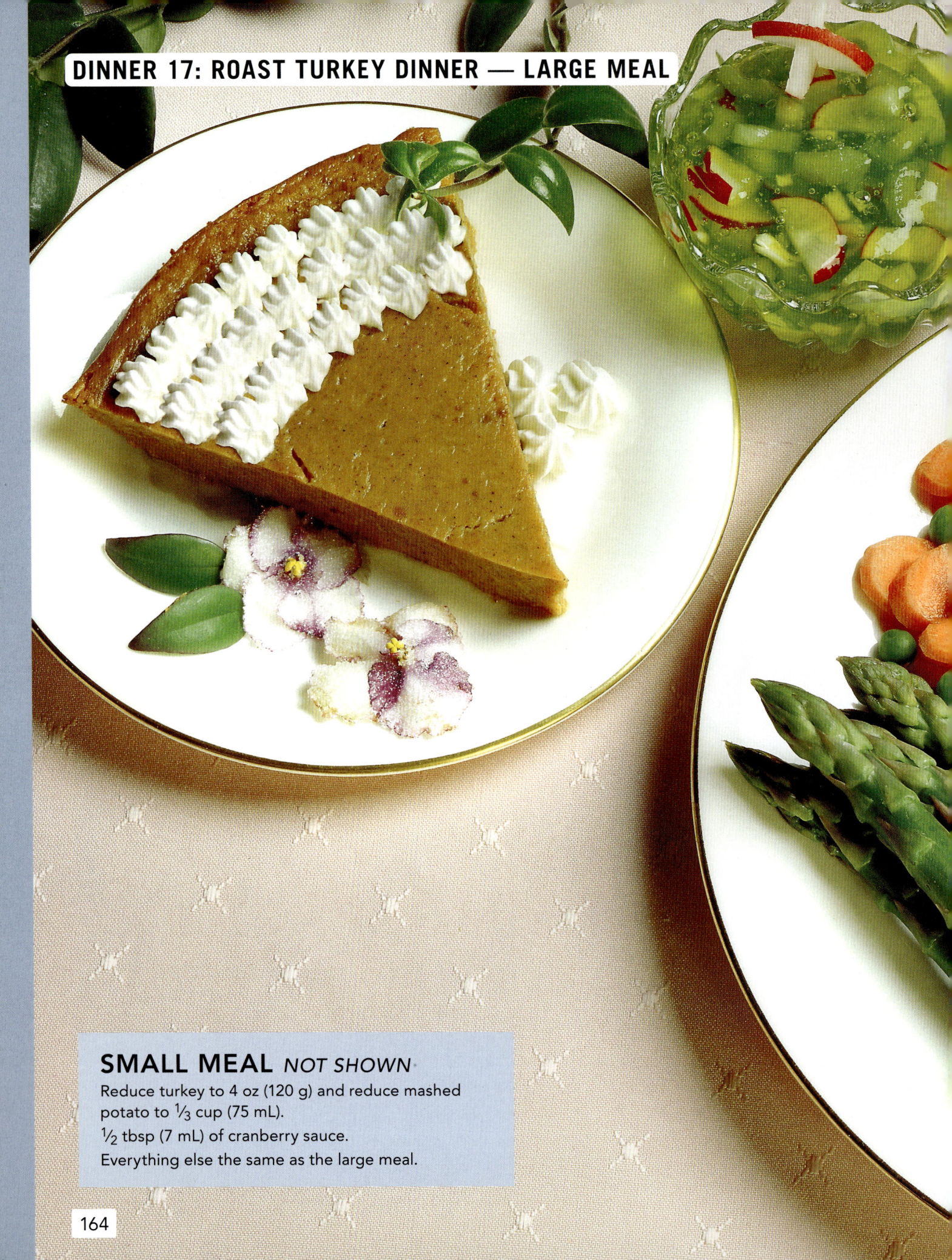

SMALL MEAL *NOT SHOWN*
Reduce turkey to 4 oz (120 g) and reduce mashed potato to 1/3 cup (75 mL).
1/2 tbsp (7 mL) of cranberry sauce.
Everything else the same as the large meal.

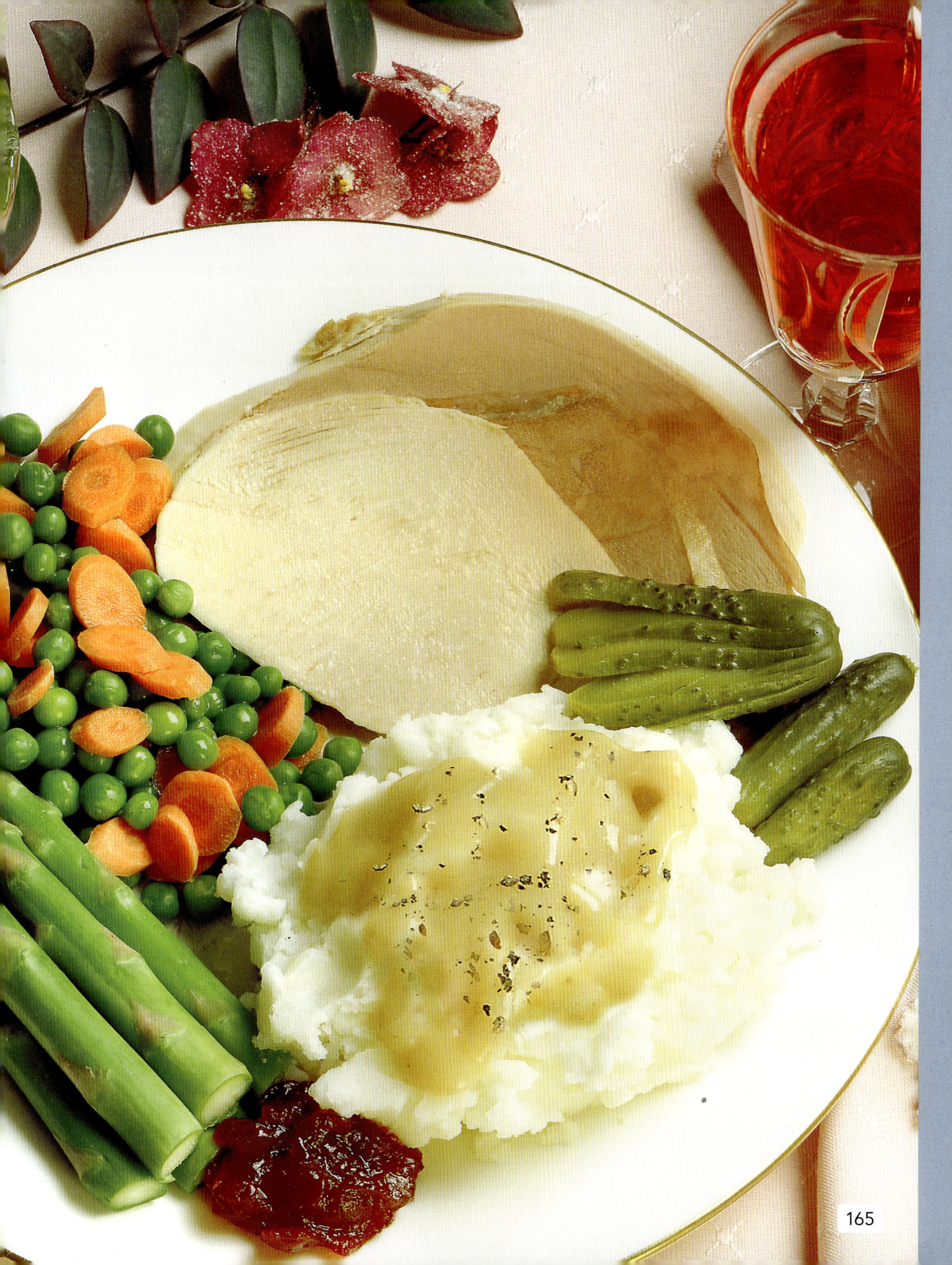

DINNER MEALS

DINNER 18

Mac & Cheese

Creamy Mac & Cheese

Makes 6 cups (4 large or 6 small servings)

Preheat oven to 350°F (180°C)

- 2 cups (500 mL)/8 oz dry elbow macaroni
- 3 tbsp (45 mL) flour
- ½ tsp (2 mL) salt
- ¼ tsp (1 mL) black pepper
- ¼ tsp (1 mL) ground cayenne pepper (or ground chili pepper)
- 3 tbsp (45 mL) butter
- 2½ cups (625 mL) 2% milk
- 2 cups (500 mL) Cheddar cheese, shredded (use sharp cheese if you have it)
- 4 slices bacon, chopped and cooked

PER 1 CUP (250 ML)	
Calories	399
Carbohydrate	38 g
Fiber	2 g
Net carbs	36 g
Protein	18 g
Fat, total	19 g
Fat, saturated	11 g
Cholesterol	58 mg
Sodium	526 mg

1. Cook pasta according to package directions (omitting salt). Drain well and place in an ungreased casserole dish about 8 by 8 inches (20 cm by 20 cm).
2. Mix flour, salt and pepper, and cayenne pepper in a small dish.
3. In a medium saucepan, melt butter over low to medium heat. Add flour mixture and whisk until foamy. Add milk and continue to whisk over medium to high heat, stirring constantly so milk doesn't burn. Once milk is steaming, cook for another 1 to 2 minutes, or until sauce thickens slightly.
4. Take off the heat and immediately add grated cheese; whisk until cheese melts. Stir cheese sauce and chopped bacon into pasta. The sauce is liquidy but will thicken with cooking.
5. Bake for 30 minutes. Let sit 15 minutes before serving.

Drink Water with Every Meal

Water helps your body digest the food you are eating. Also, importantly, sipping on water throughout your meal helps slow down how quickly you eat.

Lightly flavor the water with a slice of lemon or lime, if desired. This meal has a glass of carbonated water for a nice change.

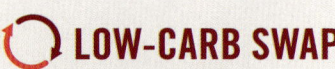

LOW-CARB SWAP

FOR CREAMY MAC & CHEESE RECIPE

Substitute whole-grain macaroni for regular macaroni.

LARGE MEAL

Swap Mac & Cheese: 2 cups (500 mL)
54 g net carbs

→ For 2 cups (500 mL) made with whole wheat macaroni: **51 g net carbs**

SMALL MEAL

Swap Mac & Cheese: 1¼ cups (300 mL)
36 g net carbs

→ For 1¼ cups (300 mL) made with whole wheat macaroni: **34 g net carbs**

See Pasta Swaps, page 275.

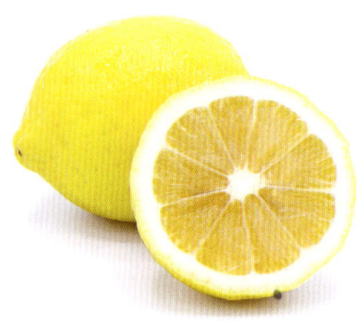

Quick-Fry Vegetables

Makes 4 cups (1 L) (2 servings)

1 to 2 tbsp (15 to 30 mL) olive or vegetable oil

2 to 3 garlic cloves, finely chopped

Sprinkle of crushed chili peppers

4 cups (1 L) of broccoli, cauliflower, onions, carrots and edamame beans, or whatever vegetables you have on hand, sliced or in chunks

PER 1½ CUP SERVING	
Calories	100
Carbohydrate	11 g
Fiber	4 g
Net carbs	7 g
Protein	5 g
Fat, total	6 g
Fat, saturated	0 g
Cholesterol	0 mg
Sodium	45 mg

1. Place oil in pan at medium heat.
2. Add garlic, crushed chili peppers and vegetables, and sauté until cooked.

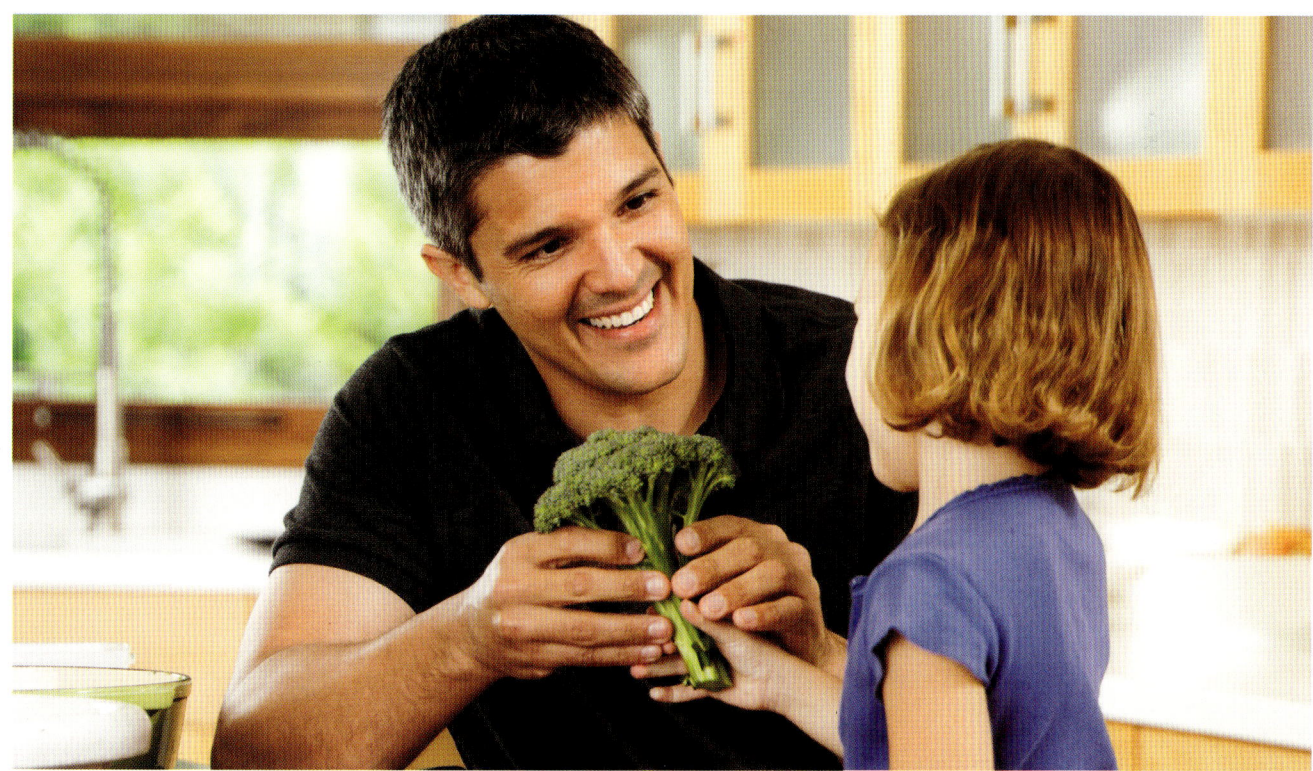

YOUR DINNER MENU	Large Meal (730 calories)	Total Carbs	NET CARBS	Small Meal (550 calories)	Total Carbs	NET CARBS
Creamy Mac & Cheese	1½ cups (375 mL): ¼ of the recipe	57	54	1 cup (250 mL): ⅙ of the recipe	38	36
Quick-Fry Vegetables	1½ cups (375 mL)	11	7	1½ cups (375 mL)	11	7
Water, plain or carbonated with lemon	12 oz	0	0	12 oz	0	0
	TOTAL CARBS	68 g	61 g	TOTAL CARBS	49 g	43 g
	Total carbs minus fiber = NET CARBS ↑			NET CARBS ↑		
	CARB CHOICES (1 carb choice = 15 g net carbs)		4	CARB CHOICES		3

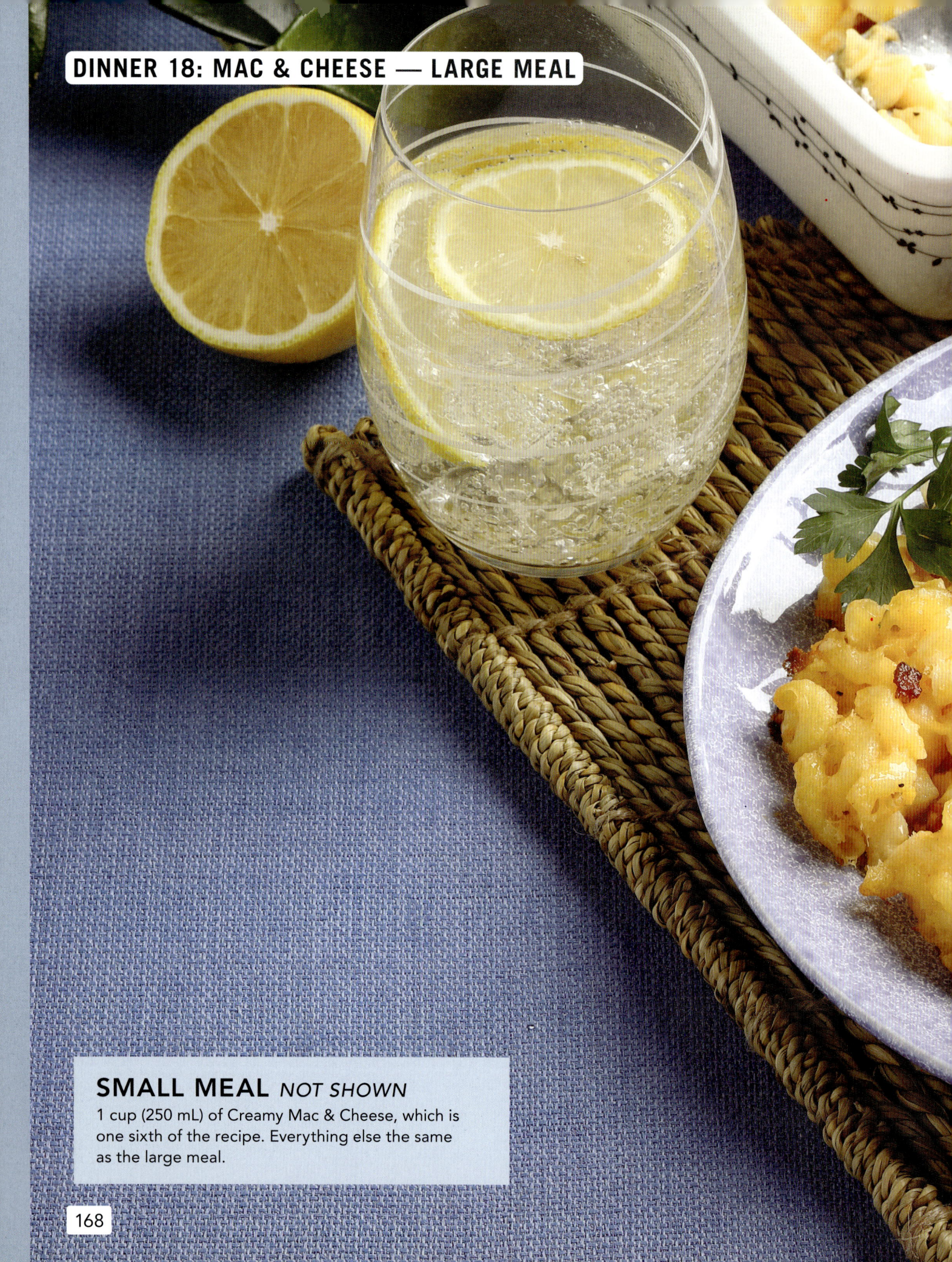

DINNER 18: MAC & CHEESE — LARGE MEAL

SMALL MEAL *NOT SHOWN*
1 cup (250 mL) of Creamy Mac & Cheese, which is one sixth of the recipe. Everything else the same as the large meal.

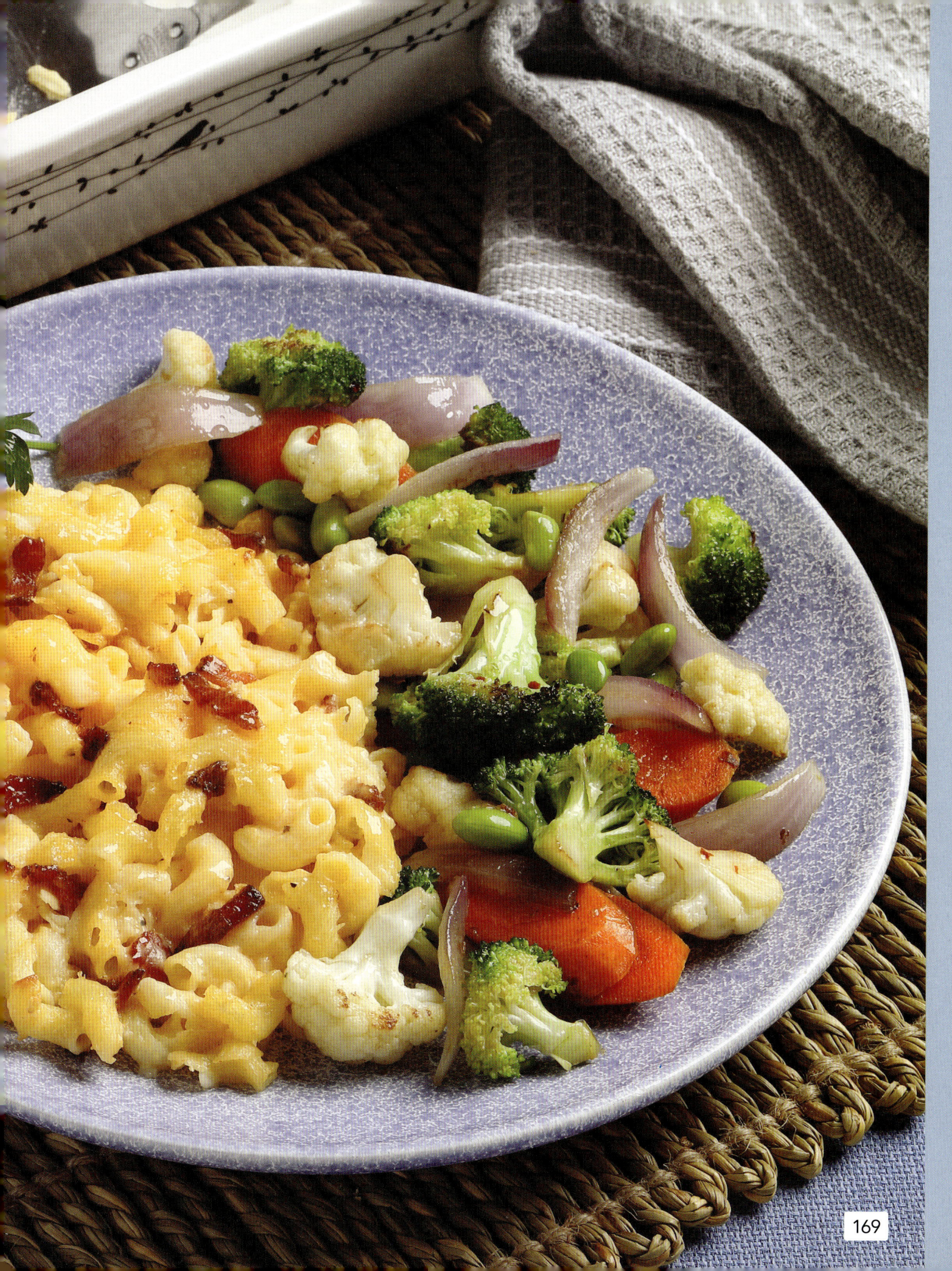

DINNER MEALS

DINNER 19

Pork Chop & Applesauce

Barbecue, broil or fry pork chops. Pork goes nicely with boiled potatoes sprinkled with fresh parsley.

A small dish of applesauce is served with the pork chop. Instead of applesauce, you could slice an apple and onion and cook them with the pork.

The German Bean Salad is not sweet at all; it has a tangy bite. This salad will keep in the fridge for a week.

German Bean Salad

Makes 4 cups (1 L)

- 4 cups (1 L) fresh yellow or green beans, cooked, or two 14 oz (398 mL) cans of cut beans (drained and rinsed)
- ½ medium onion, thinly sliced
- 1 tbsp (15 mL) vegetable or olive oil
- 2 tbsp (30 mL) vinegar or flavored vinaigrette
- ¼ tsp (1 mL) salt (no salt if using canned beans)

PER 1 CUP (250 ML)	
Calories	69
Carbohydrate	9 g
Fiber	3 g
Net carbs	6 g
Protein	2 g
Fat, total	4 g
Fat, saturated	0 g
Cholesterol	0 mg
Sodium	149 mg

1. Cut the beans into 1-inch (2.5 cm) pieces and steam to lightly cook. Cool in cold water, drain and place in a salad bowl. If you are using canned beans, drain them and place them in the bowl.
2. Mix with the other ingredients.
3. Leave to stand for 30 minutes. Serve.

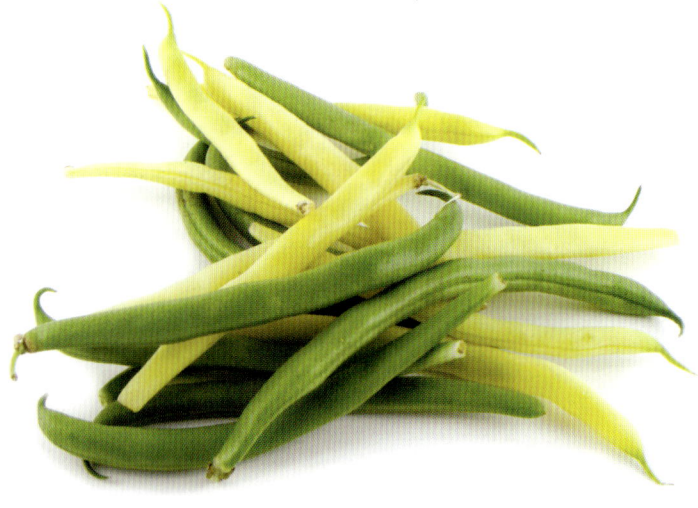

DINNER MEALS

This dessert is an old-fashioned favorite that uses minute tapioca but is adapted to be lower in carbs. Tapioca is the flour from the root of a tropical plant called casava.

Tapioca Pudding

Makes 4 servings

3 tbsp (45 mL) minute tapioca

3 tbsp (45 mL) sugar

3 tbsp (45 mL) zero-calorie sweetener that measures cup-for-cup like sugar (see page 29)

Dash of salt

3 cups (750 mL) milk

1 large egg

1 tsp (5 mL) vanilla extract

PER SERVING	
Calories	96
Carbohydrate	17 g
Fiber	0 g
Net carbs	17 g
Protein	5 g
Fat, total	1 g
Fat, saturated	0 g
Cholesterol	33 mg
Sodium	93 mg

🔄 LOW-CARB SWAP

LARGE OR SMALL MEAL

Swap Tapioca Pudding: 1 serving

17 g net carbs

→ For instead of 3 cups (750 mL) of milk, make the recipe with 1½ cups (375 mL) soy beverage and 1½ cups (375 mL) milk: **14 g net carbs**

Almond beverage does not swap well; it doesn't have the protein needed to set the pudding.

1. Place tapioca, sugar, zero-calorie sweetener, salt, milk and egg in a small, heavy pot. Let stand for 5 minutes, then stir with a whisk.
2. Cook this mixture at medium heat until it comes to a boil. Whisk it continuously. It will take about 15 minutes to come to a boil: keep whisking!
3. Once it boils, remove from heat. Add vanilla.
4. Let it cool for 20 minutes, whisking twice. The pudding will thicken as it cools.
5. Stir pudding and spoon into six dessert dishes.
6. Eat it warm or refrigerate until cool.

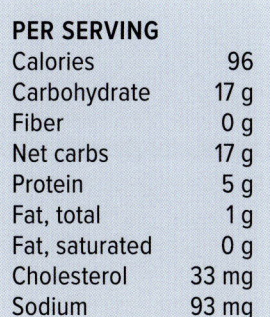

YOUR DINNER MENU	Large Meal (730 calories)	Total Carbs	NET CARBS	Small Meal (550 calories)	Total Carbs	NET CARBS
Pork chop	1 medium (5 oz/150 g, cooked)	0	0	1 medium (5 oz/150 g, cooked)	0	0
Applesauce	¼ cup (60 mL)	7	6	2 tbsp (30 mL)	4	3
Boiled potatoes with parsley	7 mini	33	31	4 mini	19	18
Margarine or butter	2 tsp (10 mL)	0	0	—	9	6
German Bean Salad	1 cup (250 mL)	9	6	1 cup (250 mL)	—	—
Tapioca Pudding	1 serving	17	17	1 serving	17	17
Coffee	1 cup (250 mL)	1	1	1 cup (250 mL)	1	1
	TOTAL CARBS	**67 g**	**61 g**	**TOTAL CARBS**	**50 g**	**45 g**
	Total carbs minus fiber = NET CARBS ↑			NET CARBS ↑		
	CARB CHOICES (1 carb choice = 15 g net carbs)		4	CARB CHOICES		3

DINNER 19: PORK CHOP & APPLESAUCE — LARGE MEAL

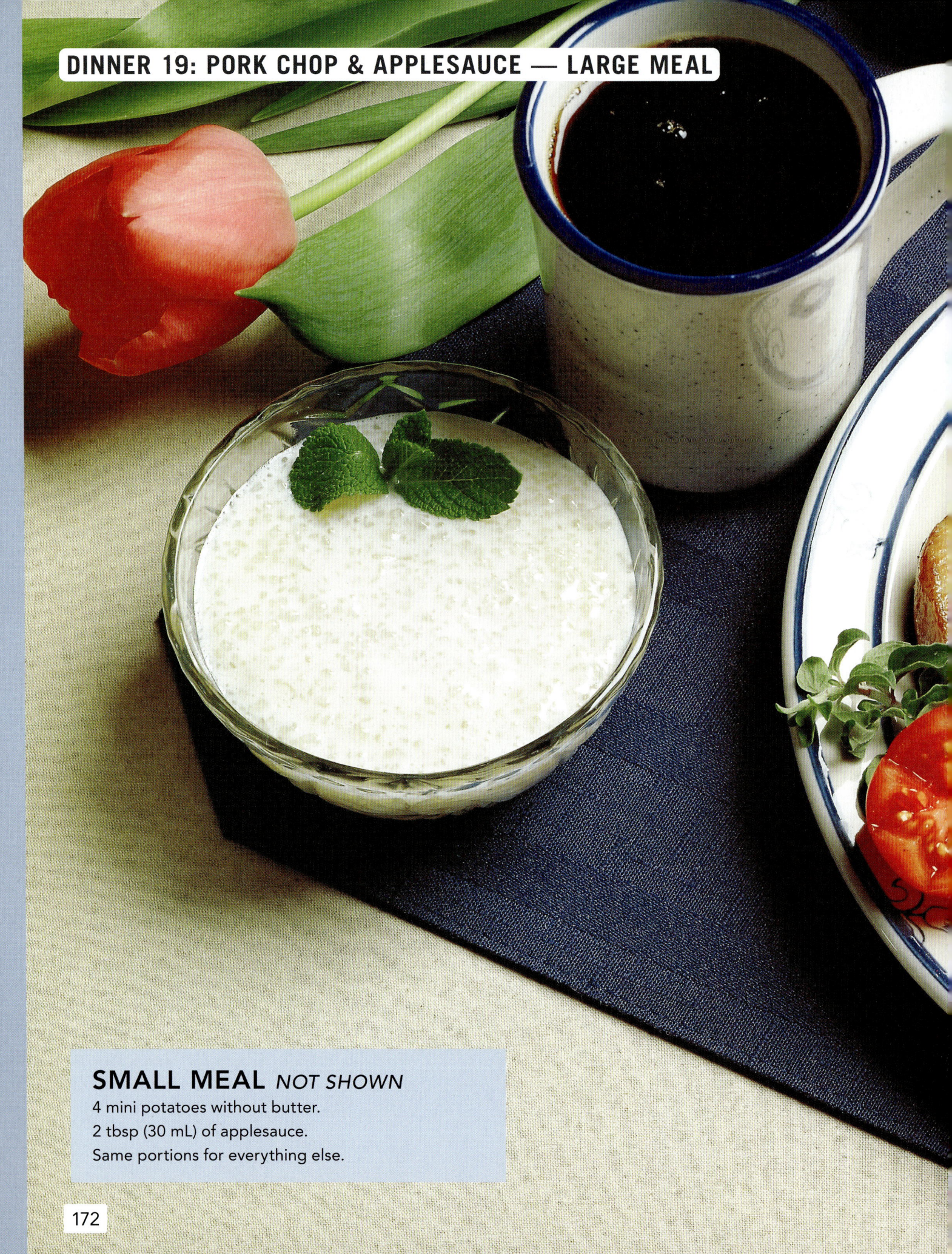

SMALL MEAL *NOT SHOWN*
4 mini potatoes without butter.
2 tbsp (30 mL) of applesauce.
Same portions for everything else.

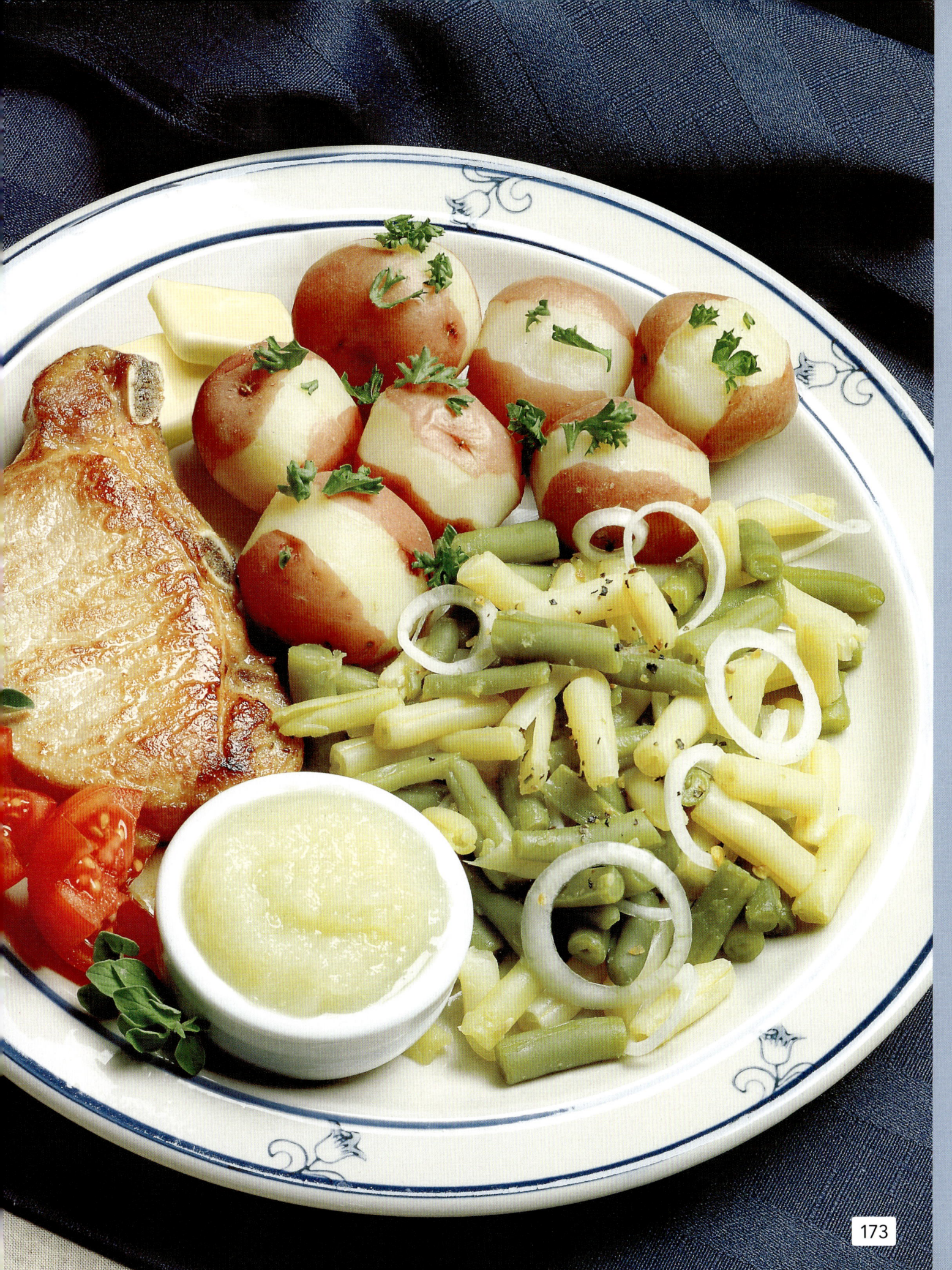

DINNER MEALS

DINNER 20

Tacos

Tacos are crunchy messes but a fun meal for kids and adults alike. Of course, you can switch the crunchy taco shells with soft 6-inch (15 cm) flour or corn tortillas.

Bean and Meat Filling

Makes 5 cups (1.25 L) (enough for 20 tacos)

1 lb (500 g) lean ground beef

SALT-FREE TACO SEASONING MIX

1 tsp (5 mL) each oregano, paprika, garlic powder and onion powder

2 tsp (10 mL) each chili powder and cumin

½ tsp (2 mL) black pepper

1 cup (250 mL) water

28 oz (796 mL) can kidney beans or white beans, drained and rinsed

1. In a medium pot, brown ground beef. Drain off the fat.
2. Stir in the Salt-free Taco Seasoning Mix and cook for a minute or two.
3. Add the water and beans. Bring to a boil, then reduce heat to medium and simmer for 10 minutes.

PER ¼ CUP (60 ML)	
Calories	74
Carbohydrate	7 g
Fiber	2 g
Net carbs	5 g
Protein	7 g
Fat, total	2 g
Fat, saturated	1 g
Cholesterol	12 mg
Sodium	84 mg

Tacos

For one taco, add these amounts of filling, cheese and vegetables:

¼ cup (60 mL) Bean and Meat Filling

2 tbsp (30 mL) cheese, shredded

Lots of raw vegetables, any kind

1. Cook tacos according to package directions.
2. Add the Bean and Meat Filling, cheese and vegetables.

PER TACO	
Calories	185
Carbohydrate	14 g
Fiber	3 g
Net carbs	11 g
Protein	12 g
Fat, total	10 g
Fat, saturated	4 g
Cholesterol	25 mg
Sodium	214 mg

Vegetable Dip

Makes 1½ cups (375 mL)

1½ cups (375 mL) Greek yogurt, 5%, plain

2 tbsp (30 mL) dried onion soup mix

1. Blend together.

PER 2 TBSP (30 ML)	
Calories	32
Carbohydrate	2 g
Fiber	0 g
Net carbs	2 g
Protein	3 g
Fat, total	2 g
Fat, saturated	1 g
Cholesterol	5 mg
Sodium	138 mg

⊘ LOW-CARB SWAP

FOR BEAN & MEAT TACOS

Swap with **Taco Salad**. Fill a large bowl with greens and salad vegetables and top with the ingredients listed below. Option: add a few slices of avocado.

LARGE MEAL

Swap 3 Bean & Meat Tacos:

34 g net carbs

→ For Taco Salad with ¾ cup (175 mL) Bean and Meat Filling, ¼ cup (60 mL) shredded cheese, 2 tbsp (30 mL) Vegetable Dip and 1 taco shell:

24 g net carbs

SMALL MEAL

Swap 2 Bean & Meat Tacos:

22 g net carbs

→ For Taco Salad with ½ cup (125 mL) Bean and Meat Filling, ¼ cup (60 mL) shredded cheese, 2 tbsp (30 mL) Vegetable Dip and 1 taco shell:

19 g net carbs

This dip is great for the fresh vegetables on the side or a topping on the Taco Salad.

DINNER MEALS

Dessert

The dessert with this meal is a 10-inch (25 cm) angel food cake cut in ten pieces, served with Greek yogurt or whipped topping, and fresh strawberries. Make the angel food cake from a mix or buy one from a bakery.

⬤ LOW-CARB SWAP RECIPE: Rice Cake Dessert

Swap angel food cake, strawberries and topping:
23 g net carbs
→ For Rice Cake Dessert:
12 g net carbs

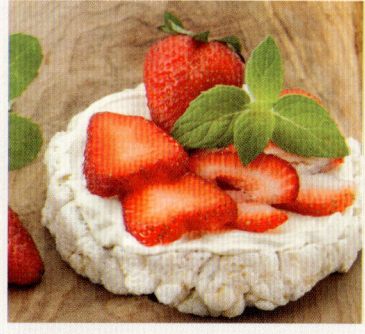

Rice Cake Dessert made from a rice cake and cream cheese is a fast and easy swap; it's also good as a snack. I also recommend you try making it with mascarpone cheese; it's more expensive but wonderfully delicious. If you don't have rice cakes on hand, you can use soda crackers.

1 DESSERT	
Calories	118
Total carbs	13 g
Net carbs	12 g

- 1 original (plain) rice cake or 4 saltine soda crackers
- 2 tbsp (30 mL) light cream cheese or mascarpone cheese
- 1 tsp (5 mL) icing sugar
- 1 tbsp (15 mL) fruit for topping (strawberry, banana, blueberries or pomegranate seeds)

1. In a small bowl, place cream cheese and icing sugar and blend with a spoon.
2. Spread cheese mixture on the rice cake and top with fruit.

YOUR DINNER MENU	Large Meal (730 calories)	Total Carbs	NET CARBS	Small Meal (550 calories)	Total Carbs	NET CARBS
Bean & Meat Tacos	3	42	34	2	28	22
Fresh vegetables on the side	2 cups (500 mL)	5	4	2 cups (500 mL)	5	4
Vegetable Dip	2 tbsp (30 mL)	2	1	2 tbsp (30 mL)	2	1
Angel food cake	1-inch (2.5 cm) piece of cake	20	19	1-inch (2.5 cm) piece of cake	20	19
Strawberries	½ cup (125 mL)	5	3	½ cup (125 mL)	5	3
Greek yogurt (5%) or non-dairy whipped topping	2 tbsp (30 mL)	1	1	2 tbsp (30 mL)	1	1
	TOTAL CARBS	75 g	62 g	TOTAL CARBS	61 g	50 g
	Total carbs minus fiber = NET CARBS ↑			NET CARBS ↑		
	CARB CHOICES (1 carb choice = 15 g net carbs)		4	CARB CHOICES		3

DINNER 20: TACOS — LARGE MEAL

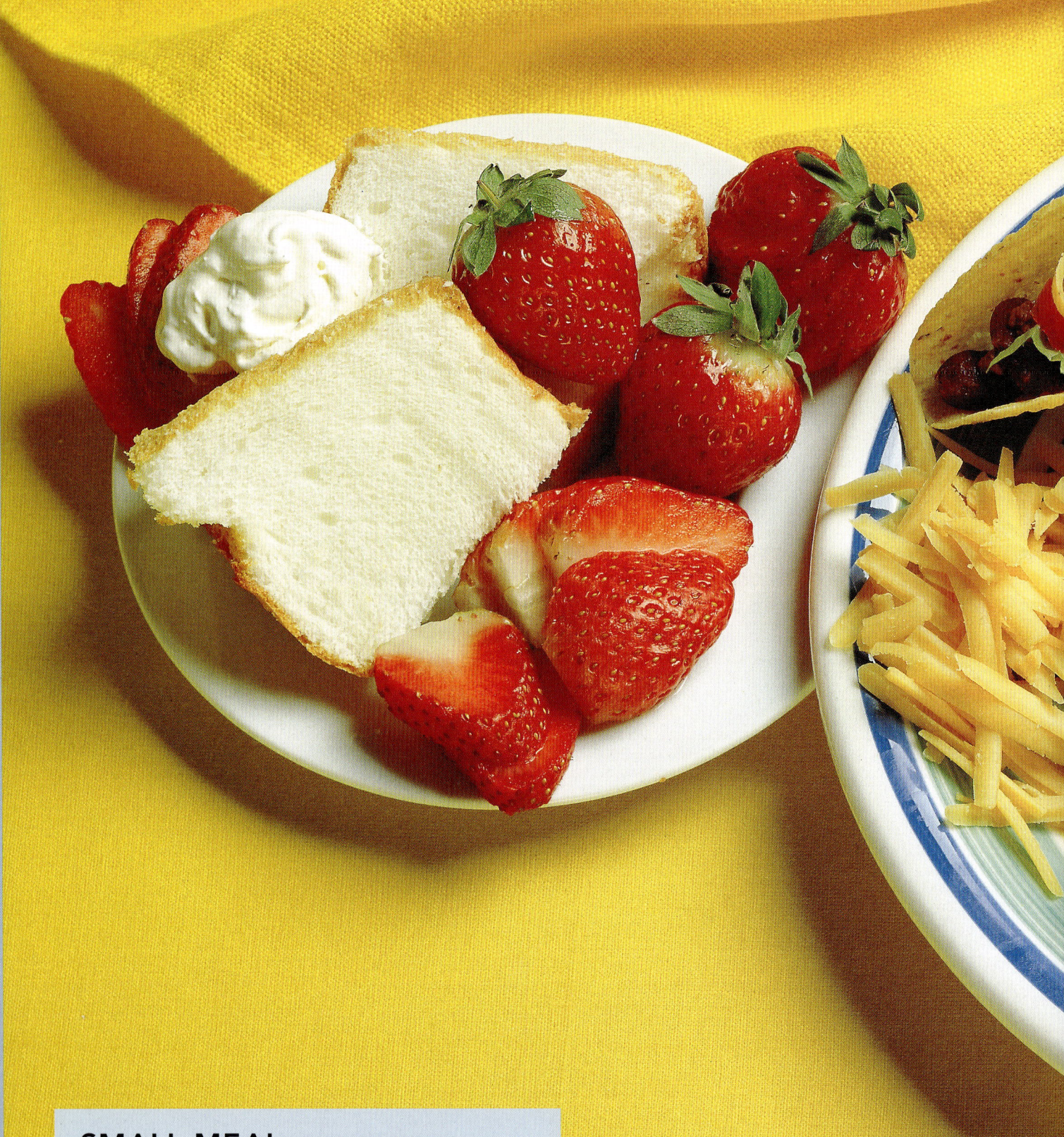

SMALL MEAL *NOT SHOWN*
2 filled tacos.
Other portions are the same as the large meal.

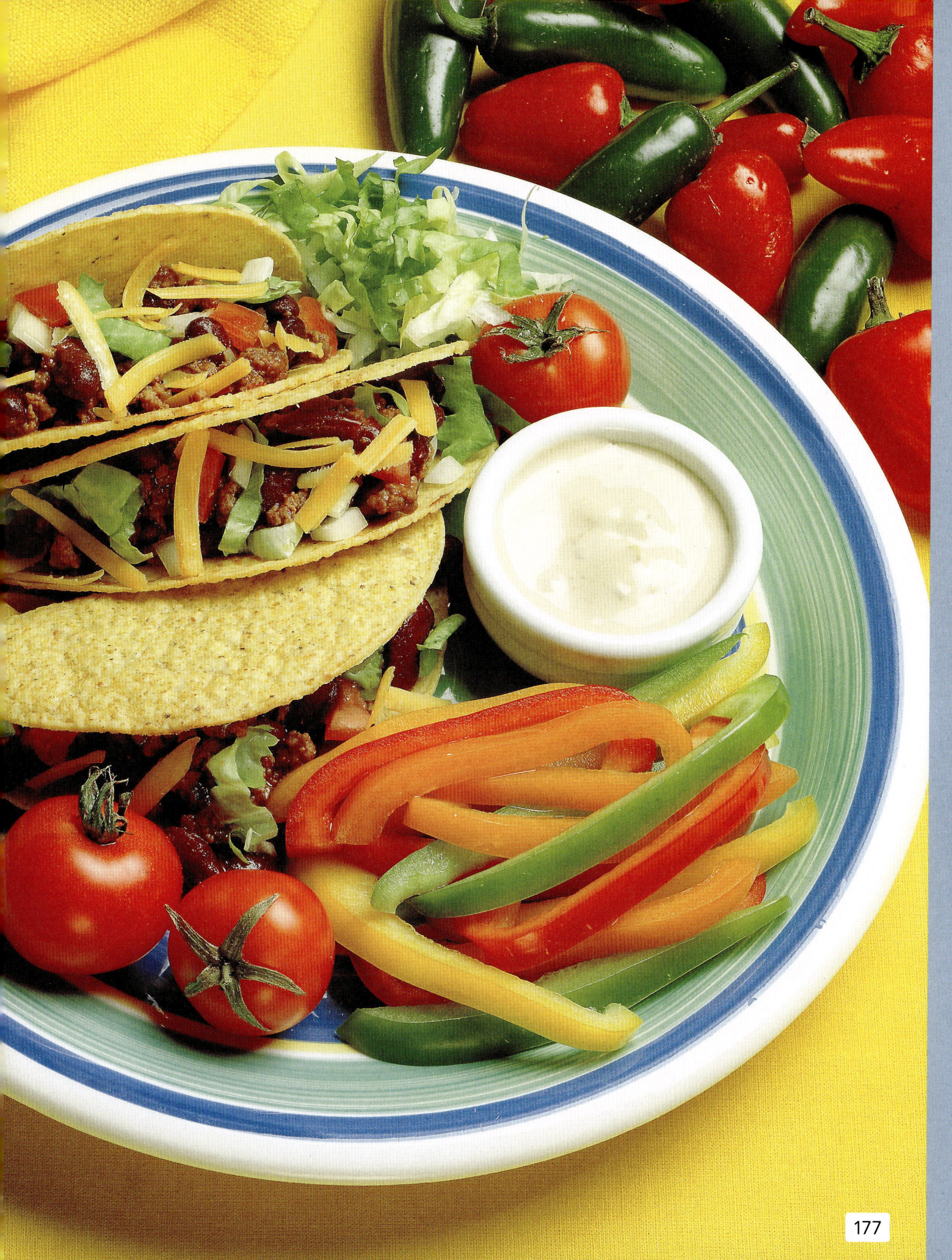

Dinner 21

DINNER MEALS

Caribbean Chicken Roti

Roti are Indian unleavened flatbread that are a staple food throughout the Caribbean. This meal is made with the popular dhalpuri roti shell that has a middle layer of seasoned yellow split pea meal or chickpea meal.

You can buy dhalpuri roti at an Indian or Caribbean store or restaurant or order them online.

For this meal, the flatbread is served with curry stew rolled up inside; the meal itself is also called a roti.

This Chicken Curry Stew is low-carb, made with chicken and cauliflower. It is best made a day ahead so the flavors blend through.

◯ LOW-CARB SWAP

FOR DHALPURI ROTI SHELL

Swap one 13-inch (90–100 g) roti shell:
45 g net carbs

→ For soft flour tortilla shell: 10 inch/25 cm (65 g):
32 g net carbs

See Bread Swaps, page 274.

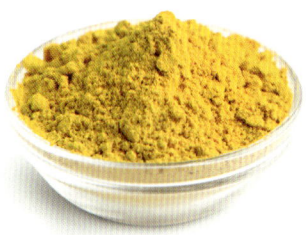

Chicken Curry Stew

Makes 7 cups (1.75 L)

- 2 tbsp (30 mL) canola oil
- 1 medium onion, chopped
- 3 cloves of garlic, minced or finely chopped
- 1 tbsp (15 mL) curry powder
- 1 tbsp (15 mL) garam masala
- 1 tsp (5 mL) cumin
- ½ tsp (2 mL) salt
- ¼ tsp (1 mL) black pepper
- Dash of hot pepper sauce
- ¾ cups (175 mL) water
- 1 package chicken bouillon, reduced salt
- 1½ lbs (680 g) boneless skinless chicken thighs or breasts, cut in 1-inch (2.5 cm) pieces
- 2 cups (500 mL) raw cauliflower (half a large head), roughly chopped

PER 1 CUP (250 ML)	
Calories	220
Carbohydrate	6 g
Fiber	2 g
Net carbs	4 g
Protein	25 g
Fat, total	12 g
Fat, saturated	3 g
Cholesterol	119 g
Sodium	393 g

1. In a large, heavy pot, heat oil over medium heat. Add onion and fry for 2 to 3 minutes or until soft. Add garlic, spices, salt and pepper, and hot sauce. Continue to stir for another minute.

2. Add water, bouillon and chicken, and bring to a boil. Let simmer covered for 5 minutes, then add cauliflower. Continue cooking, covered, until chicken is cooked and the sauce is thickened, about 20 to 30 minutes. Stir occasionally. Cool and put in the fridge overnight.

DINNER MEALS

How to fold the roti

Place a serving of Chicken Curry Stew in the middle of each dhalpuri roti shell. Fold one side over the mixture, then the other. Gently fold ends toward the center to make a neat package. Turn it over on the plate so the folds are underneath. Microwave on high for 3 minutes or until the stew is hot.

Tropical Green Salad

Makes 4 servings

4 to 6 cups (1 to 1.5 L) torn salad greens, such as Boston lettuce

¾ cup (175 mL) fresh orange sections and pineapple chunks

3 tbsp (45 mL) dried unsweetened medium coconut, plain or toasted

Squeeze of fresh lime

PER SERVING	
Calories	58
Carbohydrate	6
Fiber	2
Net carbs	4
Protein	1
Fat, total	3
Fat, saturated	3
Cholesterol	0
Sodium	5

1. In a large bowl, combine salad greens, orange and pineapple, and coconut.
2. Add the lime juice.

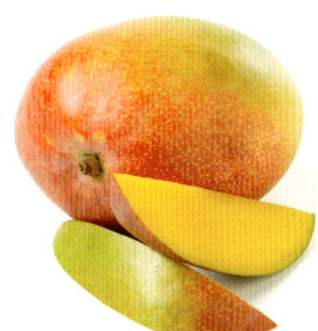

Sliced mango or papaya can be substituted for the pineapple and orange in the Tropical Green Salad.

YOUR DINNER MENU	Large Meal (730 calories)	Total Carbs	NET CARBS	Small Meal (550 calories)	Total Carbs	NET CARBS
Caribbean Chicken Roti						
• Chicken Curry Stew	1¾ cups (425 mL)	10	6	1¼ cups (310 mL)	7	5
• Dhalpuri roti shell	1 13-in (33 cm) / 90–100 g shell	48	45	two thirds of a 13-in (33 cm) / 90–100 g shell	32	30
Tropical Green Salad	1 serving	6	5	1 serving	6	5
Light coleslaw dressing	1 tbsp (15 mL)	3	3	1 tbsp (15 mL)	3	3
	TOTAL CARBS	**67 g**	**59 g**	**TOTAL CARBS**	**48 g**	**43 g**
	Total carbs minus fiber = NET CARBS ↑			NET CARBS ↑		
	CARB CHOICES (1 carb choice = 15 g net carbs)		4	CARB CHOICES		3

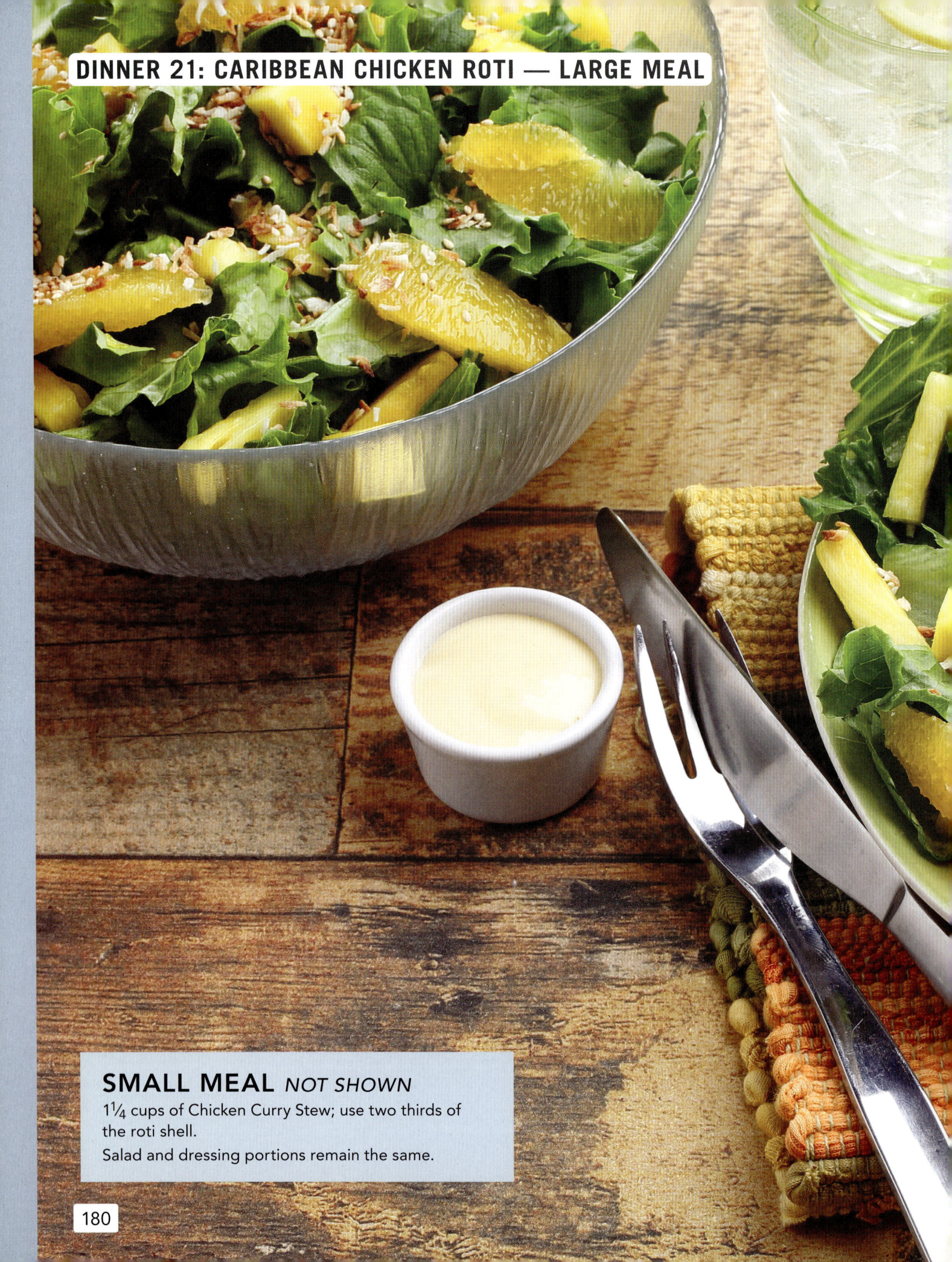

DINNER 21: CARIBBEAN CHICKEN ROTI — LARGE MEAL

SMALL MEAL *NOT SHOWN*

1¼ cups of Chicken Curry Stew; use two thirds of the roti shell.

Salad and dressing portions remain the same.

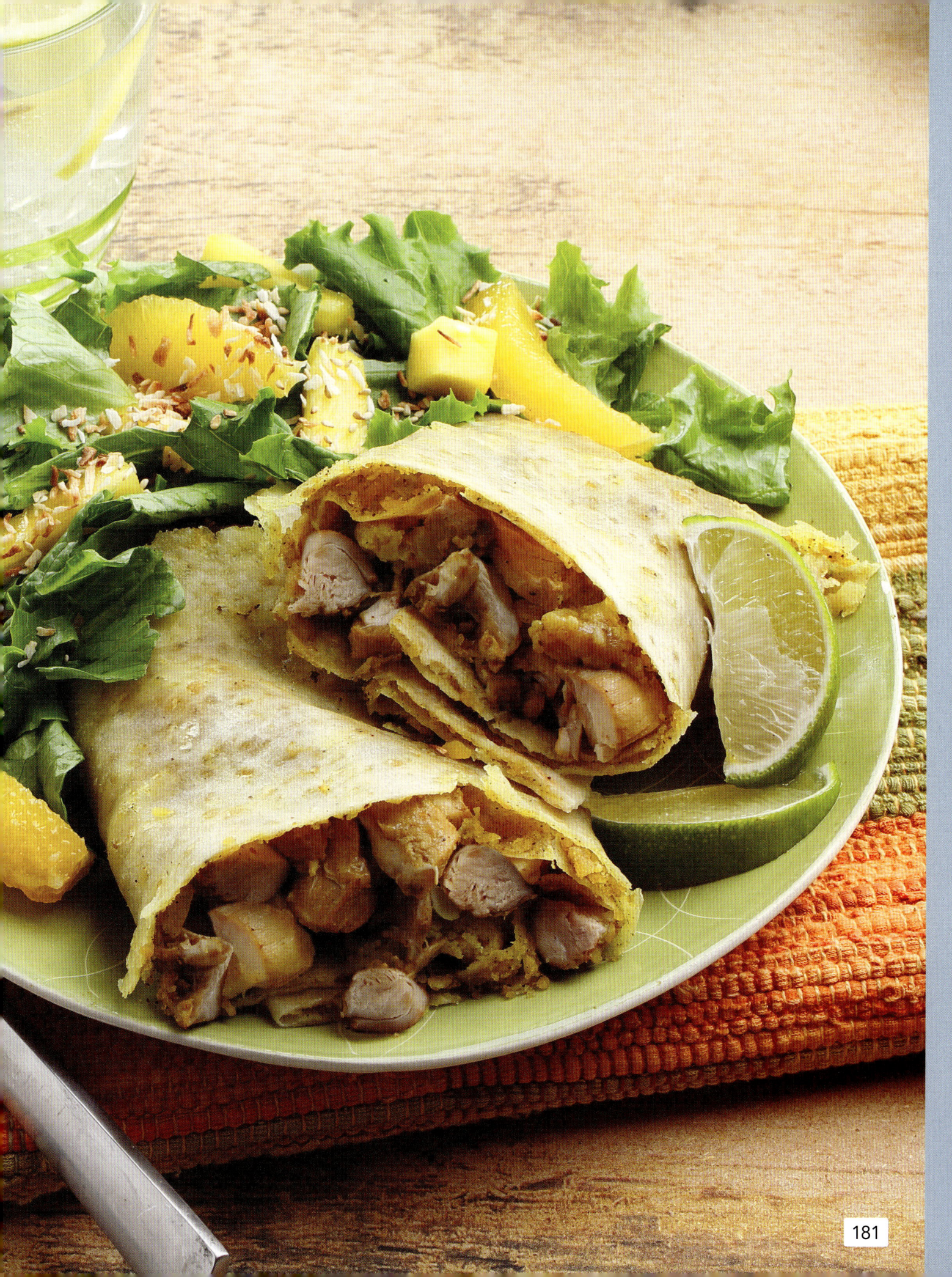

DINNER MEALS

DINNER 22

Liver & Onions

So it's all ready at one time, here are the steps to make this Liver & Onions meal.

- First, cook the rice. Keep the lid on the pot and set aside to keep warm.
- If you prefer boiled mini potatoes instead of rice: 6 for the large meal or 3 for the small meal.
- Fry the bacon and keep it warm in the oven at 200°C (95°C).
- Save a few spoonfuls of bacon fat for when you make the Liver & Onions.
- Prepare the gravy from the packaged mix. The gravy can be heated quickly in the microwave just before serving.
- Dish out the canned tomatoes. Peel and slice the carrots or use baby carrots, as shown in the photo. Put the carrots on to cook when you begin to cook the liver.

HEALTH TIP

Organ meats such as liver, kidneys and heart are rich in iron.

They are also high in cholesterol, so choose no more than once a month if your blood cholesterol level is high.

RECIPE TIP

Calf liver is more expensive and more tender and should not be pounded. Chicken liver is equally tender: 6 chicken livers equal one serving of beef liver.

Liver & Onions

Makes 3 servings

- 1 lb (500 g) beef liver, cut in pieces, lightly pounded only if pieces are thick
- 2–3 tbsp (30–45 mL) skim or 2% milk
- 2–3 tbsp (30–45 mL) flour
- Salt and pepper to taste
- 3 small onions, thinly sliced
- 2 tbsp (30 mL) butter or bacon fat

PER SMALL SERVING	
Calories	317
Carbohydrate	10 g
Fiber	1 g
Net carbs	9 g
Protein	32 g
Fat, total	14 g
Fat, saturated	7 g
Cholesterol	458 mg
Sodium	153 mg

1. Place milk in one bowl and flour, salt and pepper in another.
2. Dip liver pieces one by one first into the milk, then into the flour, salt and pepper. Place coated liver pieces on a larger platter, not overlapping. Set aside.
3. In a nonstick or cast iron pan, over low heat, cook the onion slices in butter until soft and then set aside in a bowl.
4. Increase heat to medium-high and pan fry the liver pieces. Liver cooks quickly and may need only 1 or 2 minutes on each side. The secret to tender liver is not to overcook it. Add extra fat for frying as needed.

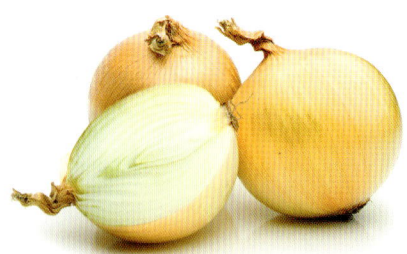

DINNER MEALS

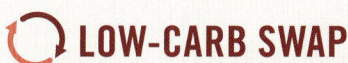
LOW-CARB SWAP

LARGE MEAL
Swap cooked white rice:
⅔ cup (150 mL)
28 g net carbs
→ For riced cauliflower:
 ⅔ cup (150 mL)
 2 g net carbs

SMALL MEAL
Swap cooked white rice:
⅓ cup (75 mL)
14 g net carbs
→ For riced cauliflower:
 ⅓ cup (75 mL)
 1 g net carbs

See Rice Swaps, page 276.

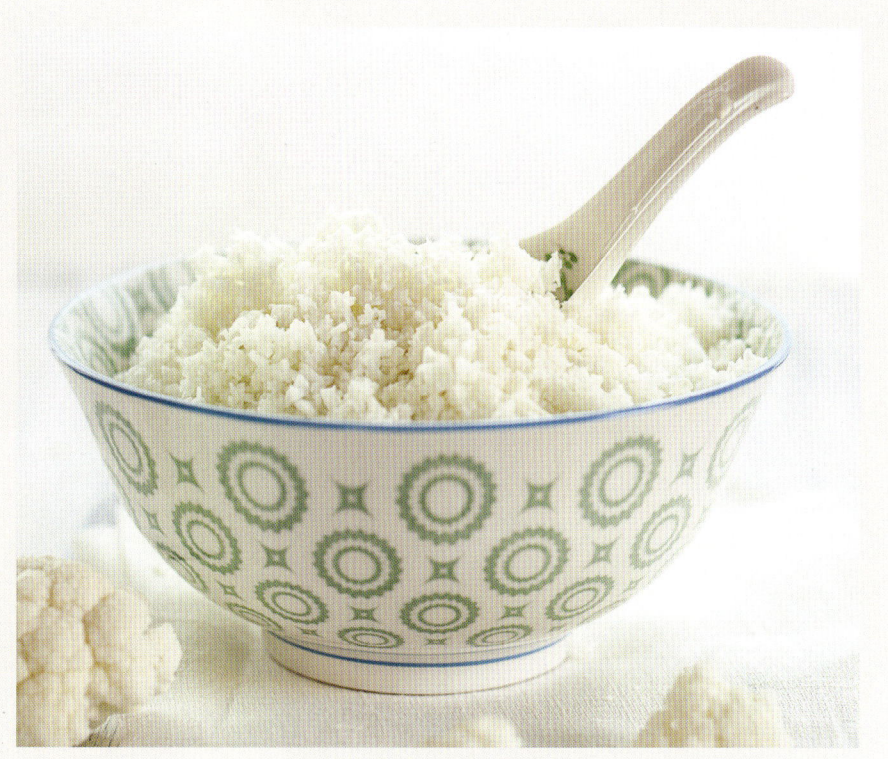

For dessert, enjoy a combo of fresh berries.

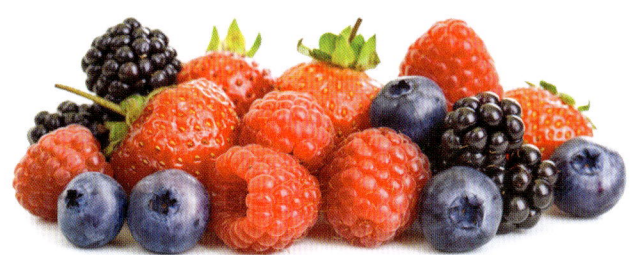

YOUR DINNER MENU	Large Meal (730 calories)	Total Carbs	NET CARBS	Small Meal (550 calories)	Total Carbs	NET CARBS
Liver & Onions	1 serving	10	9	1 serving	10	9
Rice, long-grain, converted	⅔ cup (150 mL)	29	28	⅓ cup (75 mL)	15	14
Gravy mix, regular or 25% less salt	¼ cup (60 mL)	4	4	¼ cup (60 mL)	4	4
Bacon, crisp strips	3 strips	0	0	1½ strips	0	0
Carrots	½ cup (125 mL)	8	6	½ cup (125 mL)	8	6
Canned tomatoes	1 cup (250 mL)	10	8	1 cup (250 mL)	10	8
Fresh berry combo	½ cup (125 mL)	9	7	½ cup (125 mL)	9	7
	TOTAL CARBS	**70 g**	**62 g**	**TOTAL CARBS**	**56 g**	**48 g**
	Total carbs minus fiber = NET CARBS ↑			NET CARBS ↑		
	CARB CHOICES (1 carb choice = 15 g net carbs)		4	CARB CHOICES		3

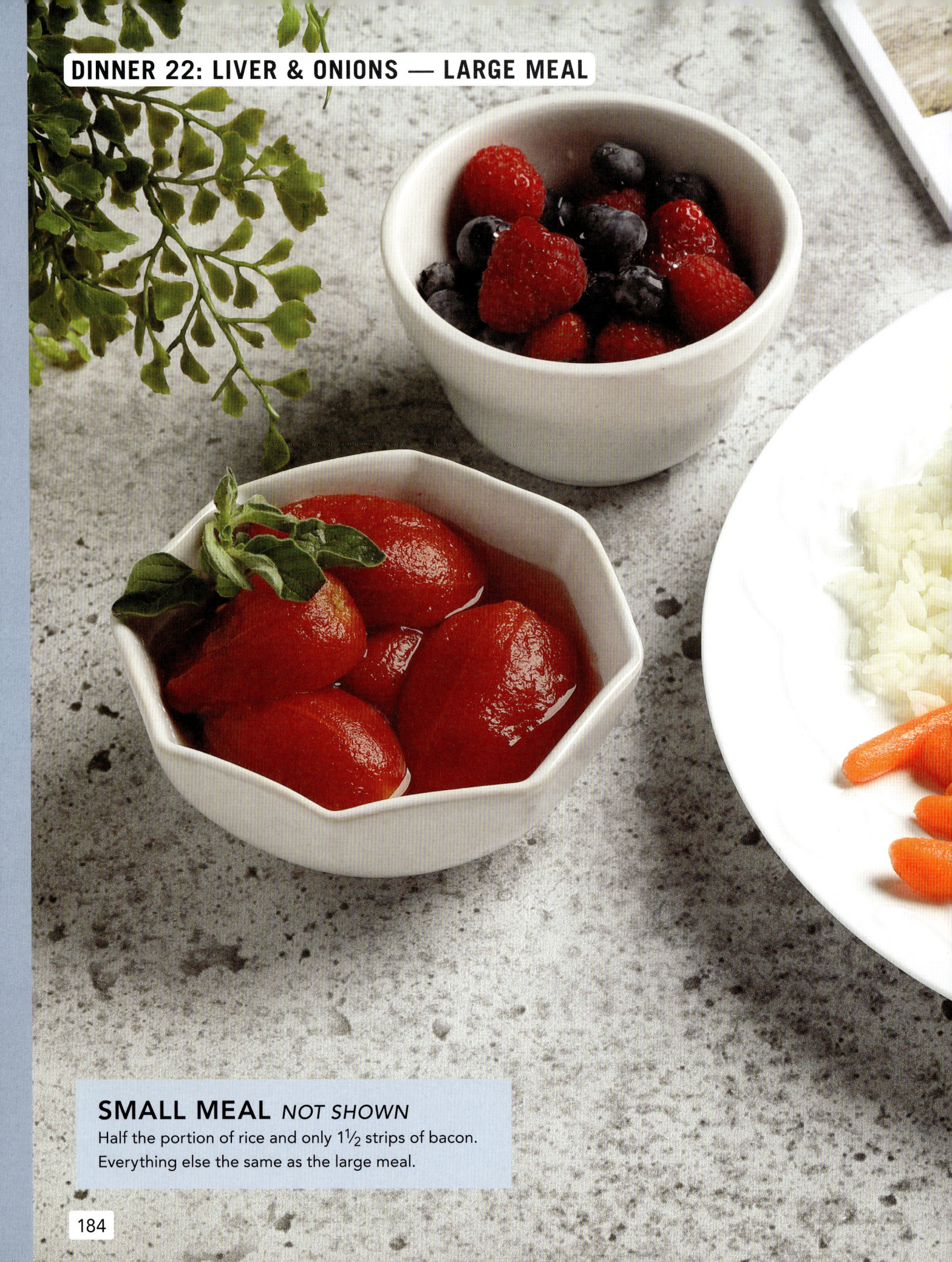

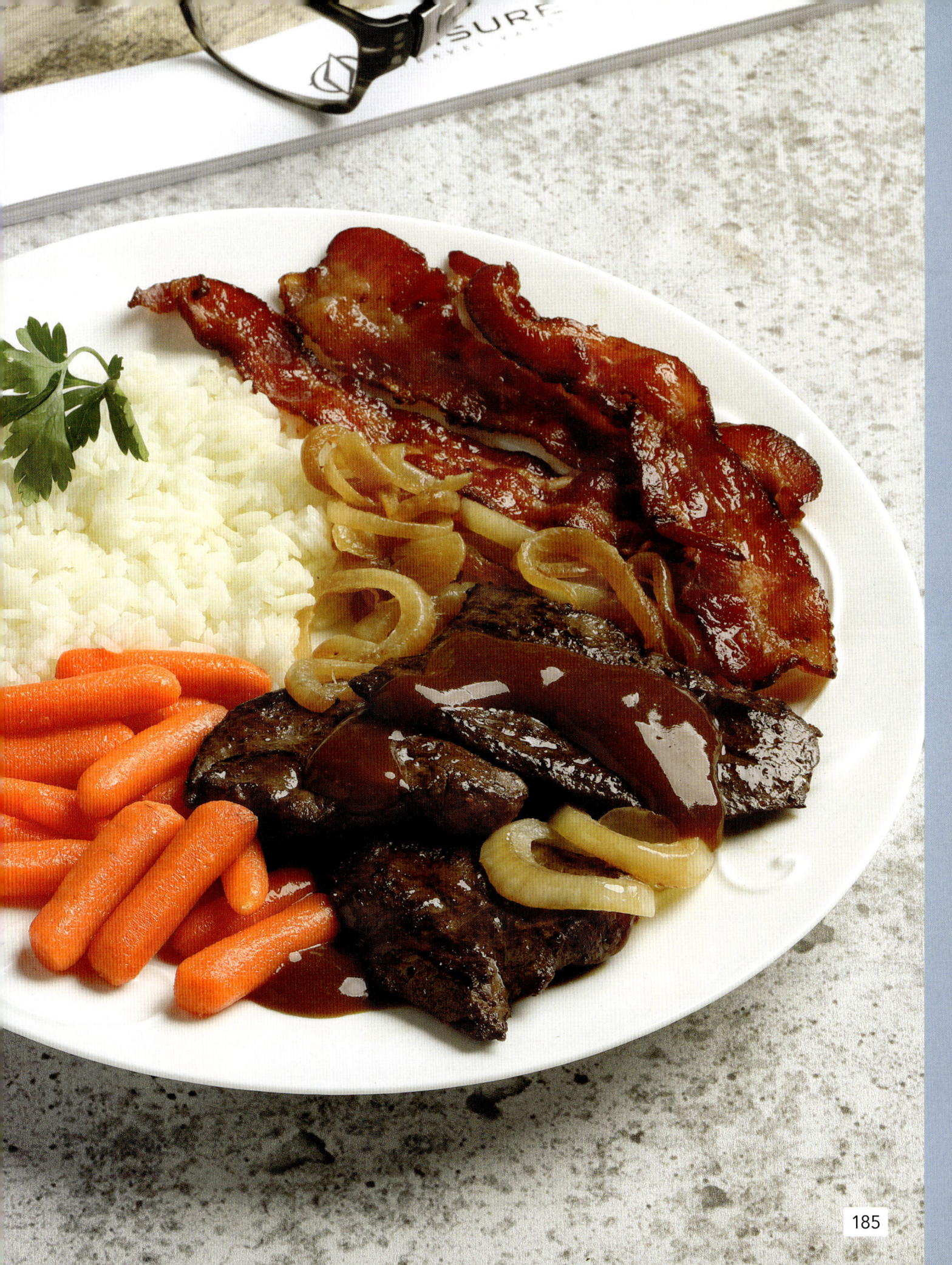

DINNER MEALS

DINNER 23

Sun Burgers

Serve these veggie burgers on a small 3-inch (7.5 cm) bagel. Be sure to add vegetable toppings to your burger such as lettuce, tomato, onion and cucumber. Spread on dill mayonnaise, a mixture of light mayo and dried dill to taste.

Sun Burgers

Makes 12 burgers

- 1 cup (250 mL) converted or long-grain cooked rice (brown or white)
- 19 oz (540 mL) can romano beans, drained (or other beans, such as pinto or kidney)
- ⅓ cup (75 mL) sesame seeds
- ⅓ cup (75 mL) sunflower seeds
- 2 tbsp (30 mL) wheat germ, ground flaxseed or chia seeds
- ½ tsp (2 mL) dried basil
- ½ tsp (2 mL) garlic powder
- ¼ tsp (1 mL) black pepper
- 1 tsp (5 mL) dried parsley
- 1 tsp (5 mL) dried dill
- 1 large egg
- 1½ cups (375 mL) mozzarella cheese, loosely packed

1. Cook rice or use leftover cold rice from a previous meal.
2. In a large bowl, mash the drained beans.
3. Add all other ingredients, including the rice, and mix well.
4. With your hands, form the mixture into 12 patties.
5. In a nonstick greased frying pan, on low to medium heat, let them cook slowly for 3 to 5 minutes on each side, until lightly browned.

PER BURGER PATTY	
Calories	148
Carbohydrate	13 g
Fiber	4 g
Net carbs	10 g
Protein	9 g
Fat, total	7 g
Fat, saturated	2 g
Cholesterol	25 mg
Sodium	139 mg

HEALTH TIP

Veggie burgers have a binder, often egg, to hold the vegetables together, while plant-based burgers are most often vegan and are considered meat substitute burgers. See page 203.

⟳ LOW-CARB SWAP

SUN BURGER RECIPE

Swap 2 Sun Burgers made with rice:

19 g net carbs

→ For 2 Sun Burgers made with quinoa: **18 g net carbs**

See Rice Swaps, page 276.

SWAP THE BAGEL FOR A WHOLE WHEAT BUN

LARGE MEAL

Swap 1 bagel: **30 g net carbs**:

→ For 1 whole wheat hamburger bun: **22 g net carbs**

SMALL MEAL

Swap ½ bagel: **15 g net carbs**

→ For ½ a whole wheat hamburger bun: **11 g net carbs**

See page 274 for more Bread Swaps.

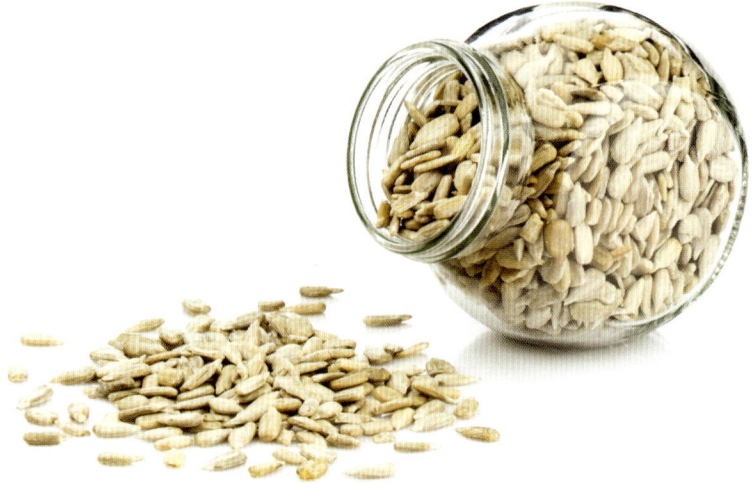

DINNER MEALS

Kale and Orange Salad

Makes 1 serving

¾ cup (175 mL) stemmed kale leaves, chopped into pieces
⅓ cup (75 mL) sliced bok choy
⅓ cup (75 mL) chopped broccoli
½ orange, broken into segments
3 strawberries, sliced

PER SERVING	
Calories	64
Carbohydrate	14 g
Fiber	4 g
Net carbs	10 g
Protein	3 g
Fat, total	1 g
Fat, saturated	0 g
Cholesterol	0 mg
Sodium	47 mg

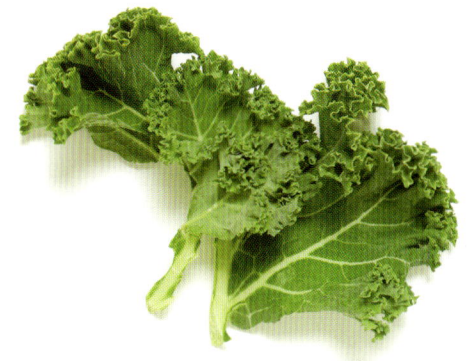

1. Combine all ingredients.

Dream Delight

Makes four 1-cup (250 mL) servings

1 pouch unflavored gelatine (Knox)
1 pouch (4-serving size) no-sugar-added flavored jelly powder (Jell-O)
1¼ cups (300 mL) boiling water
1¼ cups (300 mL) cold water
1 package dessert topping mix (enough to make 2 cups/500 mL)

PER CUP (250 ML)	
Calories	73
Carbohydrate	8 g
Fiber	0 g
Net carbs	8 g
Protein	2 g
Fat, total	4 g
Fat, saturated	4 g
Cholesterol	0 mg
Sodium	38 mg

This dessert has a fluffy texture and a delicate flavor.

1. Place unflavored gelatine and no-sugar-added jelly powder in a glass or metal bowl.
2. Stir in boiling water until powders are dissolved. Then stir in cold water. Refrigerate.
3. Remove the dessert from the fridge after about 45 minutes. It should be as thick as an unbeaten egg white. Do not allow it to get too firm.
4. Mix the topping mix as directed on the box.
5. Using the electric beater, blend topping into gelatin.
6. Pour into four dessert bowls. Refrigerate to set.

YOUR DINNER MENU	Large Meal (730 calories)	Total Carbs	NET CARBS	Small Meal (550 calories)	Total Carbs	NET CARBS
Sun Burgers	2	27	**19**	2	27	**19**
Bagel	1 (3-inch/7.5 cm)	31	**30**	½ of a 3-inch (7.5 cm)	16	**15**
Dill mayonnaise	1 tbsp (15 mL)	1	**1**	½ tbsp (7 mL)	1	**1**
Kale and Orange Salad	1 serving	14	**10**	1 serving	14	**10**
Oil and vinegar (half and half)	1 tbsp (15 mL)	0	**0**	½ tbsp (7 mL)	0	**0**
Dream Delight	1 cup (250 mL)	8	**8**	1 cup (250 mL)	8	**8**
	TOTAL CARBS	81 g	68 g	**TOTAL CARBS**	66 g	53 g
	Total carbs minus fiber = NET CARBS ↑			NET CARBS ↑		
	CARB CHOICES (1 carb choice = 15 g net carbs)		5	CARB CHOICES		4

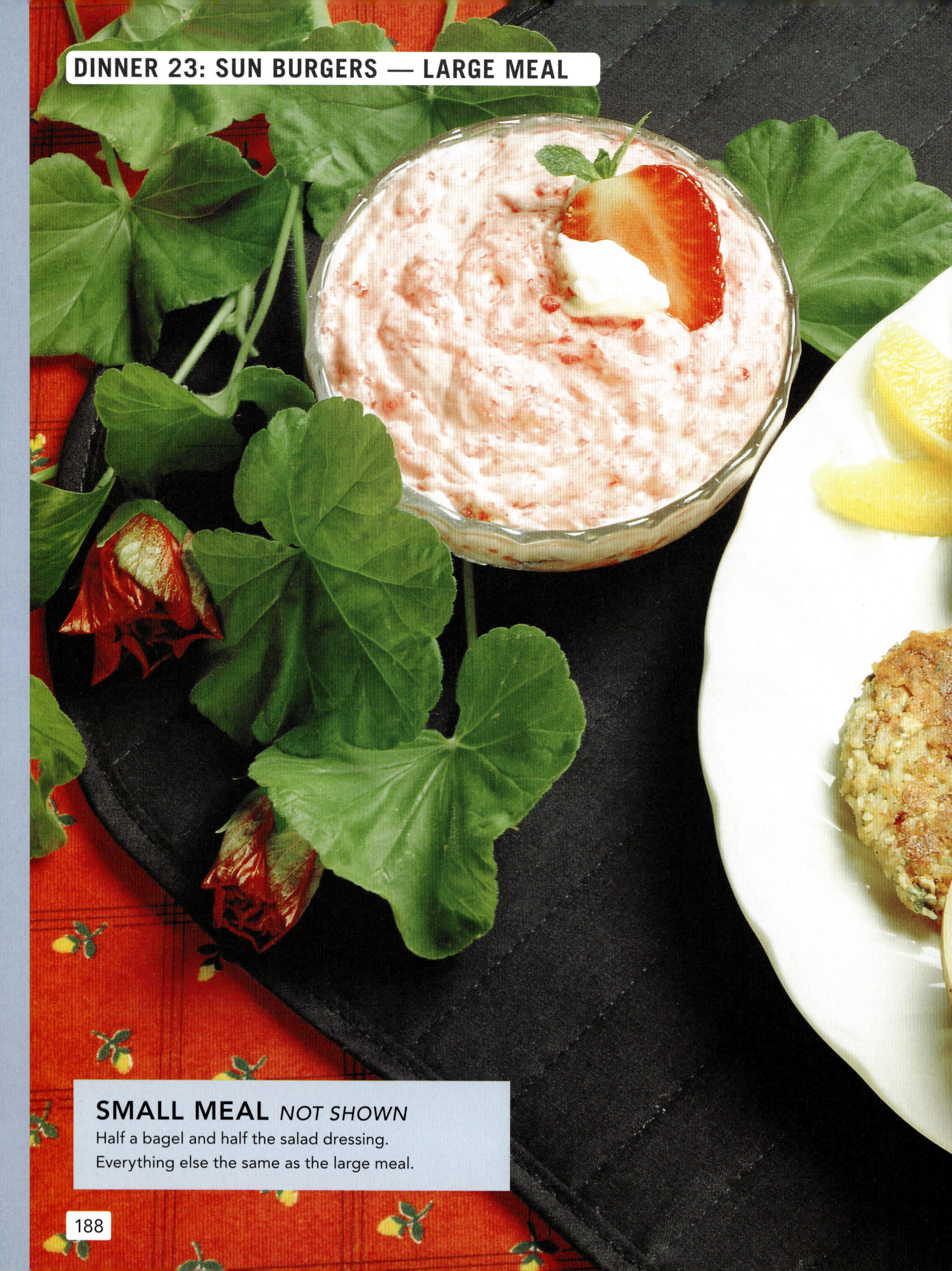

DINNER 23: SUN BURGERS — LARGE MEAL

SMALL MEAL *NOT SHOWN*
Half a bagel and half the salad dressing. Everything else the same as the large meal.

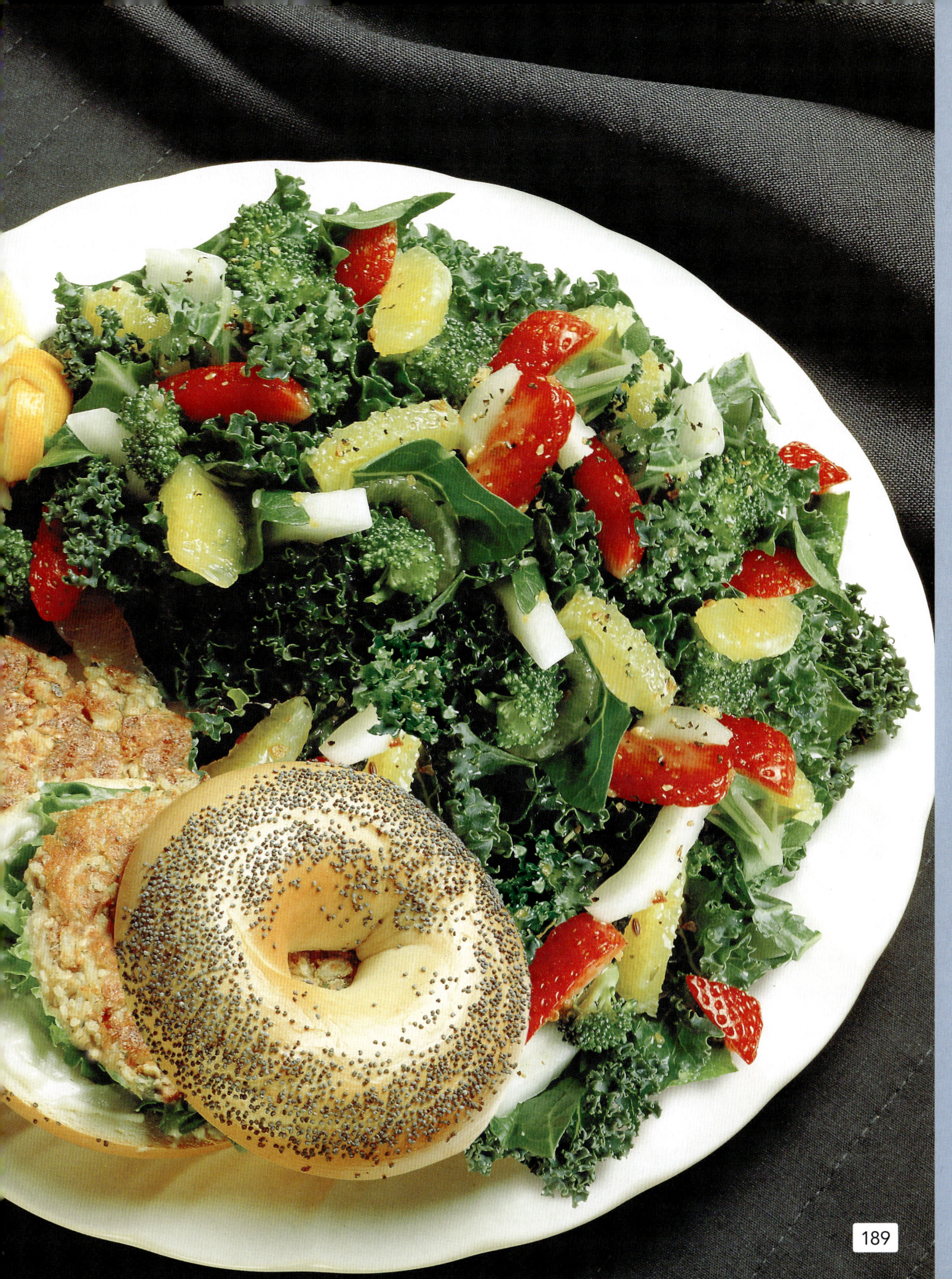

DINNER MEALS

DINNER 24

Salmon Potato Dish

Salmon Potato Dish has only three ingredients: canned salmon, mashed potato and shredded cheese. You could also make this recipe with canned tuna or leftover cooked fish equal to a can of salmon.

Salmon Potato Dish

**Makes one small baking dish
(2 large or 3 small servings)**

Preheat oven to 350°F (180°C)

1 can (7½ oz/213 g) pink or red salmon, drained

Dash of black pepper

1 cup (250 mL) Cheddar cheese, loosely packed, shredded

2 cups (500 mL) Mashed Potatoes (page 126)

1. Mash the drained salmon with the bones. Put the salmon on the bottom of a small baking dish. Sprinkle with pepper and half the shredded cheese.
2. Spread the mashed potato over the salmon and cheese.
3. Sprinkle the rest of the cheese on top.
4. Bake for 30 minutes, uncovered, or microwave for 8 minutes.

For a change, this dish can also be made into four patties. Fry in a nonstick pan with a small amount of oil or other fat. Sprinkle your favorite herbs on top.

PER LARGE SERVING	
Calories	572
Carbohydrate	40 g
Fiber	3 g
Net carbs	37 g
Protein	39 g
Fat, total	29 g
Fat, saturated	17 g
Cholesterol	148 mg
Sodium	799 mg

HEALTH TIP

If you use no-salt-added canned salmon, you will reduce the sodium per large serving to about 400 mg.

This recipe is a great way to use up leftover Mashed Potatoes.

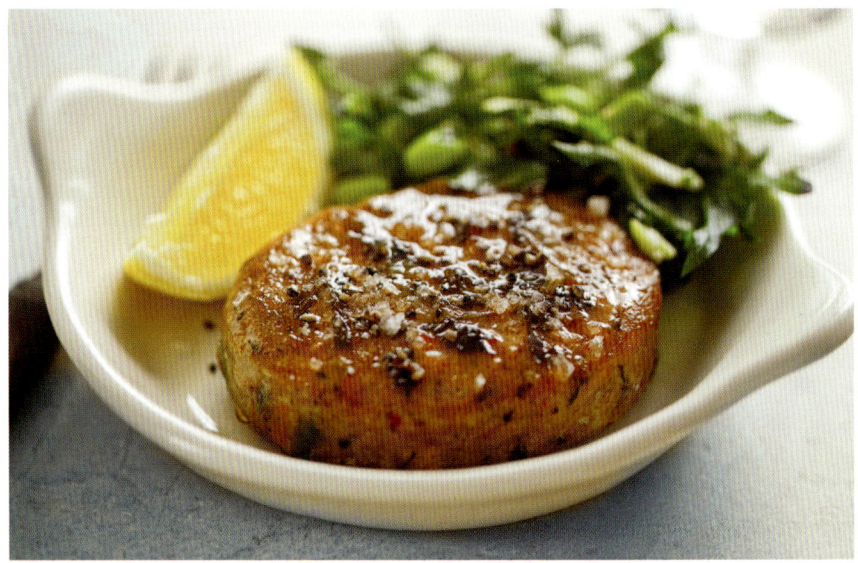

DINNER MEALS

Corn is the sweet vegetable with this meal: frozen or canned. Spinach and tomato juice are the low-calorie, low-carb vegetables. You can buy spinach fresh or frozen. Spinach, Swiss chard, beet tops and collard greens all have similar nutrition and are rich in iron, folic acid and fiber.

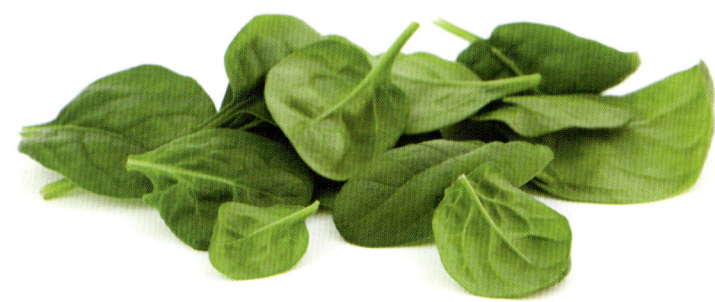

LOW-CARB SWAP

An easy swap at this meal is to replace the starchy vegetable (corn) with a second low-carb vegetable or double the serving of spinach.

LARGE MEAL
Swap corn:
¾ cup (175 mL)
22 g net carbs
→ For low-carb vegetables:
1 cup (250 mL)
1–8 g net carbs

SMALL MEAL
For corn:
⅓ cup (75 mL)
10 g net carbs
→ For low-carb vegetables:
1 cup (250 mL)
1–8 g net carbs

See page 134 for more low-carb vegetable swaps.

Sugar-Free Jelly with Berries

Makes 2 servings

1 pouch (4-serving size) no-sugar-added jelly powder, any flavor
1 cup (250 mL) boiling water
½ cup (125 mL) cold water
1 cup (250 mL) fresh sliced strawberries, blueberries or raspberries

PER SERVING	
Calories	42
Carbohydrate	5 g
Fiber	2 g
Net carbs	3 g
Protein	2 g
Fat, total	0 g
Fat, saturated	0 g
Cholesterol	0 mg
Sodium	281 mg

1. Put the jelly powder in a medium glass or metal bowl.
2. Add the boiling water and immediately stir until jelly powder is dissolved.
3. Add the cold water and fruit.
4. Pour into two dessert bowls. Refrigerate to set, about 1½ hours.

YOUR DINNER MENU	Large Meal (730 calories)	Total Carbs	NET CARBS	Small Meal (550 calories)	Total Carbs	NET CARBS
Salmon Potato Dish	½ the recipe	40	37	⅓ the recipe	26	24
Corn	¾ cup (175 mL)	24	22	⅓ cup (75 mL)	11	10
Spinach	½ cup (125 mL)	3	1	½ cup (125 mL)	3	1
Tomato juice	½ cup (125 mL)	5	4	½ cup (125 mL)	5	4
Celery	¼ stalk (in tomato juice)	1	1	¼ stalk (in tomato juice)	1	1
Sugar-Free Jelly with Berries	1 serving	5	3	1 serving	5	3
	TOTAL CARBS	78 g	68 g	**TOTAL CARBS**	51 g	43 g
	Total carbs minus fiber = NET CARBS ↑				NET CARBS ↑	
	CARB CHOICES (1 carb choice = 15 g net carbs)		5	CARB CHOICES		3

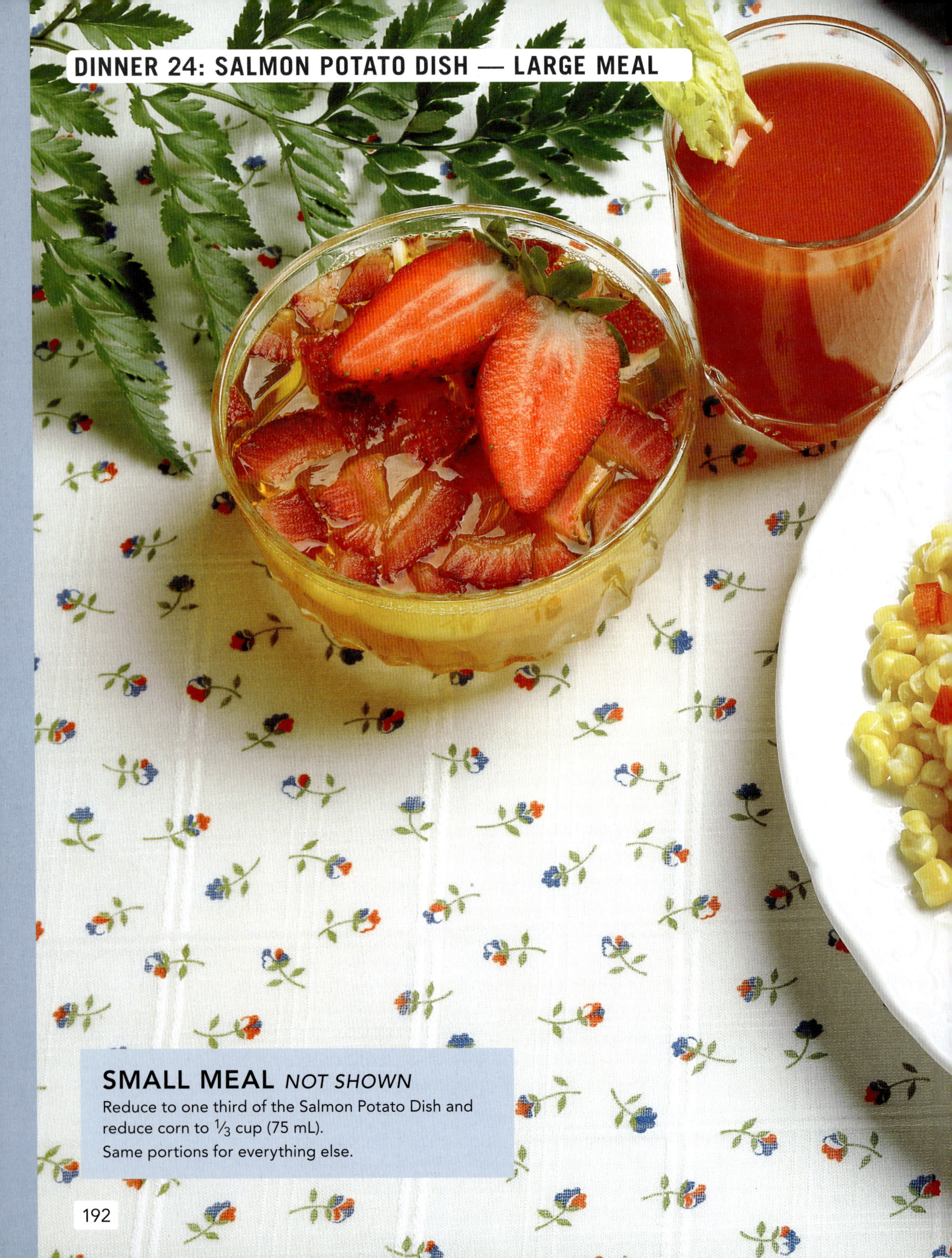

DINNER 24: SALMON POTATO DISH — LARGE MEAL

SMALL MEAL *NOT SHOWN*
Reduce to one third of the Salmon Potato Dish and reduce corn to 1/3 cup (75 mL).
Same portions for everything else.

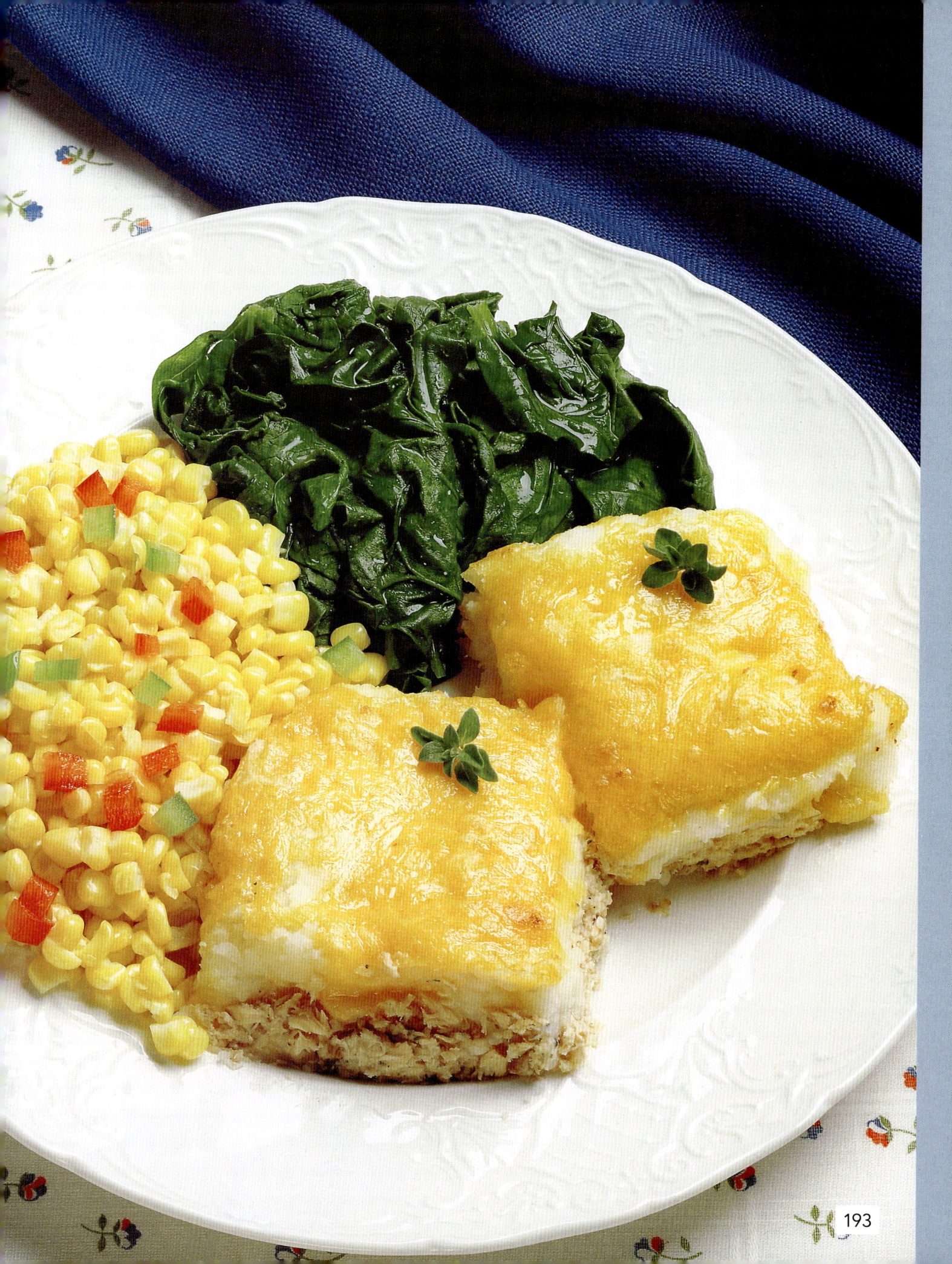

DINNER MEALS

DINNER 25

Hamburger Casserole

Cheesy Hamburger Casserole

Makes 5 cups (1.25 L)

Preheat oven to 400°F (200°C)

PER 1 CUP (250 ML)	
Calories	383
Carbohydrate	15 g
Fiber	1 g
Net carbs	14 g
Protein	29 g
Fat, total	23 g
Fat, saturated	12 g
Cholesterol	92 mg
Sodium	305 mg

1 cup (250 mL) corkscrew pasta, dry (or elbow macaroni)
1 lb (500 g) lean ground beef
1 medium onion, chopped
1 tsp (5 mL) garlic powder
½ tsp (2 mL) onion powder
¼ tsp (1 mL) black pepper
½ tsp (2 mL) ground cayenne pepper (or chili pepper)
1 cup (250 mL) Cheddar cheese, shredded
⅓ cup (75 mL) sour cream, 5%
¾ cup (175 mL) Cheddar cheese, shredded, for topping

1. Boil pasta, drain and set aside.
2. In a large, heavy pan, brown ground beef. Drain off fat.
3. Add chopped onion, garlic powder and onion powder, black pepper and cayenne pepper to the beef. Cook for 10 minutes, until onions are soft.
4. Take off the heat and stir in 1 cup (250 mL) cheese, sour cream and cooked pasta. Blend until cheese is melted.
5. Transfer to a greased 8-inch (20 cm) casserole and top with the ¾ cup (175 mL) of shredded cheese.
6. Bake for 15 minutes or until cheese melts.

Roasted Cabbage with Bacon

Makes 4 cups (1 L)

Preheat oven to 400°F (200°C)

PER 1 CUP (250 ML)	
Calories	107
Carbohydrate	11 g
Fiber	5 g
Net carbs	6 g
Protein	4 g
Fat, total	4 g
Fat, saturated	1 g
Cholesterol	7 mg
Sodium	146 mg

½ medium 6-inch (15 cm) cabbage, cored and sliced
1 tbsp (15 mL) vegetable or olive oil
Salt and pepper, to taste
3 slices (3 tbsp) cooked bacon bits

1. To a large bowl, add cabbage, oil, and salt and pepper. Mix well and spread the cabbage evenly on a greased baking sheet.
2. Bake for 30 minutes, or until tender and with slightly browned edges. Stir once or twice during cooking.
3. Top with warm precooked bacon bits.

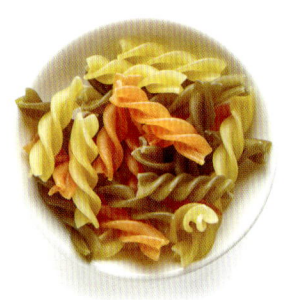

RECIPE TIP

For extra flavor in this casserole, use Old Cheddar cheese.

Old cheese has aged longer, six months to a year, to enhance and sharpen flavors.

A dash of hot sauce at the table will spice up the casserole.

RECIPE TIP

The cabbage can be topped with either the 3 tbsp (45 mL) precooked chopped bacon or ready-to-eat bacon bits, or ¼ cup (60 mL) grated cheese.

DINNER MEALS

This dessert is a surprise – it tastes as good as it looks!

Pineapple Surprise

Makes 6 servings

1½ cups (375 mL) skim milk

1 package (4-serving size) light vanilla instant pudding mix

1 cup (250 mL) frozen whipped topping (regular or light), thawed

1 cup (250 mL) canned drained crushed pineapple

2 small bananas, sliced thinly

¼ cup (60 mL) graham cracker crumbs (equal to about 4 graham crackers)

1. In a medium bowl, pour skim milk and add the pudding mix.
2. Beat with an electric mixer until thickened (about 2 minutes).
3. Fold in thawed whipped topping and drained pineapple until well blended.
4. Add sliced bananas and graham cracker crumbs to the pudding mixture. Save some bananas and crumbs for the top. If you want, you can layer the pudding mixture, bananas and crumbs.
5. Put in the fridge until ready to serve.

PER SERVING	
Calories	141
Carbohydrate	25 g
Fiber	1 g
Net carbs	24 g
Protein	3 g
Fat, total	4 g
Fat, saturated	3 g
Cholesterol	1 mg
Sodium	283 mg

LOW-CARB SWAP

FOR PINEAPPLE SURPRISE

Swap 1 serving:
24 g net carbs

→ For pineapple and pistachios: ½ cup (125 mL) fresh or canned pineapple plus 20 pistachios or other shelled nuts to equal about 2 tbsp (30 mL)

12 g net carbs

YOUR DINNER MENU	Large Meal (730 calories)	Total Carbs	NET CARBS	Small Meal (550 calories)	Total Carbs	NET CARBS
Cheesy Hamburger Casserole	1 cup (250 mL)	15	14	⅔ cup (150 mL)	10	9
Roasted Cabbage with Bacon	1 cup (250 mL) (⅕ of recipe)	11	6	1 cup (250 mL) (⅕ of recipe)	11	6
Mixed vegetables	1 cup (250 mL)	24	19	¾ cup (175 mL)	18	14
Pineapple Surprise	1 serving	25	24	1 serving	25	24
	TOTAL CARBS	75 g	63 g	**TOTAL CARBS**	64 g	53 g
	Total carbs minus fiber = NET CARBS ↑			NET CARBS ↑		
	CARB CHOICES (1 carb choice = 15 g net carbs)		4	CARB CHOICES		3

DINNER 25: HAMBURGER CASSEROLE — LARGE MEAL

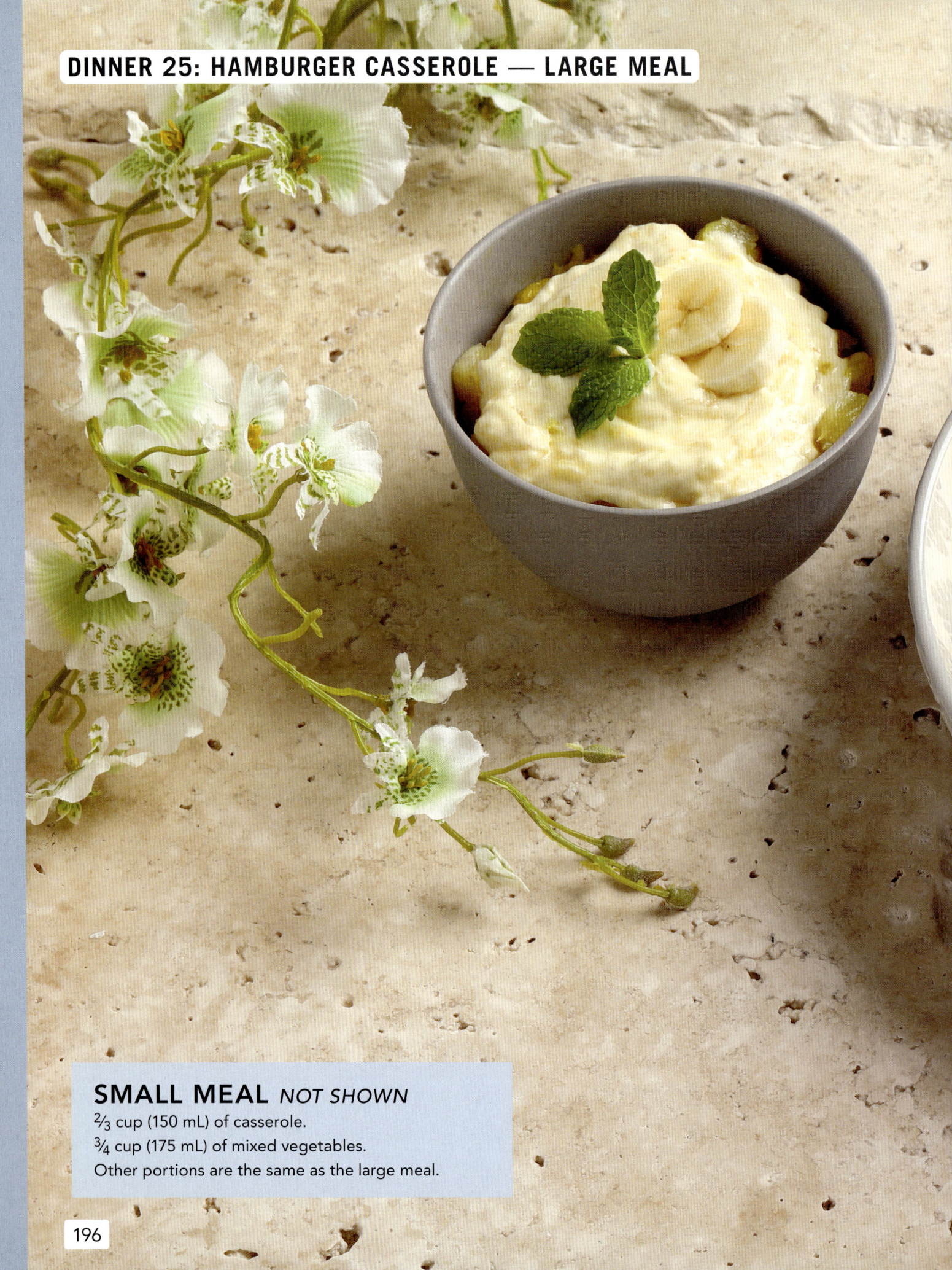

SMALL MEAL *NOT SHOWN*
⅔ cup (150 mL) of casserole.
¾ cup (175 mL) of mixed vegetables.
Other portions are the same as the large meal.

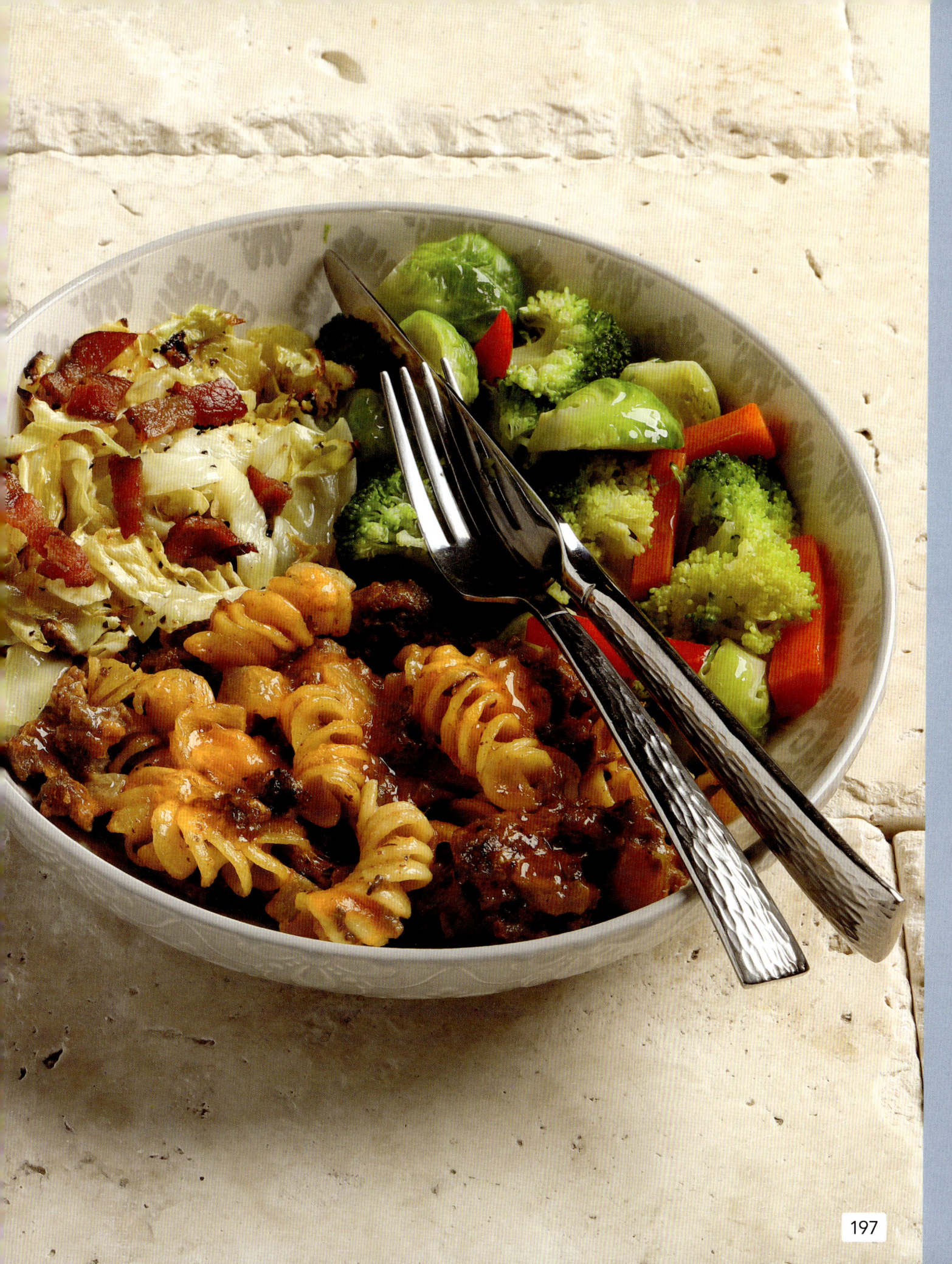

DINNER MEALS

DINNER 26

Pizza

Homemade Thin-Crust Pizza

Makes one 12-inch (30 cm) pizza (6 slices)

Preheat oven to temperature on pizza shell package

- 12-inch (150 g) thin-crust pizza shell
- ½ cup (125 mL) pizza sauce
- 3 oz (90 g) thinly sliced pepperoni, ham, sausage or cooked hamburger
- 1 cup (250 mL) raw or sautéed vegetables
- Fresh or dried herbs, as desired
- 1 cup (250 mL) mozzarella cheese, shredded

1. Spread pizza sauce on the pizza shell.
2. Top with the meat, vegetables, herbs and cheese.
3. Bake according to the instructions on the pizza shell package until the cheese bubbles, about 10 minutes.

PER 1 SLICE	
Calories	206
Carbohydrate	17 g
Fiber	1 g
Net carbs	16 g
Protein	9 g
Fat, total	12 g
Fat, saturated	6 g
Cholesterol	26 mg
Sodium	537 mg

HEALTH TIP

Three pieces of thin-crust pizza has about the same carbs as two pieces of thick crust.

RECIPE TIP

Vegetables on pizza: Try onions, mushrooms, cherry tomatoes, bell peppers or jalapeno peppers, eggplant or zucchini.

◯ LOW-CARB SWAP RECIPE: Low-Carb Cauliflower Pizza Crust

LARGE OR SMALL MEAL

Swap standard thin-crust pizza:
1 slice of crust of 12-inch (30 cm)
13 g net carbs

→ For Low-Carb Cauliflower Pizza Crust:
1 slice of crust of 11-inch (27 cm)
6 g net carbs

Makes one 11-inch pizza crust

Preheat oven to 425°F (220°C)

- 3 cups (750 mL) frozen riced cauliflower
- 2 large eggs, beaten
- ¼ cup (60 mL) flour
- ¼ cup (60 mL) almond flour
- ¼ tsp (1 mL) baking powder
- ¼ cup (60 mL) mozzarella cheese, shredded

1 SLICE OF CRUST	
Calories	106
Total carbs	9 g
Net carbs	6 g

1. Place frozen riced cauliflower in a large, dry nonstick pan at medium-high heat. Once sizzling, cook for 7 minutes, uncovered, stirring frequently to release moisture.
2. Take cauliflower off the heat to cool. Once cooled, add the beaten eggs.
3. Mix flour, almond flour and baking powder in a medium bowl.
4. Add the dry ingredients to the cauliflower mixture, and blend well.
5. Place the mixture on a parchment-lined baking sheet (so the crust doesn't stick).
6. Use a spatula or your hands to flatten the dough and shape into an oval.
7. Bake for 25 minutes, or until lightly browned.
8. Remove from the oven. Add your favorite toppings and bake again for another 10 minutes, or until cheese bubbles.

DINNER MEALS

This delightful deep green salad has a splash of red and light green from the added fruit.

Arugula Pear Salad

Makes 4 servings

4 cups arugula or other leafy greens

¼ cup (60 mL) blue cheese, crumbled (or other soft cheese such as feta or goat cheese)

1 medium pear, sliced

2 tbsp (30 mL) walnuts, chopped or halves

¼ cup (60 mL) pomegranate seeds or sliced strawberries (or 1½ tbsp/22 mL dried cranberries)

SALAD DRESSING

1 tbsp (15 mL) olive oil or vegetable oil

1 tbsp (15 mL) light syrup (40% less sugar), see page 29

Fresh lemon juice from half a lemon (about 2 tbsp/30 mL)

Dash of salt

Dash of black pepper

PER SERVING	
Calories	115
Carbohydrate	11 g
Fiber	2 g
Net carbs	9 g
Protein	3 g
Fat, total	7 g
Fat, saturated	2 g
Cholesterol	4 mg
Sodium	113 mg

1. In a large bowl, combine arugula, crumbled blue cheese, pear slices, walnut pieces and pomegranate seeds.
2. In a small bowl, mix salad dressing ingredients and add to salad.

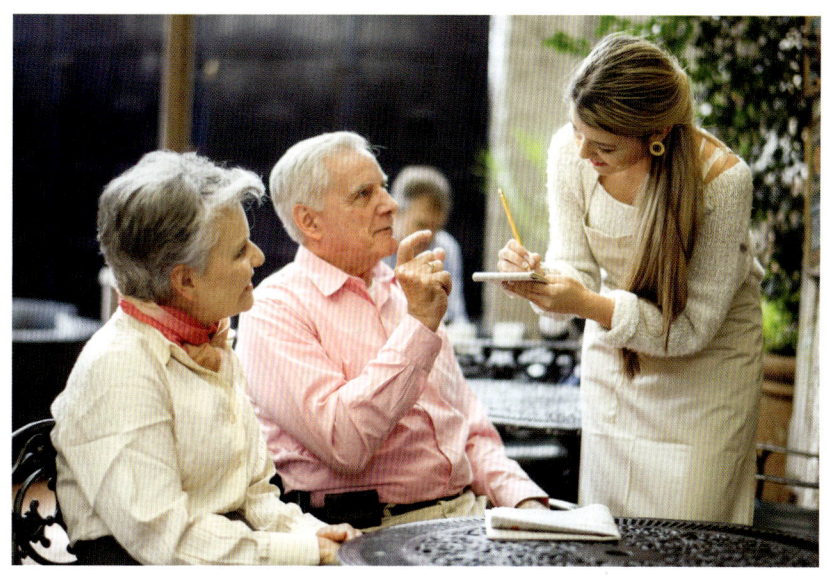

YOUR DINNER MENU	Large Meal (730 calories)	Total Carbs	NET CARBS	Small Meal (550 calories)	Total Carbs	NET CARBS
12-inch (30 cm) Pizza, thin crust	3 slices (½ pizza)	51	48	2 slices (⅓ pizza)	34	32
Arugula Pear Salad with dressing	1 serving	11	9	1 serving	11	9
Diet soft drink	Large	1	1	Large	1	1
	TOTAL CARBS	63 g	58 g	TOTAL CARBS	46 g	42 g
Total carbs minus fiber = NET CARBS ↑				NET CARBS ↑		
CARB CHOICES (1 carb choice = 15 g net carbs)			4	CARB CHOICES		3

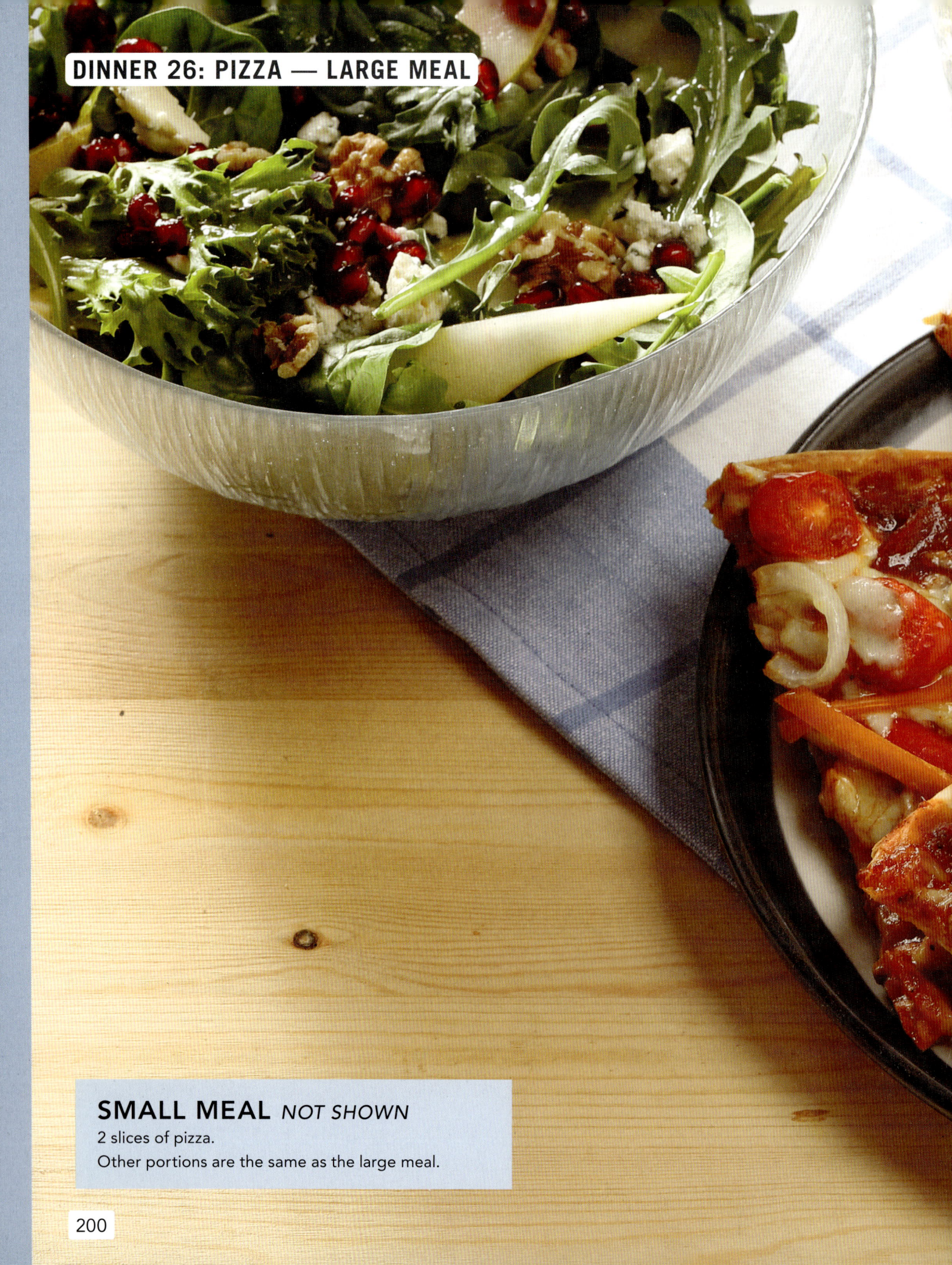

DINNER 26: PIZZA — LARGE MEAL

SMALL MEAL *NOT SHOWN*
2 slices of pizza.
Other portions are the same as the large meal.

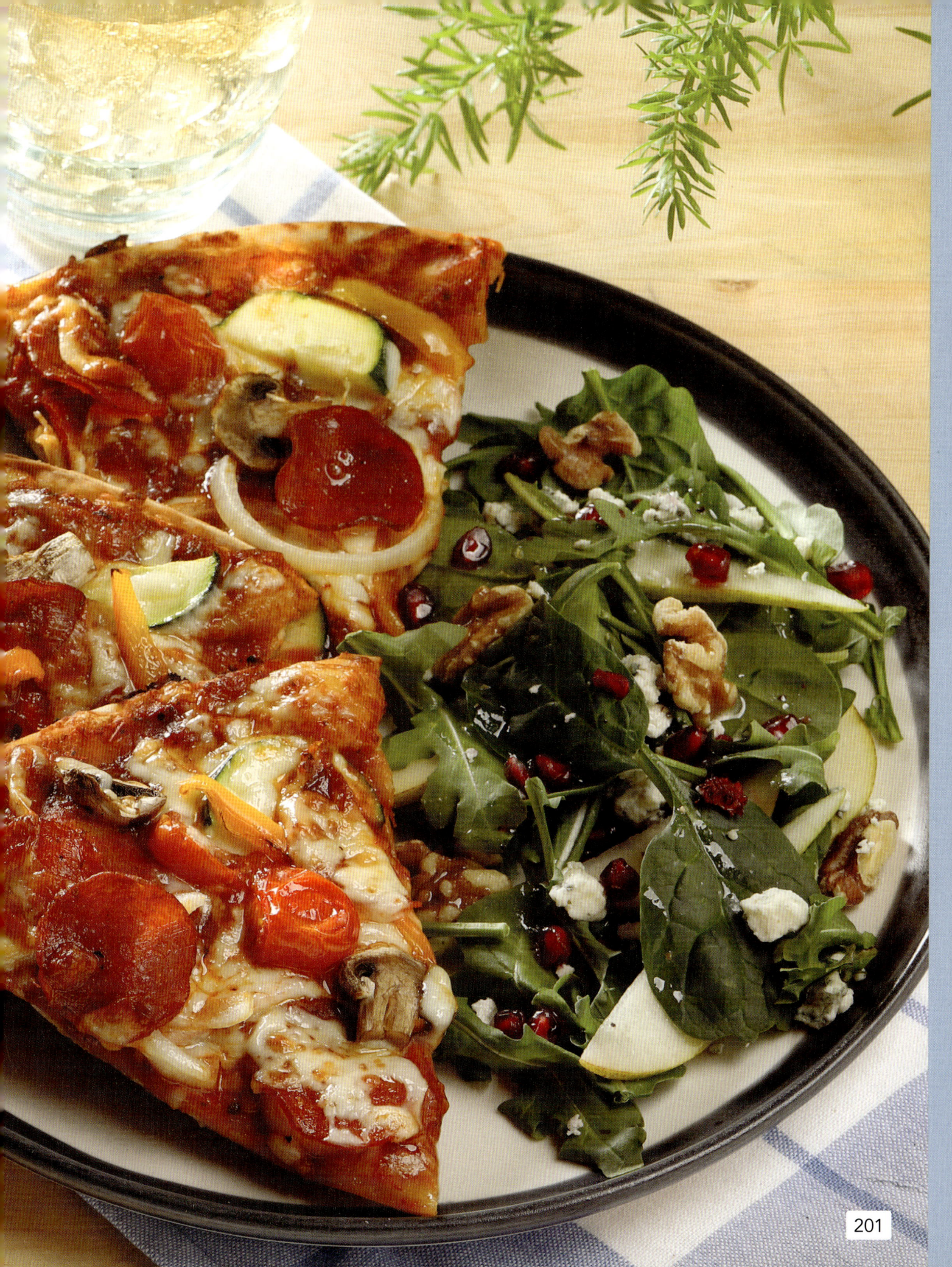

DINNER MEALS

DINNER 27

Fast-Food Dinner

For the best diabetes health, enjoy a fast-food takeout meal only occasionally. We know these meals are high in carbs, fat and sodium and low in fiber. They have few vegetables, so you don't get a balanced, nutritious meal.

Check Websites

Review nutrition information on restaurant websites, decide what choices fit for you, work out the carbs and calories, and try to stick to those choices.

◯ **LOW-CARB SWAP**

Swap double cheeseburger:
32 g net carbs

→ For double cheeseburger, discard top of bun and exchange for extra cheese slice:
19 g net carbs

Order the extra slice of cheese to be separate and uncooked.

Three Examples of Fast-Food Burgers with All Toppings

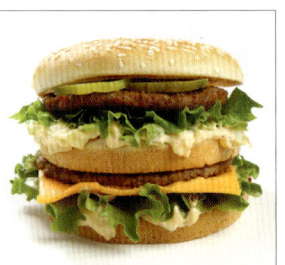

Big Mac-type: two 1 oz (28 g) burgers with cheese and middle bun

Calories	Carbs	Fiber	Net carbs	Protein	Fat	Sodium
550	45 g	3 g	42 g	25 g	30 g	1010 mg

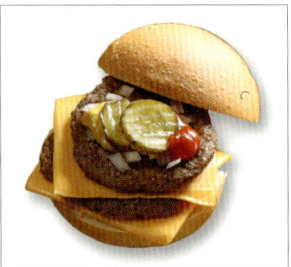

Double cheeseburger: 3 oz (90 g) burger with double cheese (see Dinner Menu)

Calories	Carbs	Fiber	Net carbs	Protein	Fat	Sodium
420	34 g	2 g	32 g	24 g	21 g	1010 mg

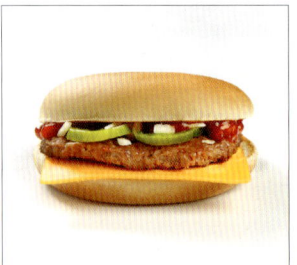

Cheeseburger: 1 oz (28 g) burger with cheese

Calories	Carbs	Fiber	Net carbs	Protein	Fat	Sodium
300	32 g	2 g	30 g	15 g	13 g	720 mg

DINNER MEALS

Skip the regular soft drinks

Research tells us about half of American youth and adults (a bit less in Canada) drink a sugary soft drink or other sugar-sweetened beverage daily. That can add up to an extra 3,500 calories in a month, enough to gain one pound in a month or 10 pounds in a year. Seniors tend to drink less sugar-sweetened beverages.

HEALTH TIP

Plant-based burgers

These are a good option to decrease how much meat you eat. The main ingredients are a combination of soybeans, legumes, wheat gluten and potato starch. However, as these burgers are designed to mimic meat, they are highly processed. They have color additives, preservatives and flavor enhancers, including sugar, salt and oils, so the burgers look and taste like meat.

They often have the same calories and more salt than a meat burger.

A great option is a Sun Burger, page 186: a home-made veggie burger that is definitely worth a try.

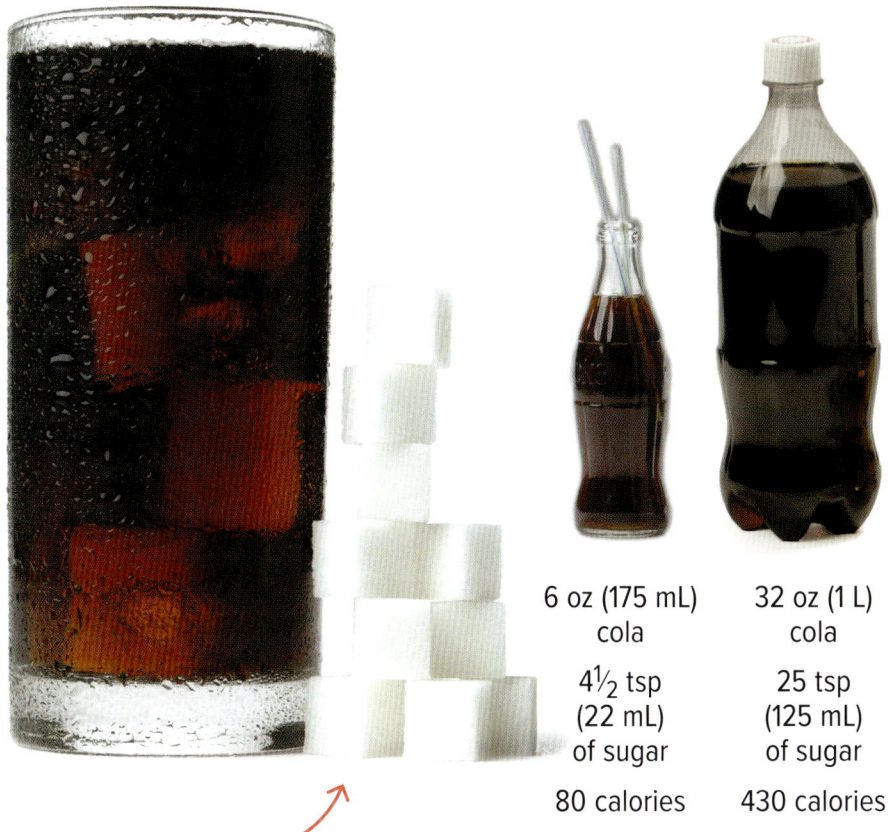

6 oz (175 mL) cola
4½ tsp (22 mL) of sugar
80 calories

32 oz (1 L) cola
25 tsp (125 mL) of sugar
430 calories

Every time you drink a 12 oz (355 mL) can of soda, you get 10 tsp (50 mL) of sugar that you don't need.

YOUR DINNER MENU	Large Meal (730 calories)	Total Carbs	NET CARBS	Small Meal (550 calories)	Total Carbs	NET CARBS
Double cheeseburger	1 burger (about 420 calories)	34	32	1 burger (about 420 calories)	34	32
French fries	1 small order	31	28	½ small order	16	14
Ketchup	2 tbsp (30 mL)	6	6	1 tbsp (15 mL)	3	3
Diet soft drink	Medium (570 mL/19 oz)	1	1	Medium (570 mL/19 oz)	1	1
	TOTAL CARBS	72 g	67 g	**TOTAL CARBS**	54 g	50 g
	Total carbs minus fiber = NET CARBS ↑			NET CARBS ↑		
	CARB CHOICES (1 carb choice = 15 g net carbs)		4	CARB CHOICES		3

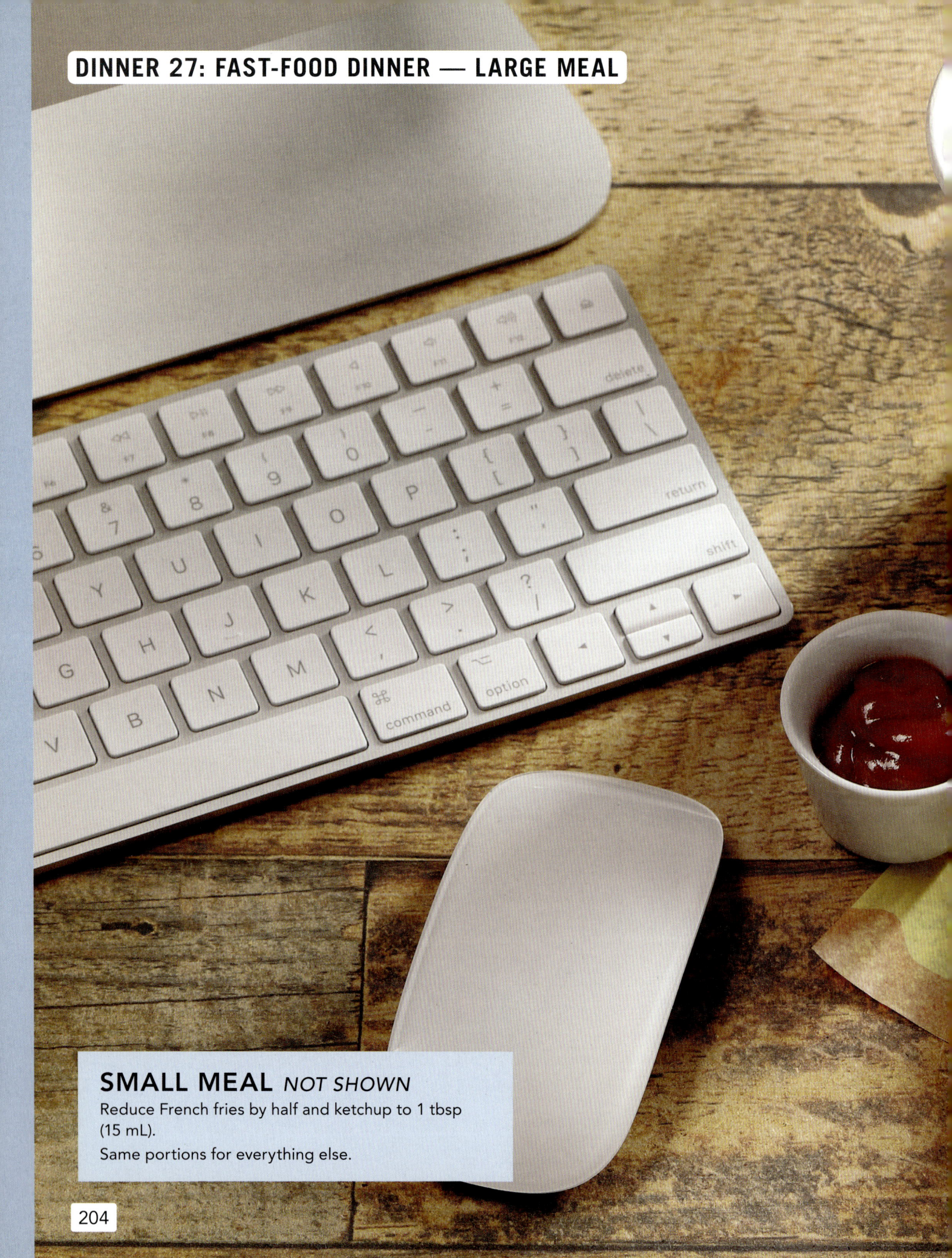

DINNER 27: FAST-FOOD DINNER — LARGE MEAL

SMALL MEAL *NOT SHOWN*
Reduce French fries by half and ketchup to 1 tbsp (15 mL).
Same portions for everything else.

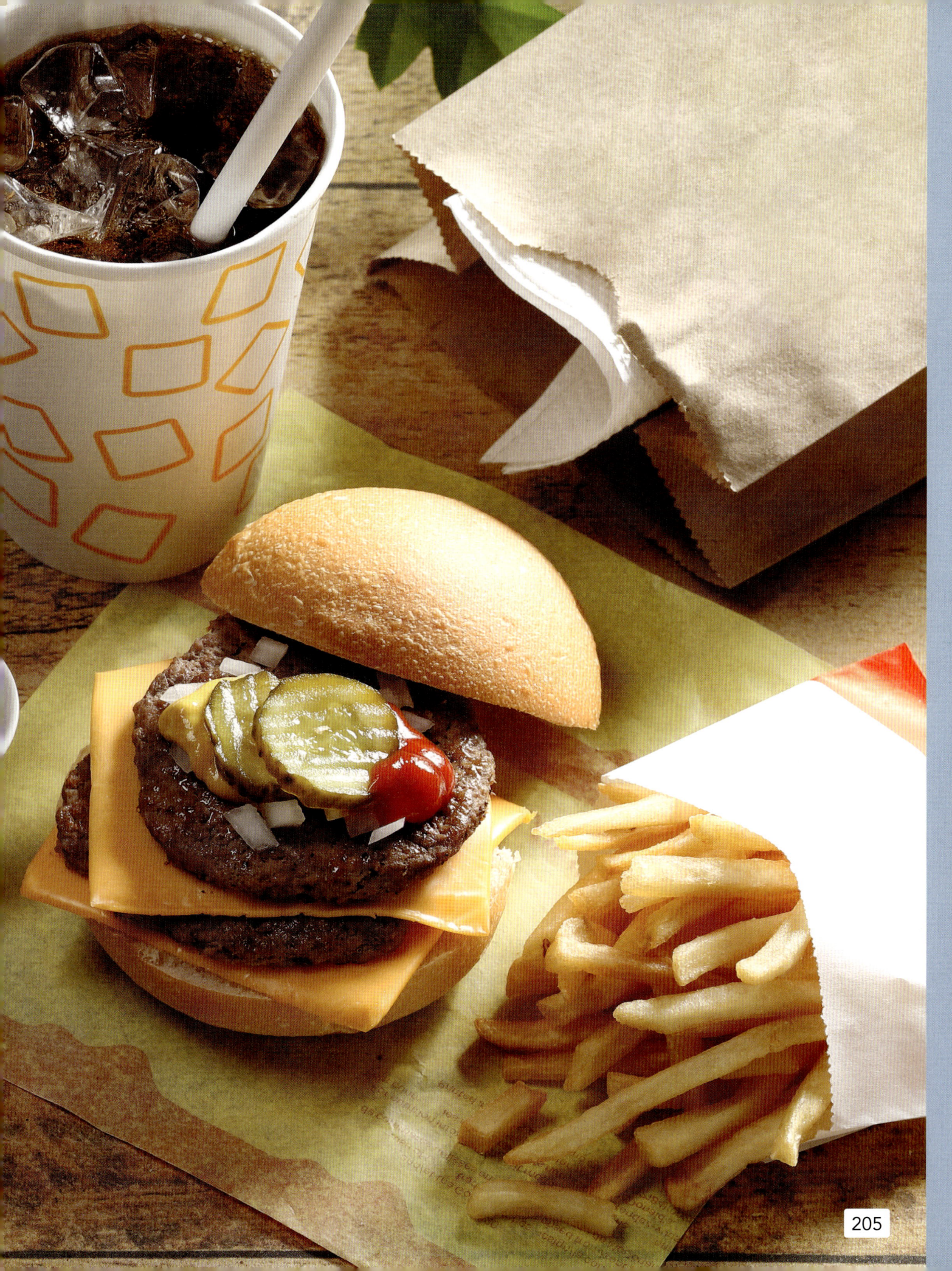

DINNER MEALS

DINNER 28

RECIPE TIPS

SEAFOOD OPTION

6 oz (175 g) of meat can be replaced with 23 large shrimp (7 oz/200 g)

VEGETARIAN OPTION

6 oz (175 g) of meat can be replaced with tofu, edamame beans or cashews. These are nutritious but will have more carbs than meat, as listed below:

- ½ cup (125 mL) firm tofu chunks
  1 g net carbs
- 1 cup (250 mL) edamame beans
  6 g net carbs
- 20 cashews
  9 g net carbs

Try a combination of all three: ¼ cup of tofu, ½ cup edamame beans and 10 cashews for a total of 8 g net carbs.

Marinate your tofu in advance as you would the meat.

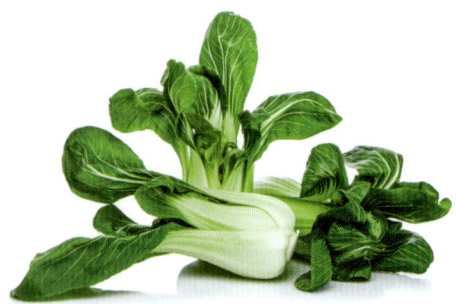

Stir-Fry

Stir-Fry

Makes 4 cups (1 L) (2 servings)

¾ cup/175 mL (or 6 oz/175 g) raw lean pork, beef or chicken, thinly sliced

MEAT MARINADE:

- ¼ tsp (1 mL) salt
- 1 tsp (5 mL) sugar
- 2 tsp (10 mL) cornstarch
- 1 tbsp (15 mL) wine or wine vinegar
- 1 tsp (5 mL) reduced-sodium soy sauce
- 1 tsp vegetable oil

3 cloves garlic, peeled and finely chopped

1-inch (2.5 cm) piece of fresh ginger, peeled and finely chopped

1 medium carrot, sliced

4 cups (1 L) loosely packed low-carb shredded vegetables or pieces (celery, bok choy, cabbage, broccoli, green or red pepper, zucchini, snow peas, mushrooms or onions)

2 tbsp (30 mL) vegetable oil

1 tbsp (15 mL) reduced-sodium soy sauce

PER 1 CUP (250 ML)	
Calories	169
Carbohydrate	11 g
Fiber	3 g
Net carbs	8 g
Protein	12 g
Fat, total	10 g
Fat, saturated	2 g
Cholesterol	18 mg
Sodium	328 mg

1. Mix the Meat Marinade in a medium bowl. Add meat, stir well and let sit for 30 minutes.
2. Prepare garlic and ginger and put in a small bowl on its own. Prepare the other vegetables, separating the ones that need more cooking time, such as carrots, celery and broccoli pieces. Set aside.
3. In a wok or large frying pan, heat oil over medium to high heat. Once it is sizzling, add vegetables that need more cooking time. Once cooked to tender, remove from the pan.
4. Add meat strips and quickly stir until lightly cooked on the outside. Add garlic and ginger, precooked vegetables and raw vegetables.
5. Stir at medium-high heat for 1–2 minutes or until cooked.
6. Add soy sauce, then serve.

DINNER MEALS

Fried Rice

Makes 3 cups

- 2 cups (500 mL) precooked long-grain rice (converted brown rice is a good choice). Day-old rice makes the best fried rice because it is less sticky.
- 2 tbsp (30 mL) vegetable oil
- 1 cup (250 mL) frozen peas or mixed vegetables
- 2 large eggs, beaten
- 2 tbsp (30 mL) reduced-sodium soy sauce (or combination of soy sauce and oyster sauce)
- 4 green onions, tops and stems, sliced

1. Cook the rice a day ahead, cool and refrigerate overnight.
2. On medium-high heat in a wok or frying pan, heat oil.
3. Add beaten eggs and stir, breaking into pieces, until cooked. Transfer cooked eggs to a clean plate.
4. Break up the cold rice with your hands or a spoon, then add to the pan. Add frozen vegetables. Stir until heated through. Add the cooked eggs back to the pan.
5. Stir in soy sauce and top with green onions.

PER 1 CUP (250 ML)	
Calories	329
Carbohydrate	40 g
Fiber	5 g
Net carbs	35 g
Protein	11 g
Fat, total	14 g
Fat, saturated	3 g
Cholesterol	124 mg
Sodium	413 mg

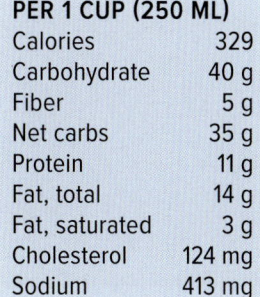

LOW-CARB SWAP

Make Low-Carb Fried Rice: Make the recipe with 1 cup (250 mL) cooked rice and 2 cups (500 mL) frozen veggies.

LARGE MEAL

Swap Fried Rice:
1¼ cups (300 mL)
44 g net carbs
→ For Low-Carb Fried Rice:
1¼ cups (300 mL)
33 g net carbs

SMALL MEAL

Swap Fried Rice:
¾ cup (175 mL)
26 g net carbs
→ For Low-Carb Fried Rice:
¾ cup (175 mL)
20 g net carbs

See Rice Swaps, page 276.

HEALTH TIP

The glycemic index (GI) of rice is a way to measure how quickly the starch is digested and turned into blood sugar (see page 276).

Ginger Tea

Here is an easy homemade ginger tea for two. Slice a 2-inch (5 cm) piece of ginger into a saucepan with 3 cups (750 mL) of water and bring to a boil. Cover the pan and let steep for 15 minutes. Use a fork to press the ginger against the side of the saucepan to release the flavor.

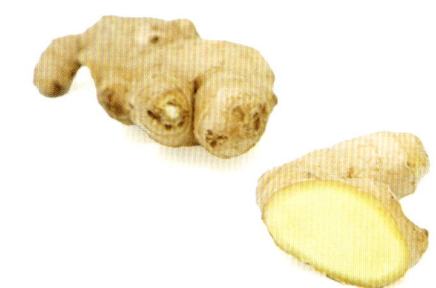

YOUR DINNER MENU	Large Meal (730 calories)	Total Carbs	NET CARBS	Small Meal (550 calories)	Total Carbs	NET CARBS
Stir-Fry	2 cups (500 mL)	22	17	2 cups (500 mL)	22	17
Fried Rice	1¼ cups (300 mL)	50	44	¾ cup (175 mL)	30	26
Ginger Tea	1 cup (250 mL)	1	1	1 cup (250 mL)	1	1
	TOTAL CARBS	73 g	62 g	**TOTAL CARBS**	53 g	44 g
	Total carbs minus fiber = NET CARBS ↑			NET CARBS ↑		
	CARB CHOICES (1 carb choice = 15 g net carbs)		4	CARB CHOICES		3

DINNER 28: STIR-FRY — LARGE MEAL

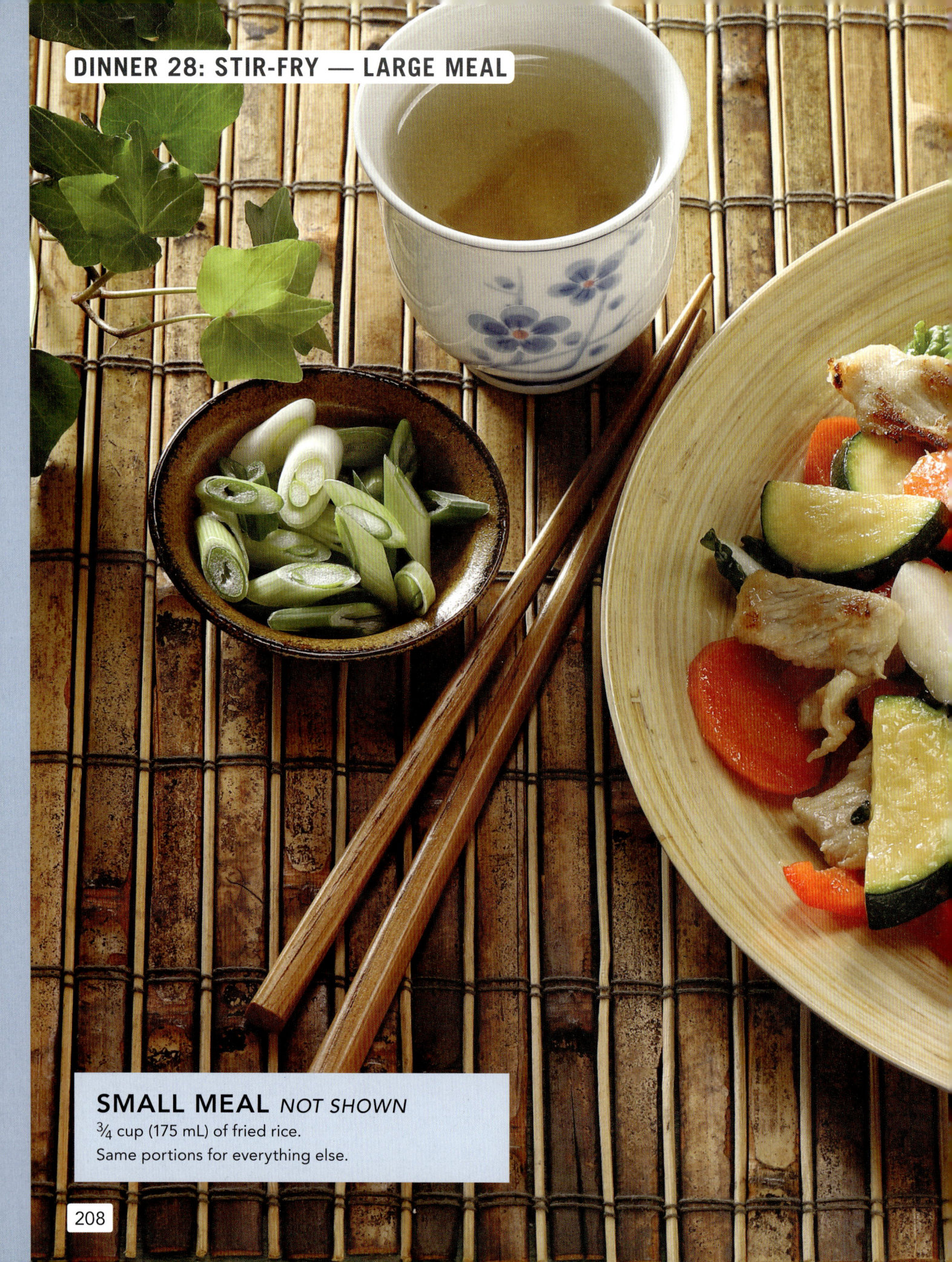

SMALL MEAL *NOT SHOWN*
¾ cup (175 mL) of fried rice.
Same portions for everything else.

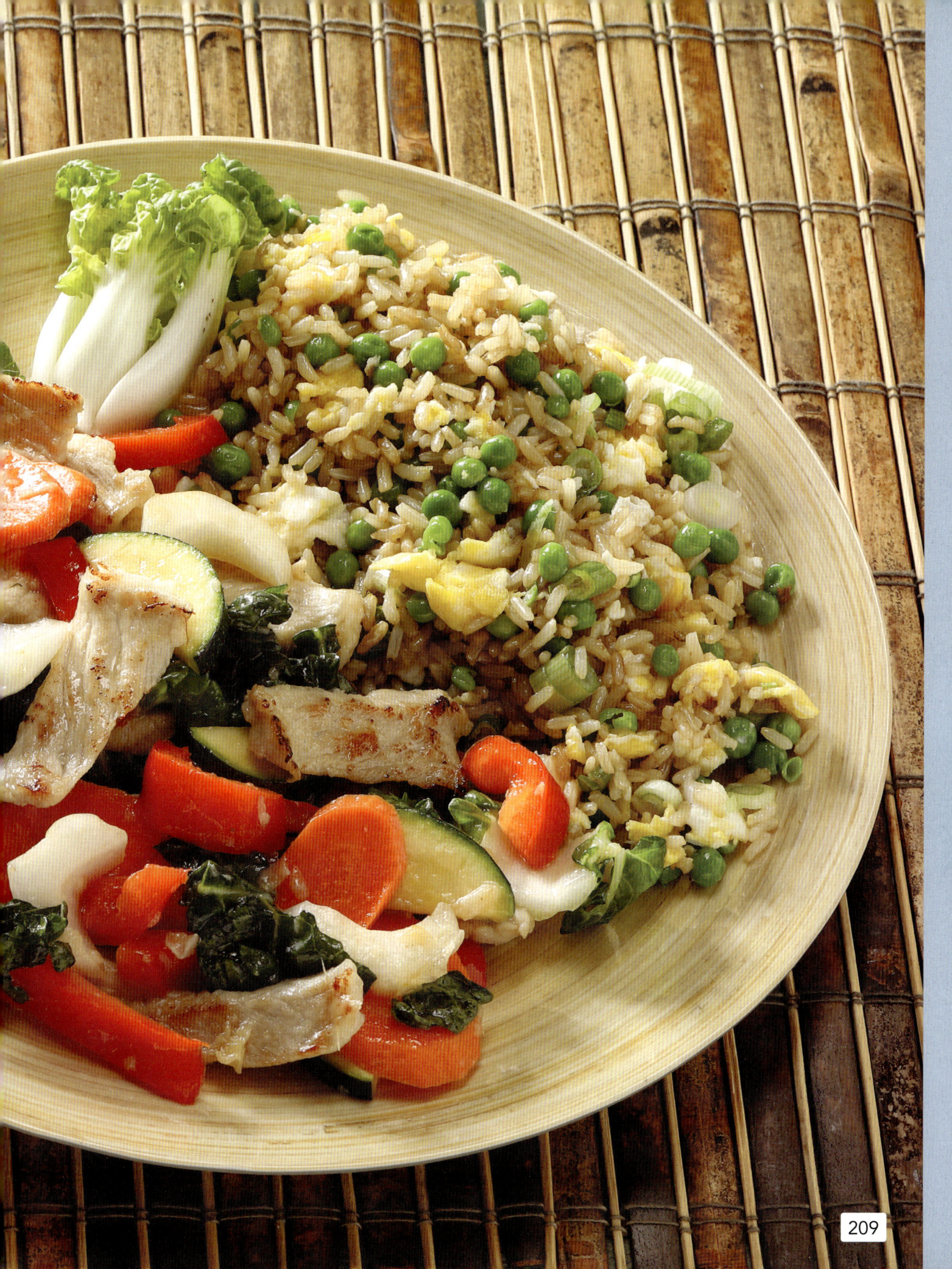

DINNER MEALS

Dinner 29

Denver Sandwich & Soup

This meal includes a Denver Sandwich with a salad, and soup with bread sticks. A Denver sandwich is also known as a Western sandwich. It is always made with scrambled eggs, with additions such as ham or bacon, onion or green pepper.

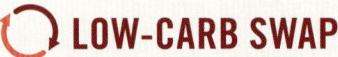
LOW-CARB SWAP

Swap the whole wheat bread (toasted) shown in photo for a bread marked as low-carb.

Swap whole wheat bread:
1 slice
12 g of net carbs
→ For low-carb bread:
1 slice
2 g net carbs

See Bread Swaps, page 274.

Note: Low-carb breads may spoil faster and should be kept in the fridge.

HEALTH TIP

1 cup (250 mL) canned condensed tomato soup prepared with water has about 700 mg sodium; a lower-salt canned-soup version has about one third less sodium.

Denver Sandwich

Makes 1 sandwich

1 slice bacon or 1 oz (30 g) ham, chopped

2 large eggs

1 tbsp (15 mL) green onion tops or chives, chopped

Black pepper to taste

2 slices toast, each spread with 1 tsp (5 mL) margarine or butter, or 2 tsp (10 mL) light mayonnaise

Lettuce

PER SANDWICH	
Calories	397
Carbohydrate	27 g
Fiber	4 g
Net carbs	23 g
Protein	21 g
Fat, total	23 g
Fat, saturated	6 g
Cholesterol	381 mg
Sodium	712 mg

1. In a nonstick pan, fry chopped bacon. Drain off the fat. If you are using chopped ham instead of bacon, you don't need to cook it first.
2. In a small bowl, beat eggs with a fork. Add bacon or ham and green onion tops or chives.
3. Cook in the nonstick pan. Stir on and off.
4. Place egg mixture on the toast.
5. Bulk up the sandwich with lettuce or other vegetables.

Bread Stick Alternatives

(each equals 1 bread stick, with about 4 g net carbs)

- 2 soda crackers
- 1 Ryvita-type snackbread cracker
- 1½ melba toasts
- 2 Ritz-type party crackers

DINNER MEALS

Walking after a meal makes you feel better and helps to bring down your blood sugar.

Your blood sugar goes up after a meal. Taking a short walk an hour or so after eating will help bring down your blood sugar. Even a 10- or 15-minute walk can help bring down your blood sugar and blood pressure after you've eaten.

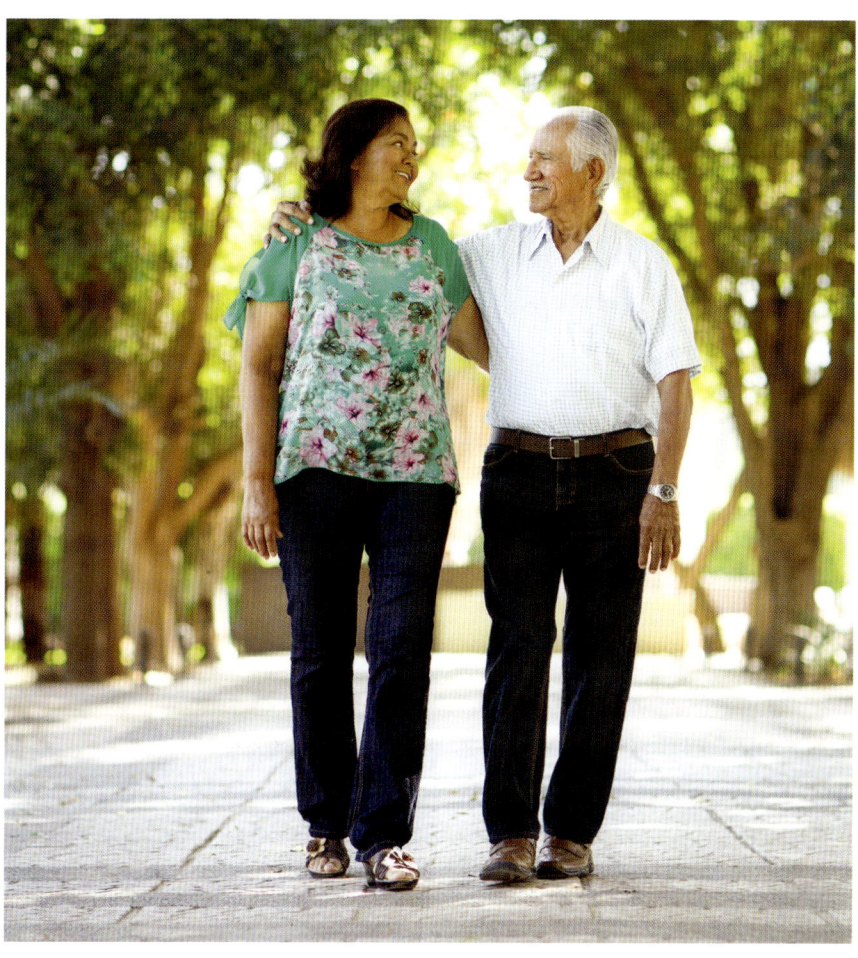

HEALTH TIP

Exercise helps your body's insulin work better for 12 to 24 hours.

YOUR DINNER MENU	Large Meal (730 calories)	Total Carbs	NET CARBS	Small Meal (550 calories)	Total Carbs	NET CARBS
Tomato soup (made with water)	1 cup (250 mL)	17	16	1 cup (250 mL)	17	16
Bread sticks	1½	7	7	1	5	5
Denver Sandwich	1½ sandwiches	40	34	1 sandwich	27	23
Salad	Medium	3	2	Medium	3	2
Ranch salad dressing, light	1 tbsp (15 mL)	4	3	1 tbsp (15 mL)	4	3
	TOTAL CARBS	71 g	62 g	TOTAL CARBS	56 g	49 g
	Total carbs minus fiber = NET CARBS ↑				NET CARBS ↑	
	CARB CHOICES (1 carb choice = 15 g net carbs)		4	CARB CHOICES		3

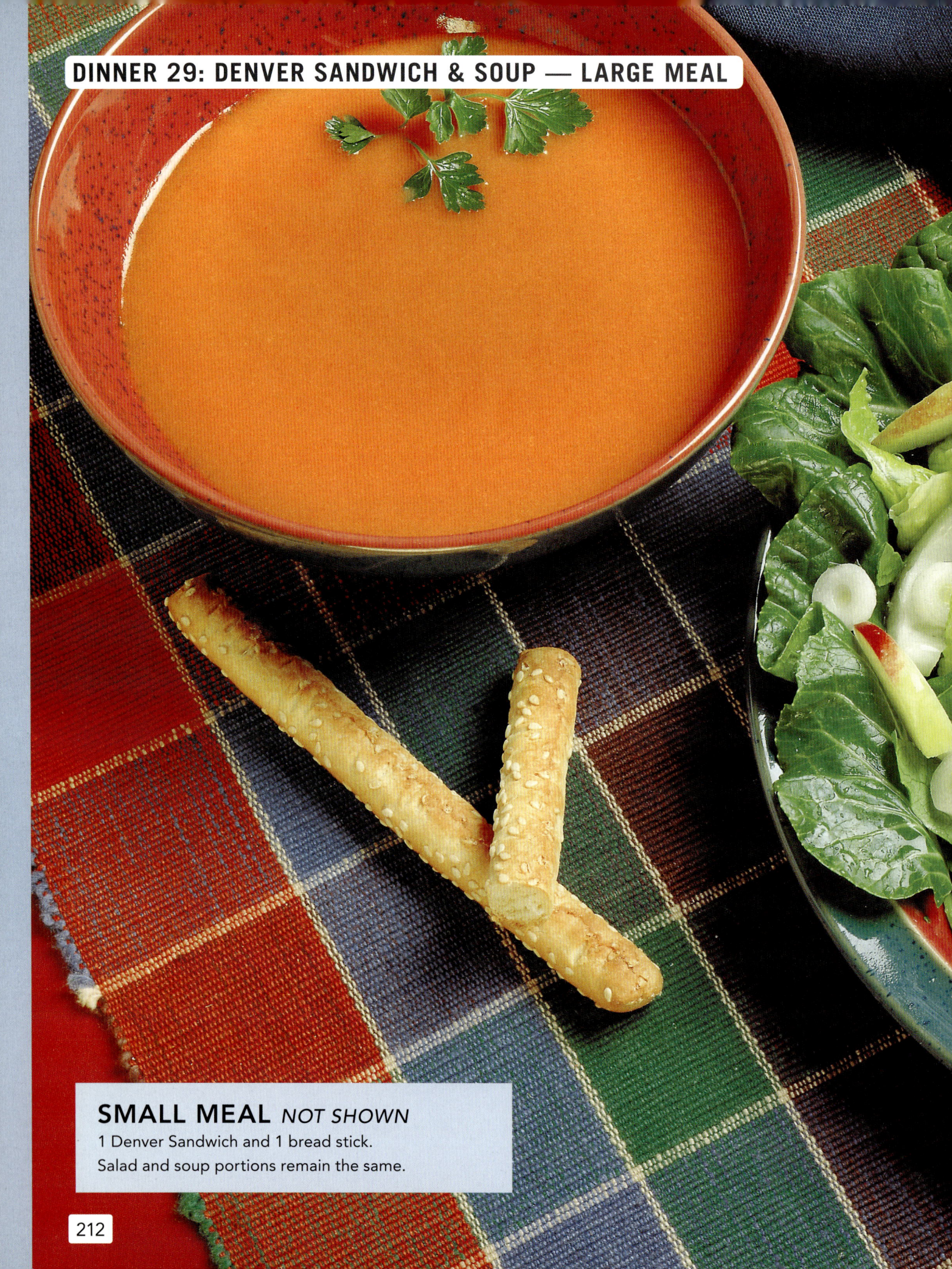

DINNER 29: DENVER SANDWICH & SOUP — LARGE MEAL

SMALL MEAL *NOT SHOWN*
1 Denver Sandwich and 1 bread stick.
Salad and soup portions remain the same.

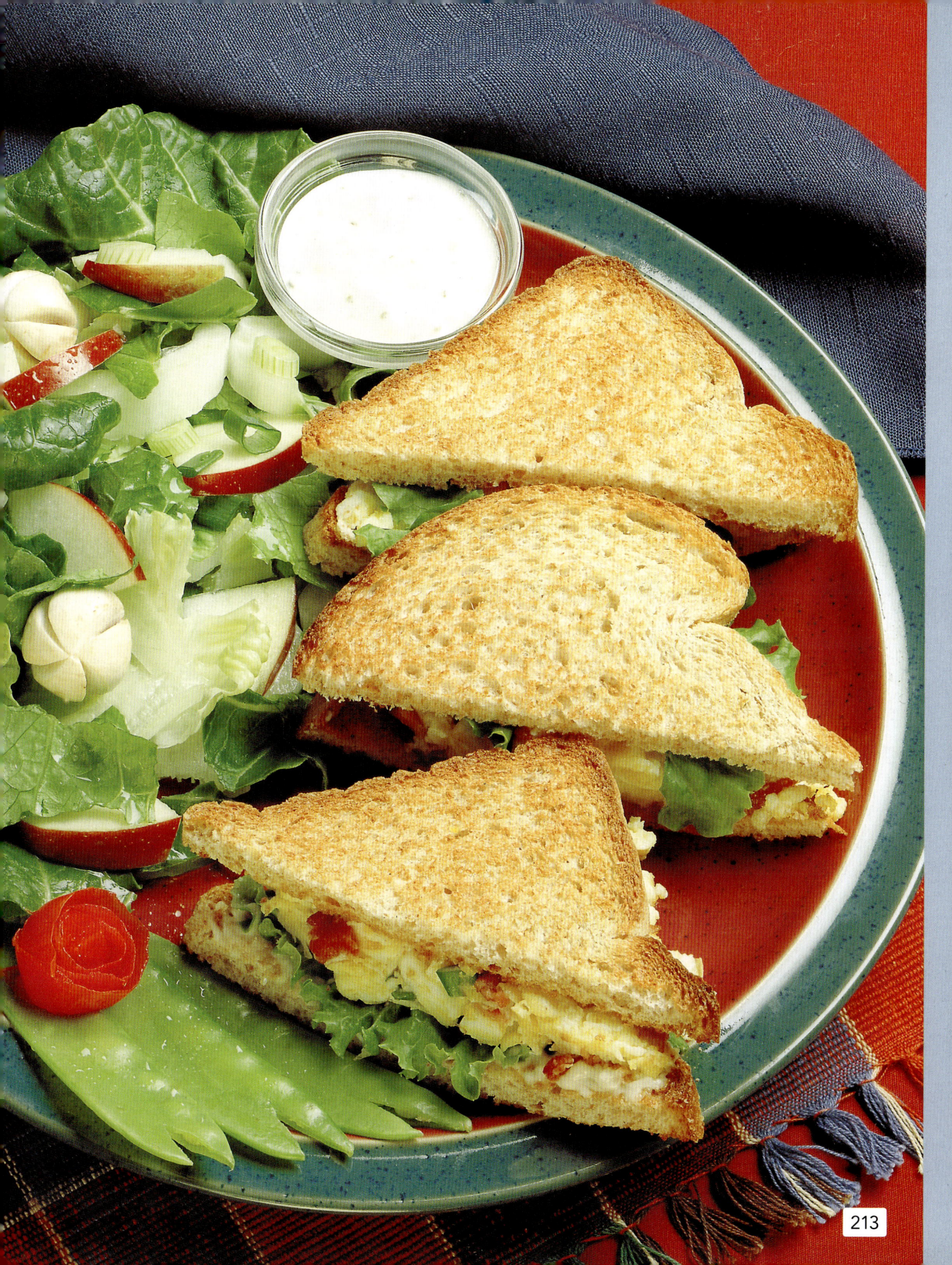

DINNER MEALS

DINNER 30

⟳ LOW-CARB SWAP

LARGE MEAL

Swap cooked white rice, converted:
2/3 cup (150 mL)
28 g net carbs

→ For cooked couscous or quinoa:
2/3 cup (150 mL)
22 g net carbs

SMALL MEAL

Swap cooked white rice, converted:
1/3 cup (75 mL)
14 g net carbs

→ For cooked couscous or quinoa:
1/3 cup (75 mL)
11 g net carbs

See Rice Swaps, page 276.

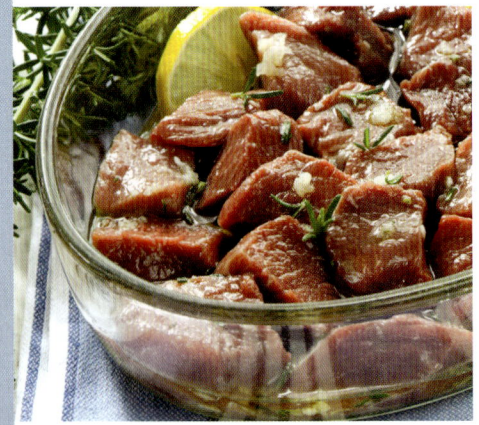

Shish Kebabs

Shish kebabs are cubes of marinated meat placed on skewers and grilled on a barbecue or on a rimmed baking sheet in the oven. With this meal they are served with rice and Greek Salad. Shish kebabs originate in Mediterranean and Middle Eastern countries and are now popular around the world. The key to tasty and tender shish kebabs is to marinate the meat for several hours or overnight.

In our book *Diabetes Essentials*, you'll find another skewered meat recipe: Chicken Souvlaki served with Tzatziki (cucumbers and yogurt).

Shish Kebabs

Makes 2 shish kebabs (2 servings)

12 oz/350 g raw lean beef or lamb, cut into 8 large cubes (or 10 medium cubes), best with a tender cut of meat such as sirloin, sirloin tip or filet

MEAT MARINADE

1 tbsp (15 mL) olive oil
1 tbsp (15 mL) lemon juice
2 tbsp (30 mL) dry wine (or wine vinegar)
1 clove garlic, crushed or finely chopped
1 tsp (5 mL) oregano, dried
1/2 tsp (2 mL) rosemary, dried
1/2 tsp (2 mL) salt
1/4 tsp (1 mL) black pepper

PER SHISH KEBAB	
Calories	272
Carbohydrate	5 g
Fiber	1 g
Net carbs	4 g
Protein	32 g
Fat, total	13 g
Fat, saturated	10 g
Cholesterol	161 mg
Sodium	304 mg

Vegetables: whole fresh mushrooms, chunks of green pepper, whole small onion (or chunks of onion), zucchini, eggplant or any other vegetables you like.

1. Mix the marinade recipe above in a bowl, and stir in the meat. Marinate for several hours or overnight.
2. Soak wooden skewers in water for 30 minutes to prevent them from burning.
3. Preheat barbecue grill to medium.
4. Remove meat cubes from marinade. Thread meat and vegetables on skewers, as shown in the meal photo. Brush veggies with marinade. Discard leftover marinade.
5. Grill kebabs for 5 to 10 minutes or until cooked to desired doneness. Turn skewers occasionally to cook meat on all sides.

DINNER MEALS

Greek Salad

Makes 2 servings

- 2 large tomatoes, cut into wedges
- ½ medium red onion, sliced
- ½ green pepper, cut into chunks
- ½ small cucumber, cut into chunks
- 12 small black olives (or 4 large)
- ¼ cup (60 mL) feta cheese, crumbled or chunks
- 1 tbsp (15 mL) olive oil
- 1 tbsp (15 mL) red wine vinegar
- 1 tsp (5 mL) dried oregano

PER SERVING	
Calories	198
Carbohydrate	16 g
Fiber	4 g
Net carbs	12 g
Protein	5 g
Fat, total	14 g
Fat, saturated	4 g
Cholesterol	17 mg
Sodium	439 mg

HEALTH TIP

If you are having a Greek salad in a restaurant, ask for the salad dressing on the side. Use less than the amount provided.

1. In a large bowl, combine tomatoes, onions, green pepper, cucumber, olives and feta cheese.
2. In a small bowl, whisk together oil, vinegar and oregano. Pour over salad and toss to coat.

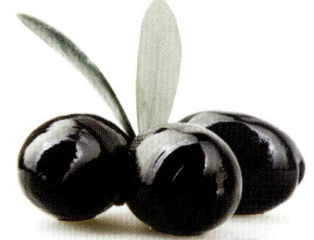

Cinnamon Apple Slices

Apple slices sprinkled with cinnamon and icing sugar add fresh sweetness to the meal. They are also very nice as a dessert after the meal. You can replace the apples with an orange or ½ cup (125 mL) of cantaloupe, melon or grapes.

This meal serving is ½ medium apple with ½ tsp (2 mL) icing sugar plus ground cinnamon.

YOUR DINNER MENU	Large Meal (730 calories)	Total Carbs	NET CARBS	Small Meal (550 calories)	Total Carbs	NET CARBS
Shish Kebab	1 serving	5	4	1 serving	5	4
White or brown rice, converted	⅔ cup (150 mL)	29	28	⅓ cup (75 mL)	14	14
Greek Salad with dressing	1 serving	16	12	1 serving	16	12
Crusty white bun	1	15	14	—	—	—
Butter or margarine	1 tsp (5 mL)	0	0	—	—	—
Cinnamon Apple Slices	1 serving	12	11	1 serving	12	11
	TOTAL CARBS	77 g	69 g	**TOTAL CARBS**	47 g	41 g
	Total carbs minus fiber = NET CARBS ↑			NET CARBS ↑		
	CARB CHOICES (1 carb choice = 15 g net carbs)		5	CARB CHOICES		3

DINNER 30: SHISH KEBABS — LARGE MEAL

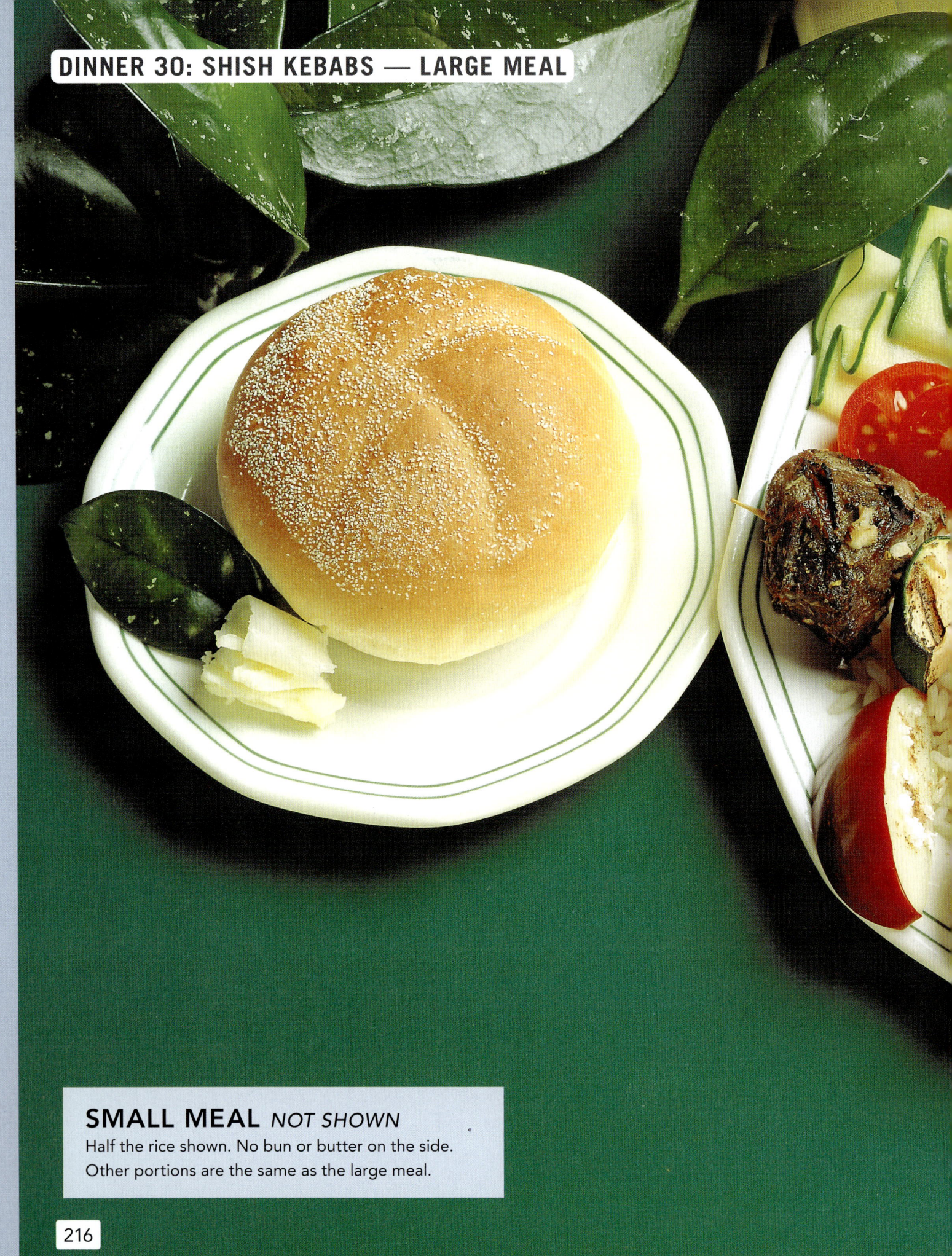

SMALL MEAL *NOT SHOWN*
Half the rice shown. No bun or butter on the side.
Other portions are the same as the large meal.

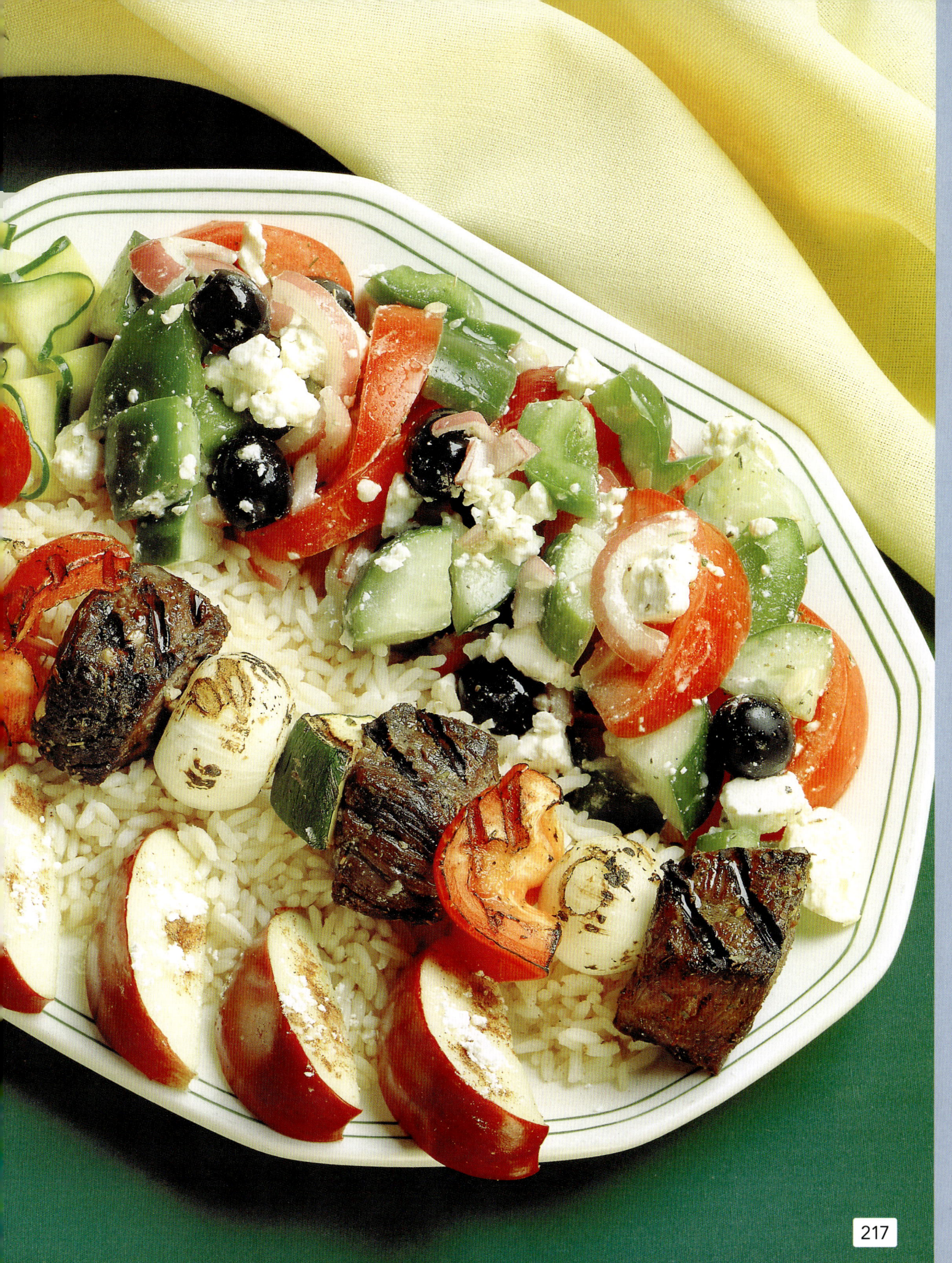

Dinner 31

Tandoori Chicken & Rice

Tandoori chicken is a traditional meal from India that has become a world favorite. The chicken is marinated overnight which sets the flavor in the meat.

Tandoori Chicken and Sauce

Makes 5 servings and 1 cup (250 mL) cooked sauce

Preheat oven to 350°F (180°C)

TANDOORI SAUCE

- 1½ cups (375 mL) Greek yogurt, 0–2%, plain
- 1½ tbsp (22 mL) tandoori spice mix (or curry powder)
- 1½ tbsp (22 mL) vinegar
- 1½ tbsp (22 mL) lemon juice

2½ lbs (1 kg) chicken pieces (weight with bones and skin), skin removed; this equals 5 large legs (as shown) or 12 drumsticks

1. In a large casserole dish, mix all the marinade ingredients.
2. Make small cuts in each chicken piece; this allows the marinade to flavor throughout the meat. Place the chicken in the dish and cover with marinade. Cover the dish and refrigerate overnight.
3. The next day, remove the chicken and brush off extra sauce into a small pot for cooking. Lay the chicken on parchment paper on a rimmed baking sheet.
4. Bake for 45 minutes until done.
5. The last step is to broil the chicken for a couple of minutes on each side to give that charred look and flavor.
6. The marinade that held the raw chicken will need to be brought to a boil on the stove and cooked for a full 5 minutes before it is safe to eat. The cooked marinade is like gravy that can be served on rice or as a side for dipping the chicken.

Poppadoms (papadums)

Cook without oil: grill or microwave according to package directions.

PER 1 TBSP (15 ML) SAUCE	
Calories	18
Carbohydrate	1 g
Fiber	0 g
Net carbs	1 g
Protein	2 g
Fat, total	1 g
Fat, saturated	0 g
Cholesterol	2 mg
Sodium	8 mg

⟳ LOW-CARB SWAP

Swap basmati rice with Cilantro Riced Cauliflower (see below). Or do a half-and-half blend of rice and cauliflower.

CILANTRO RICED CAULIFLOWER

Add 2 tsp (10 mL) oil to frying pan and heat to sizzling. Then add 1 finely chopped clove of garlic, ¼ tsp (1 mL) ground cumin, 2 tbsp (30 mL) chopped cilantro and 2 cups (500 mL) frozen riced cauliflower. At medium heat, stir quickly until heated.

Add the yummy Tandoori Sauce, and you will hardly notice you've swapped cauliflower for rice.

LARGE MEAL

Swap cooked basmati rice: ¾ cup (175 mL)
33 g net carbs
→ For Cilantro Riced Cauliflower: 1 cup (250 mL)
3 g net carbs

SMALL MEAL

Swap cooked basmati rice: ½ cup (125 mL)
22 g net carbs
→ For Cilantro Riced Cauliflower: 1 cup (250 mL)
3 g net carbs

See Rice Swaps, page 276.

Chai Latte

Makes five 1-cup (250 mL) servings

2 chai tea bags

4 cups (1 L) boiling water

1¼ cups (310 mL) hot 3.25% milk

PER 1 CUP (250 ML)	
Calories	40
Carbohydrate	3 g
Fiber	0 g
Net carbs	3 g
Protein	2 g
Fat, total	2 g
Fat, saturated	1 g
Cholesterol	7 mg
Sodium	27 mg

1. Place tea bags in a teapot. Add boiling water and let them steep for 4 minutes.
2. Heat the milk on the stove, or in the microwave, or in a milk steamer.
3. Remove the tea bags from the teapot and add the hot milk.
4. Sweeten with zero-calorie sweetener. If using honey or sugar, limit to 1 tsp (5 mL) per cup.

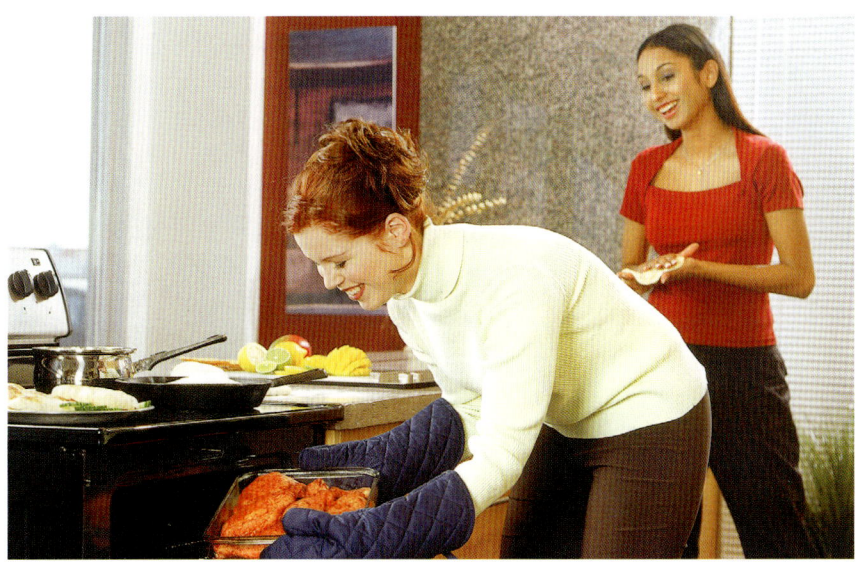

YOUR DINNER MENU	Large Meal (730 calories)	Total Carbs	NET CARBS	Small Meal (550 calories)	Total Carbs	NET CARBS
Tandoori Chicken	1 large leg	0	0	1 large leg	0	0
Tandoori Sauce	4 tbsp (60 mL)	5	5	2 tbsp (30 mL)	3	3
Rice (basmati)	¾ cup (175 mL)	34	33	½ cup (120 mL)	22	22
Lettuce, tomato and cucumber	As desired	3	2	As desired	3	2
Poppadoms	2	10	8	2	10	8
Mango	½ medium	17	15	½ medium	17	15
Chai Latte	1 cup (250 mL)	3	3	1 cup (250 mL)	3	3
	TOTAL CARBS	72 g	66 g	TOTAL CARBS	58 g	53 g
	Total carbs minus fiber = NET CARBS ↑			NET CARBS ↑		
	CARB CHOICES (1 carb choice = 15 g net carbs)		4	CARB CHOICES		3

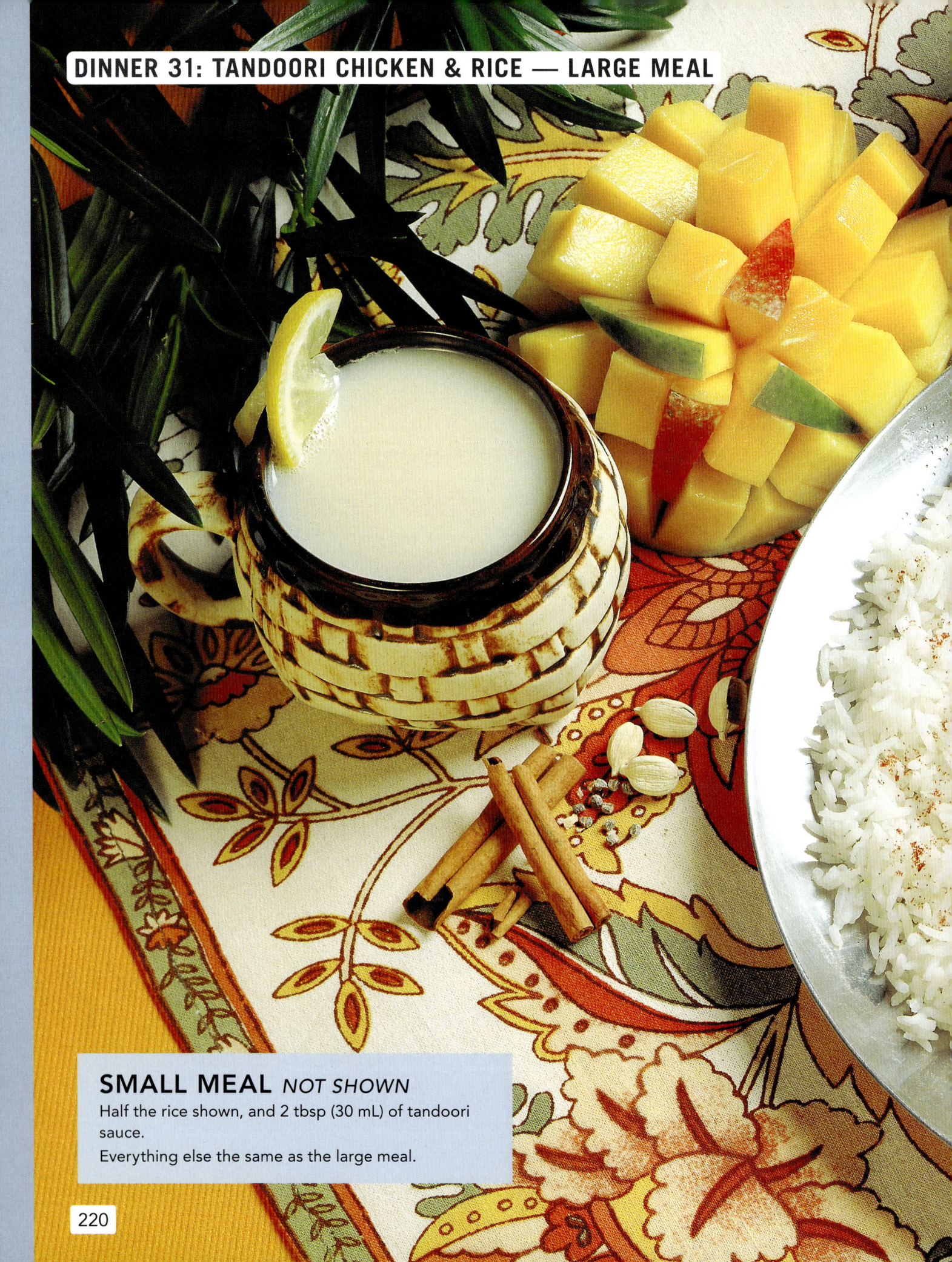

DINNER 31: TANDOORI CHICKEN & RICE — LARGE MEAL

SMALL MEAL *NOT SHOWN*

Half the rice shown, and 2 tbsp (30 mL) of tandoori sauce.

Everything else the same as the large meal.

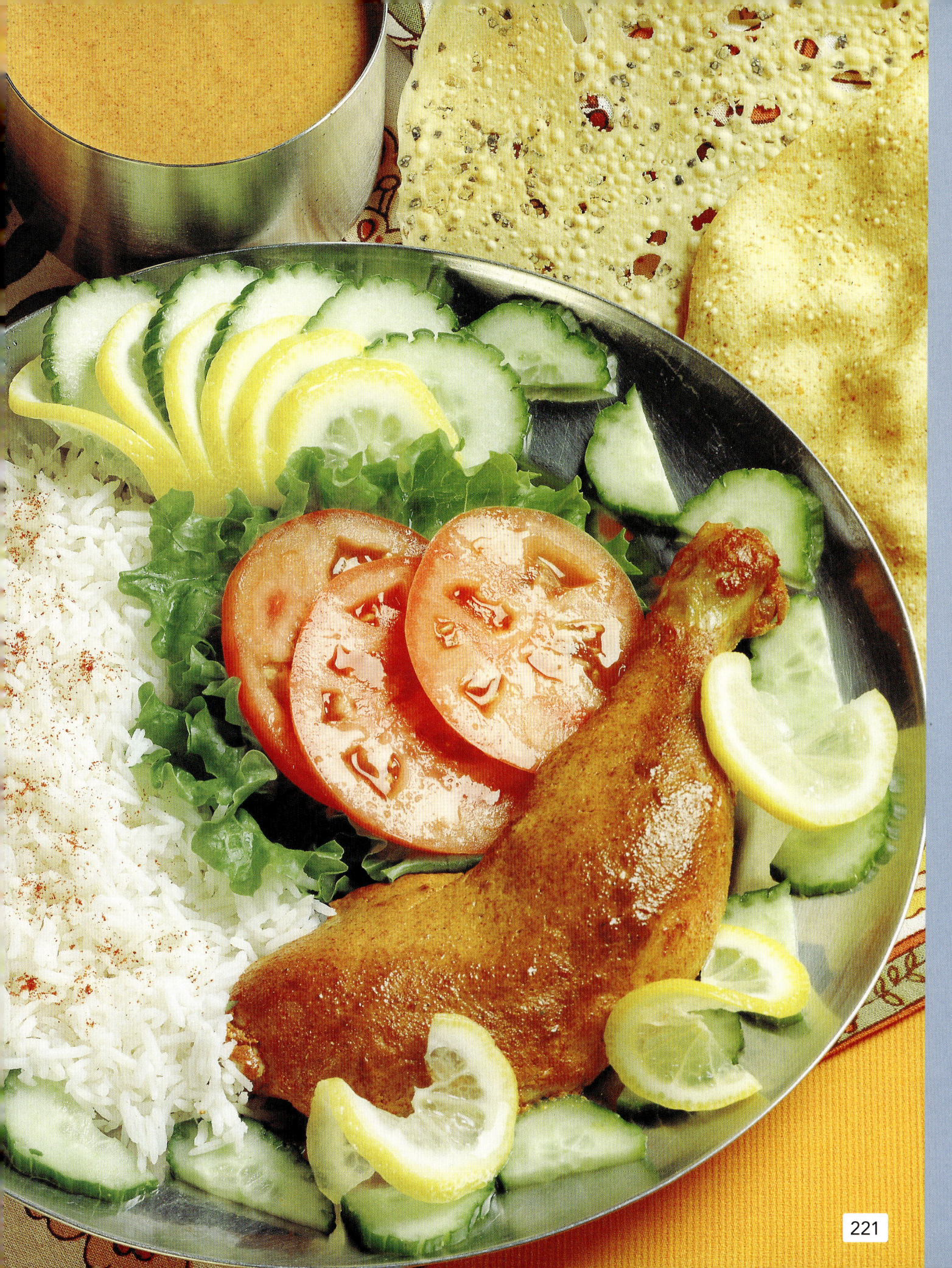

DINNER MEALS

DINNER 32

Swiss Steak

This old family recipe for Swiss Steak has been adapted to have less butter and to use a dry wine. It is made with sirloin tip steak and is so tender, it gets rave reviews every time.

Grandma's Swiss Steak

Makes 6 servings

Preheat oven to 325°F (160°C)

- 3 lbs (1.5 kg) sirloin tip steaks
- 1 tsp (5 mL) Hy's Seasoning Salt
- ¼ tsp (1 mL) black pepper
- 2 tbsp (30 mL) butter
- 1 large onion, chopped or sliced
- 5 cups (1.25 L) washed and sliced fresh mushrooms
- 1 tbsp (15 mL) butter
- ¼ cup (60 mL) dry red or white wine
- ¾ cup (175 mL) water

PER LARGE SERVING (⅙ OF RECIPE)	
Calories	324
Carbohydrate	5 g
Fiber	1 g
Net carbs	4 g
Protein	47 g
Fat, total	11 g
Fat, saturated	5 g
Cholesterol	121 mg
Sodium	361 mg

1. Pound the steak on both sides with a meat pounder (or use the edge of a small plate to flatten the meat). Trim off visible fat. Poke holes in the meat with a fork. Cut the meat into pieces the size of a deck of cards or smaller. Place meat on a baking sheet.
2. Sprinkle Hy's Seasoning Salt and pepper on both sides of the meat, and rub it in with the back of a spoon.
3. In a large, heavy pan or nonstick frying pan, fry onions and mushrooms in the 2 tbsp (30 mL) of butter until the onions are soft. Set aside in a bowl.
4. Add another 1 tbsp (15 mL) of butter to the pan, and fry the seasoned meat on medium, browning both sides.
5. Move the meat to a casserole dish (or roasting pan) and cover with wine, cooked onions and mushrooms.
6. Add the water to the frying pan to stir up any brown bits and seasoning, then add this meat juice to the casserole.
7. Put the lid on the casserole and bake the steak in the oven for 2 hours, or longer, until it is fork-tender. Add a small amount of water as necessary to keep the meat cooking in juice.

Serve the Swiss Steak with boiled potatoes, peas and carrots, and red pepper strips, either roasted or fresh.

RECIPE TIP

Tenderizing steak

Swiss Steak recipes involve tenderizing and slow-cooking. This recipe is tenderized by pounding the meat and adding seasoning salt and wine.

Some Swiss Steak recipes use a lower-cost meat, such as round steak, and may include tomatoes which have acid that helps to break down the tough muscle fibers.

RECIPE TIP

Seasoning for steak

One important tenderizing and flavor-enhancing ingredient in this recipe is the Hy's Seasoning Salt, a Canadian favorite. Of course, you can always substitute your own favorite steak seasoning salt.

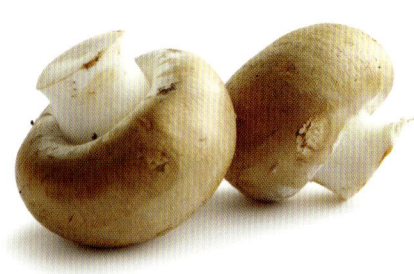

DINNER MEALS

Roasted Pepper Strips

Cut whole peppers in half and remove seeds. Place the cut side down on a baking sheet and grill for 5 to 8 minutes, until the skin chars and blackens. Then place in a Ziploc or small paper bag and let them sit for a few minutes. Peel off the blackened skin and cut the peppers into strips.

This recipe does not use oil or spices. It is a bit messy, but these soft and sweet-tasting pepper strips are worth it.

Lemon Pear-fection

Makes 1 serving

3 small (or 2 medium) canned pear halves, with 3 tbsp (45 mL) of Lemon Sauce

LEMON SAUCE (ENOUGH FOR 4 SERVINGS)

¾ cup (175 mL) pear juice (remaining juice in a 14 oz/398 mL can)

1 tbsp (15 mL) cornstarch

1 tsp (5 mL) lemon zest and 1 tbsp (15 mL) lemon juice (from ½ lemon)

1 tbsp (15 mL) sugar

PER SERVING	
Calories	88
Carbohydrate	23 g
Fiber	2 g
Net carbs	21 g
Protein	0 g
Fat, total	0 g
Fat, saturated	0 g
Cholesterol	0 mg
Sodium	7 mg

⟲ LOW-CARB SWAP

Swap Lemon Pear-fection: 1 serving
20 g net carbs
→ For fresh pear with pecans or walnuts: ½ pear with 4 pecan or walnut halves
11 g net carbs

1. Place pear halves in a dessert dish.
2. Pour pear juice into a small pot. Add cornstarch and blend well with a whisk so there are no lumps. Add lemon zest, lemon juice and sugar, and mix.
3. With the pot on medium heat, stir constantly until the lemon sauce has thickened and the color has lightened.
4. Pour 3 tbsp (45 mL) of the warm Lemon Sauce over the pears, and serve immediately.

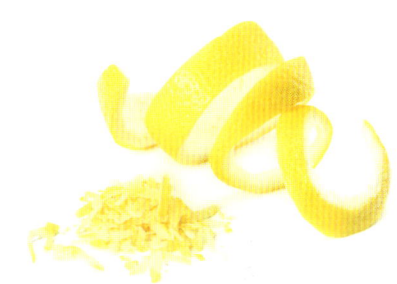

YOUR DINNER MENU	Large Meal (730 calories)	Total Carbs	NET CARBS	Small Meal (550 calories)	Total Carbs	NET CARBS
Grandma's Swiss Steak	1 serving = 4 oz (125 g) steak, plus sauce	5	4	1 serving = 4 oz (125 g) steak, plus sauce	5	4
Boiled potatoes	7 mini	33	31	4 mini	19	18
Margarine or butter	1 tsp (5 mL)	0	0	—	—	—
Peas and carrots	¾ cup (175 mL)	12	8	¾ cup (175 mL)	12	8
Red pepper, roasted or fresh	6 strips	2	2	6 strips	2	2
Almond beverage	1 cup (250 mL)	1	0	1 cup (250 mL)	1	0
Lemon Pear-fection	3 small pear halves + 3 tbsp (45 mL) sauce	22	20	3 small pear halves + 3 tbsp (45 mL) sauce	22	20
	TOTAL CARBS	**75 g**	**65 g**	**TOTAL CARBS**	**61 g**	**52 g**
	Total carbs minus fiber = NET CARBS ↑			NET CARBS ↑		
	CARB CHOICES (1 carb choice = 15 g net carbs)		4	CARB CHOICES		3

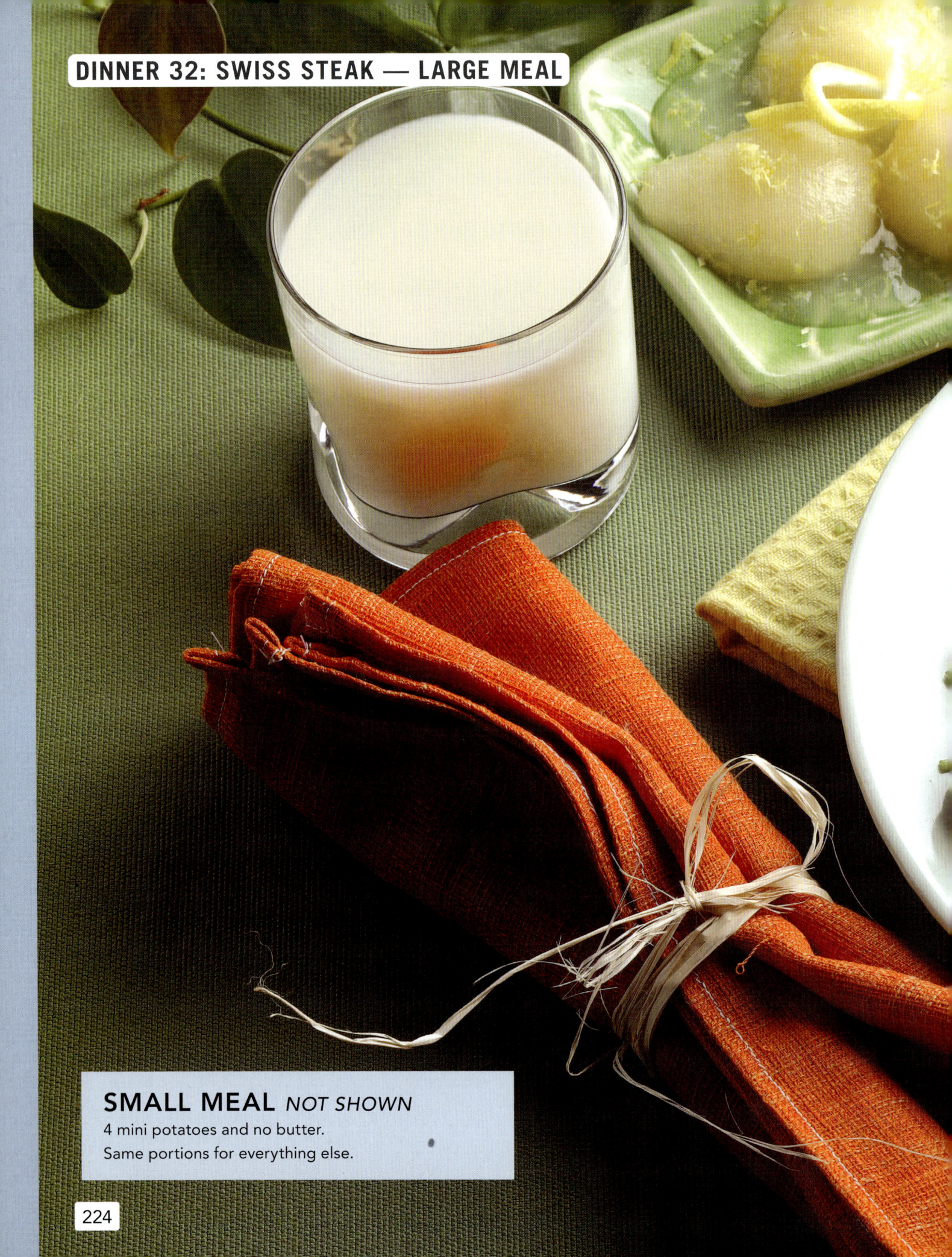

DINNER 32: SWISS STEAK — LARGE MEAL

SMALL MEAL *NOT SHOWN*
4 mini potatoes and no butter.
Same portions for everything else.

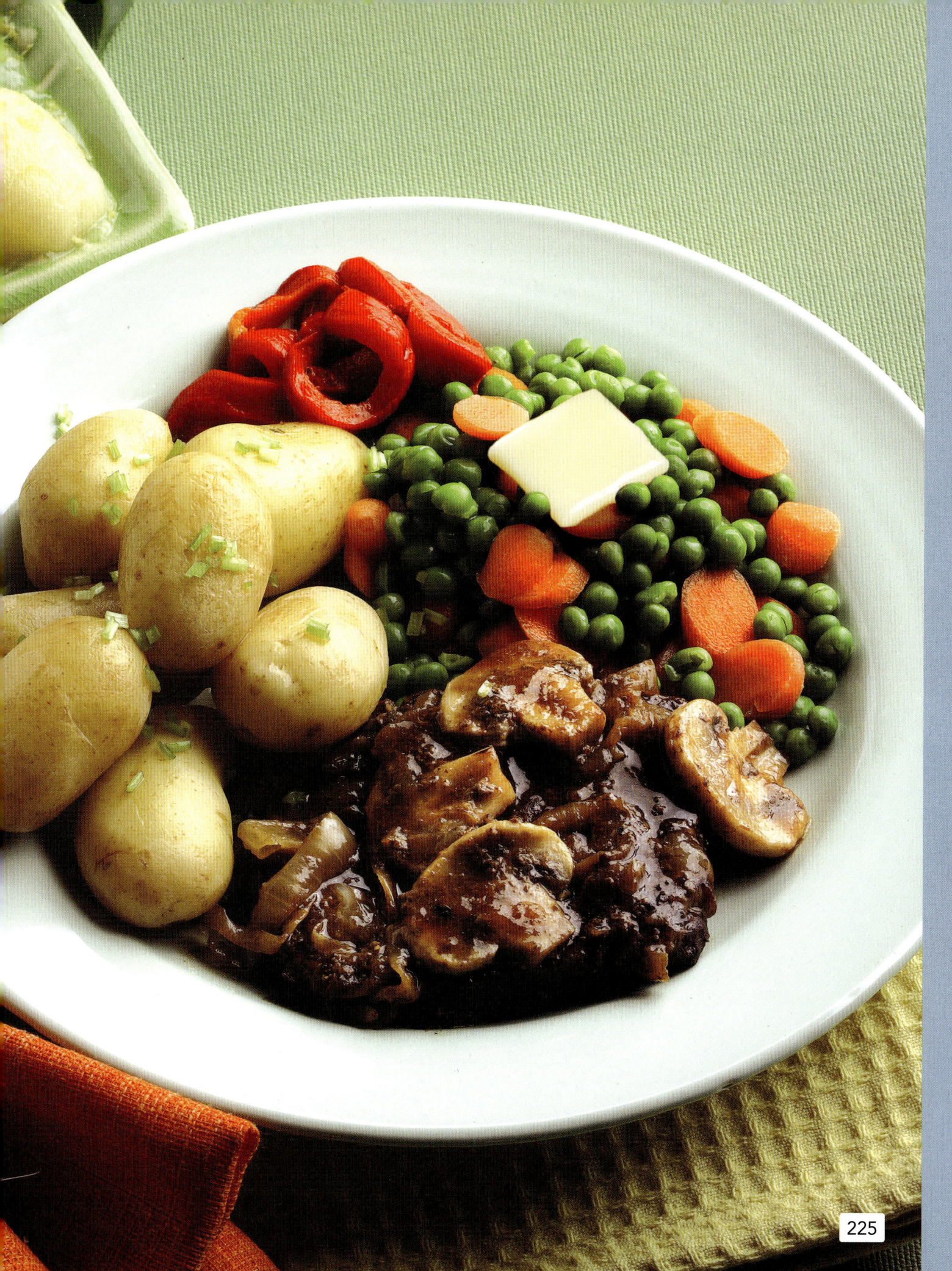

DINNER MEALS

DINNER 33

Thai Chicken

The chicken is cooked in water and not with the traditional method using oil. The cornstarch thickens the sauce, so it's a one-pan chicken meal. If you like peanut butter, you'll enjoy this pleasant mix of flavors. Complete this meal with a fresh spinach salad that is balanced with red onion and fresh fruit.

Thai Chicken

Makes 4 cups (1 L) (4 large or 5 small servings)

- 7 chicken thighs or 4 medium chicken breasts, skin, fat and bones removed, cut into chunks or strips
- 1 small onion, chopped
- 2 tbsp (30 mL) water
- ¾ cup (175 mL) salsa (mild or hot)
- 2 tbsp (30 mL) chopped fresh cilantro
- 3 tbsp (45 mL) peanut butter
- 1 tbsp (15 mL) oyster sauce
- 1 cup (250 mL) skim (non-fat) evaporated canned milk
- 1 tsp (5 mL) cornstarch
- Cilantro or lime wedges, for garnish

1. In a large nonstick frying pan, add the water, chicken pieces and onions. Stir over medium heat until there is no pink inside the chicken.
2. In one bowl, mix the salsa, cilantro, peanut butter and oyster sauce.
3. In another bowl, whisk the cornstarch into the evaporated milk until well blended.
4. Then add the salsa mixture to the cooked chicken, followed by the milk mixture. Stir until the sauce boils and thickens.

PER 1 CUP (250 ML)	
Calories	302
Carbohydrate	15 g
Fiber	2 g
Net carbs	13 g
Protein	32 g
Fat, total	12 g
Fat, saturated	3 g
Cholesterol	87 mg
Sodium	474 mg

LOW-CARB SWAP

Swap cooked rice noodles:
⅓ cup (75 mL)
20 g net carbs

→ For konjac noodles:
⅓ cup (75 mL)
0 g net carbs

OR

→ For edamame (soybean) spaghetti:
⅓ cup (75 mL)
6 g net carbs

Double portions for the large meal.

See Pasta Swaps, page 275.

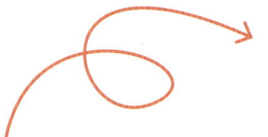

Konjac noodles are a low-carb swap for rice noodles.

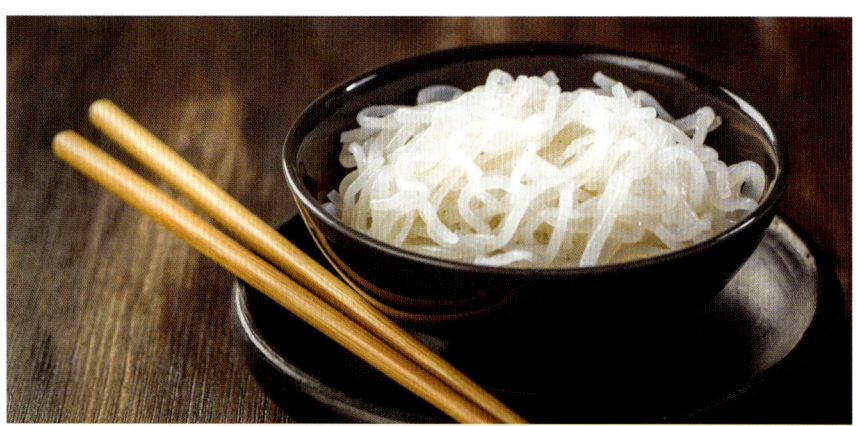

DINNER MEALS

Poppy Seed Spinach Salad

Makes 2 servings

⅓ of a 10 oz (300 g) bag of fresh washed spinach

1 medium tomato, cut in wedges

½ cup (125 mL) sliced fresh strawberries or other fruit

2 tbsp (30 mL) sliced almonds, toasted

¼ small red onion, sliced into rings

Sprinkle of poppy seeds

PER SERVING	
Calories	70
Carbohydrate	8 g
Fiber	4 g
Net carbs	4 g
Protein	3 g
Fat, total	4 g
Fat, saturated	0 g
Cholesterol	0 mg
Sodium	39 mg

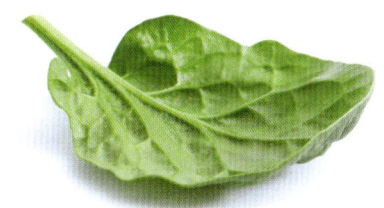

1. Wash spinach and arrange in two salad bowls.
2. Place the other ingredients on top of the spinach.

Sour Cream and Fruit

Makes 2 servings

1 cup (250 mL) fresh fruit, or canned fruit, drained

1 tbsp (15 mL) zero-calorie sweetener, brown sugar replacement

¼ tsp (1 mL) cinnamon

⅓ cup (75 mL) sour cream, 5%

PER SERVING	
Calories	89
Carbohydrate	12 g
Fiber	2 g
Net carbs	10 g
Protein	2 g
Fat, total	2 g
Fat, saturated	1 g
Cholesterol	7 mg
Sodium	40 mg

HEALTH TIP

Healthy desserts

Fruit-based dessert is not just a sweet treat to end a meal: it contributes to your day's nutrition.

1. Divide the fruit into two dessert dishes.
2. Mix the sweetener, cinnamon and sour cream, and place on the fruit.
3. For a change, use oven-safe bowls and grill your dessert until caramelized on top.

YOUR DINNER MENU	Large Meal (730 calories)	Total Carbs	NET CARBS	Small Meal (550 calories)	Total Carbs	NET CARBS
Thai Chicken	1 cup (250 mL)	15	13	¾ cup (175 mL)	11	10
Rice noodles, cooked	⅔ cup (150 mL)	28	26	⅓ cup (75 mL)	21	20
Poppy Seed Spinach Salad	1 serving	8	4	1 serving	8	4
Creamy poppy seed salad dressing	2 tbsp (30 mL)	8	8	1 tbsp (15 mL)	4	4
Sour Cream and Fruit	1 serving	18	10	1 serving	18	10
	TOTAL CARBS	77 g	61 g	TOTAL CARBS	62 g	48 g
	Total carbs minus fiber = NET CARBS ↑			NET CARBS ↑		
	CARB CHOICES (1 carb choice = 15 g net carbs)		4	CARB CHOICES		3

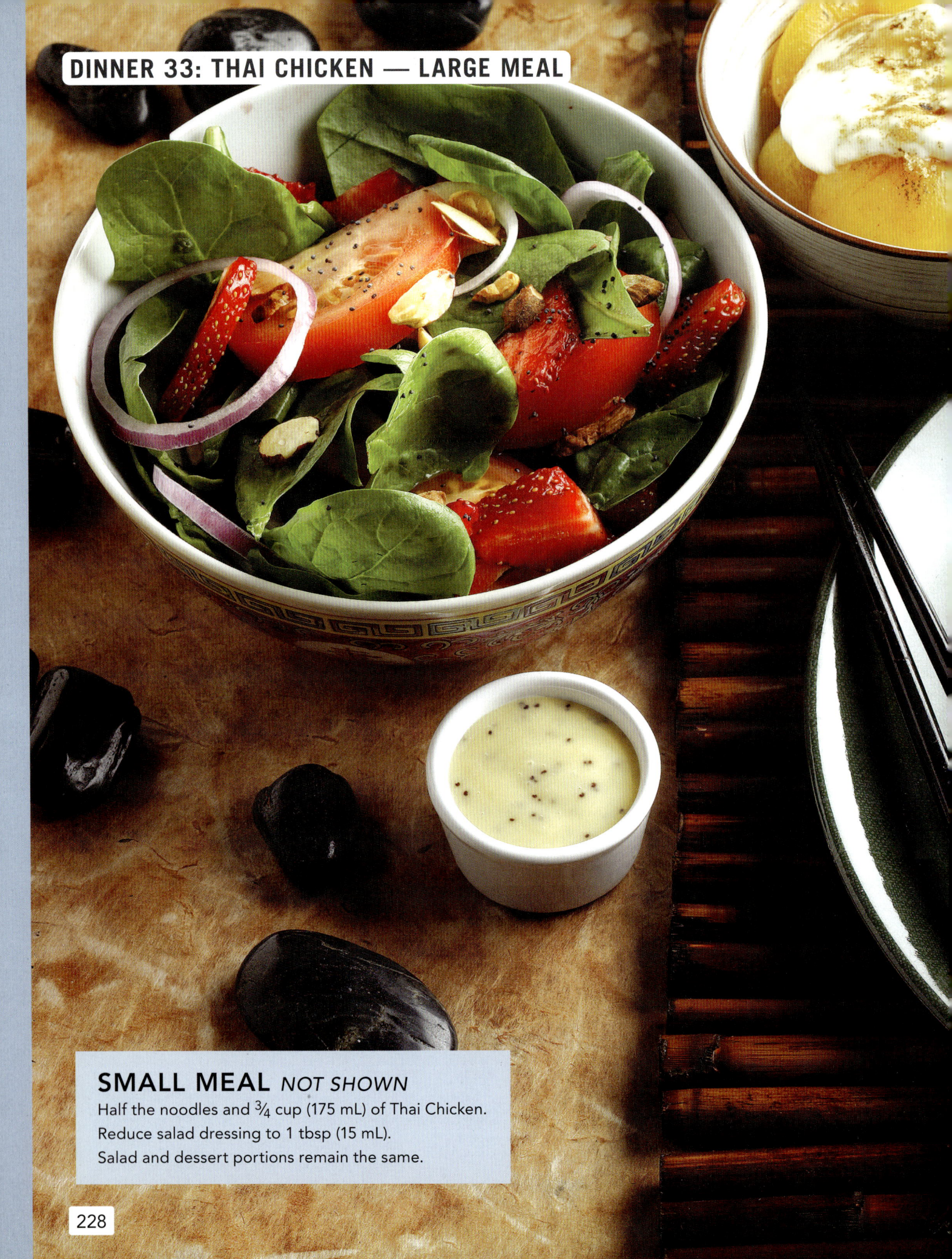

DINNER 33: THAI CHICKEN — LARGE MEAL

SMALL MEAL *NOT SHOWN*
Half the noodles and ¾ cup (175 mL) of Thai Chicken.
Reduce salad dressing to 1 tbsp (15 mL).
Salad and dessert portions remain the same.

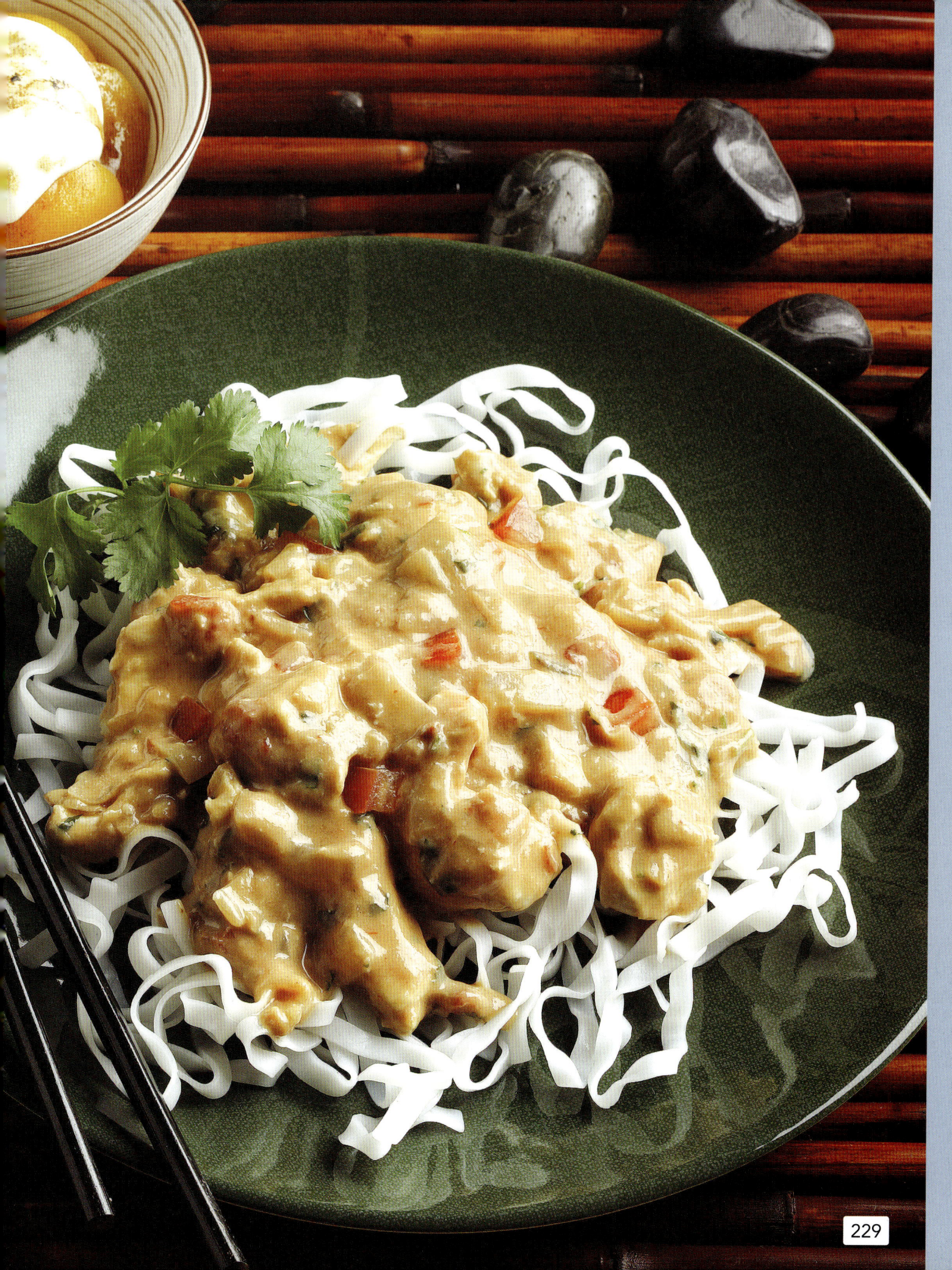

DINNER MEALS

DINNER 34

HEALTH TIP

For a list of low-fat and high-fat fish, see page 106.

Poached Salmon with Dill

This meal is a combination of omega-3 oil-rich fish spruced up with tangy pickled beets and green beans. In addition, the Walnut Barley Medley adds crunchy nut texture and sweet currants for a savory blend of flavors. Enjoy the glass of milk with your meal or as part of your dessert.

How to poach fish

Poaching means to simmer at a low temperature in water, low-salt broth or milk. The fluid is usually flavored with lemon juice or white wine, along with peppercorns, garlic, cloves and bay leaves.

1. Bring a pan of water with flavorings to a gentle simmer and place the fish in, skin-side down. The water should just cover the fish.
2. Cover with a lid and let it continue to simmer for 5 to 10 minutes, until fish is white, firm and flaky.
3. Remove fish with a slotted spoon.

Dill Topping

Makes ¼ cup (60 mL)

¼ cup (60 mL) low-fat/light mayonnaise

1 tsp (5 mL) dried dill or 1 tbsp (15 mL) finely chopped fresh dill

1. Combine ingredients, and serve with the fish.

PER 1 TBSP (15 ML)	
Calories	13
Carbohydrate	2 g
Fiber	0 g
Net carbs	2 g
Protein	0 g
Fat, total	0 g
Fat, saturated	0 g
Cholesterol	1 mg
Sodium	126 mg

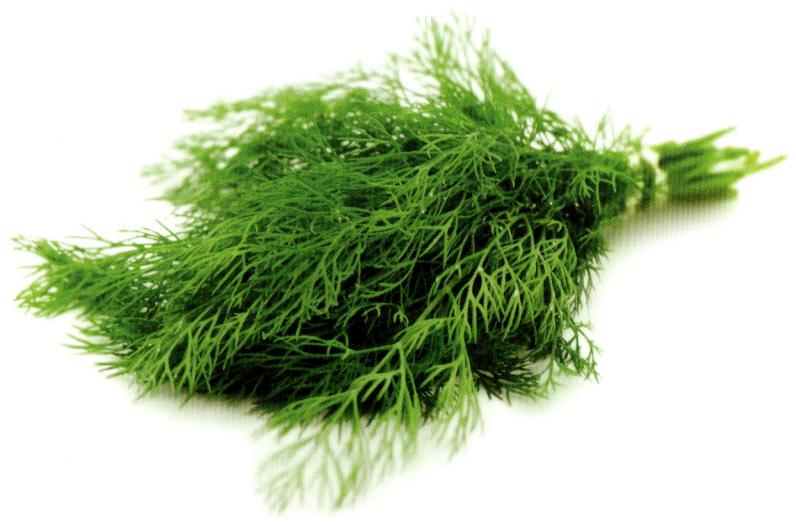

DINNER MEALS

You can cook the Walnut Barley Medley a day ahead and keep it covered in the fridge. This helps enrich the flavors. The next day, reheat in the microwave for dinner. This dish is also tasty eaten cold.

Walnut Barley Medley

Makes 2½ cups (625 mL)

½ cup (125 mL) pot barley
1 tbsp (15 mL) wild rice
1 packet (4.5 g) reduced-salt beef or chicken bouillon powder
1½ cups (375 mL) water
¼ cup (60 mL) chopped walnuts
¼ cup (60 mL) currants

PER ½ CUP (125 ML)	
Calories	138
Carbohydrate	24 g
Fiber	3 g
Net carbs	21 g
Protein	4 g
Fat, total	4 g
Fat, saturated	1 g
Cholesterol	0 mg
Sodium	108 mg

1. In a small pot over medium-high heat, bring barley, wild rice, bouillon and water to a boil. As soon as it boils, reduce the heat to low, cover with a lid and simmer for 1 hour, until the liquid has been absorbed. It will still be slightly moist.
2. Once the barley is cooked, stir in walnuts and currants. Remove from the heat and serve, or refrigerate for the next day.

Cookies for Dessert (Large Meal)

Look for cookies that are labeled as about 100 calories for three cookies. These cookies will be thinner or smaller than super-sized bakery cookies.

HEALTH TIP
Benefits of barley

Barley is rich in soluble fiber, which helps absorb the bad cholesterol from your bloodstream. Soluble fiber also helps to slow the absorption of carbohydrates into your blood. Pot barley is higher in soluble fiber and has a lower glycemic index (GI) than pearl barley or quick-cooking barley.

↻ LOW-CARB SWAP

LARGE MEAL

Swap thin cookies:
2 cookies
8 g net carbs

→ For a serving of light gelatin:
0 g net carbs

SMALL MEAL

Light gelatin can also be part of the small meal.

YOUR DINNER MENU	Large Meal (730 calories)	Total Carbs	NET CARBS	Small Meal (550 calories)	Total Carbs	NET CARBS
Poached Salmon	3½ oz (105 g)	0	0	3½ oz (105 g)	0	0
Dill Topping	2 tbsp (30 mL)	4	4	2 tbsp (30 mL)	4	4
Walnut Barley Medley	¾ cup (175 mL)	37	33	½ cup (125 mL)	24	21
Green beans	1 cup (250 mL)	10	6	1 cup (250 mL)	10	6
Margarine	1 tsp (5 mL)	0	0	—	—	—
Pickled beets	½ cup (125 mL)	13	12	½ cup (125 mL)	13	12
Skim or 1% milk	¾ cup (175 mL)	9	9	¾ cup (175 mL)	9	9
Thin cookies	2	8	8	—	—	—
	TOTAL CARBS	81 g	72 g	**TOTAL CARBS**	60 g	52 g
	Total carbs minus fiber = NET CARBS ↑			NET CARBS ↑		
	CARB CHOICES (1 carb choice = 15 g net carbs)		5	CARB CHOICES		3

DINNER 34: POACHED SALMON WITH DILL — LARGE MEAL

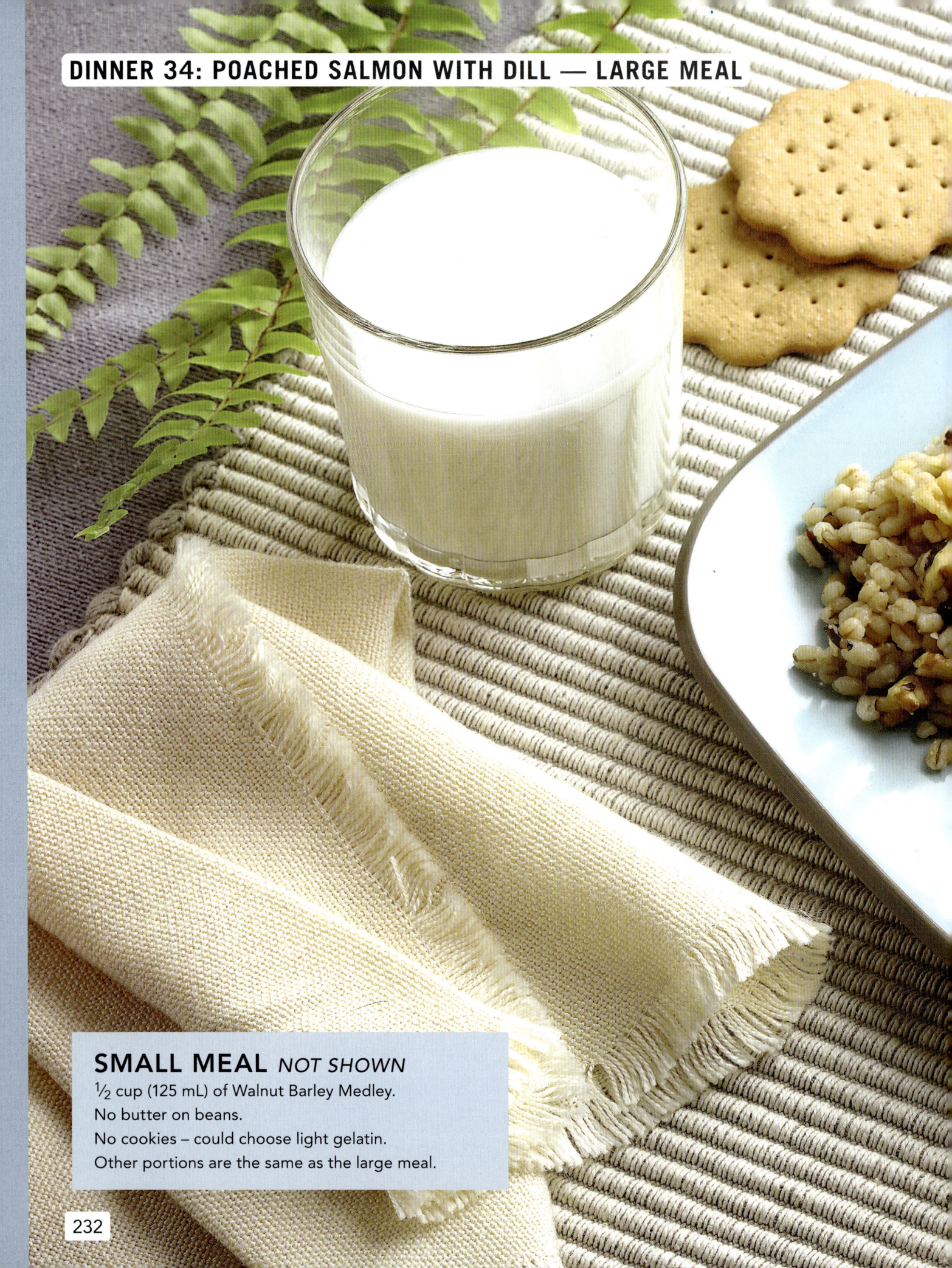

SMALL MEAL *NOT SHOWN*
½ cup (125 mL) of Walnut Barley Medley.
No butter on beans.
No cookies – could choose light gelatin.
Other portions are the same as the large meal.

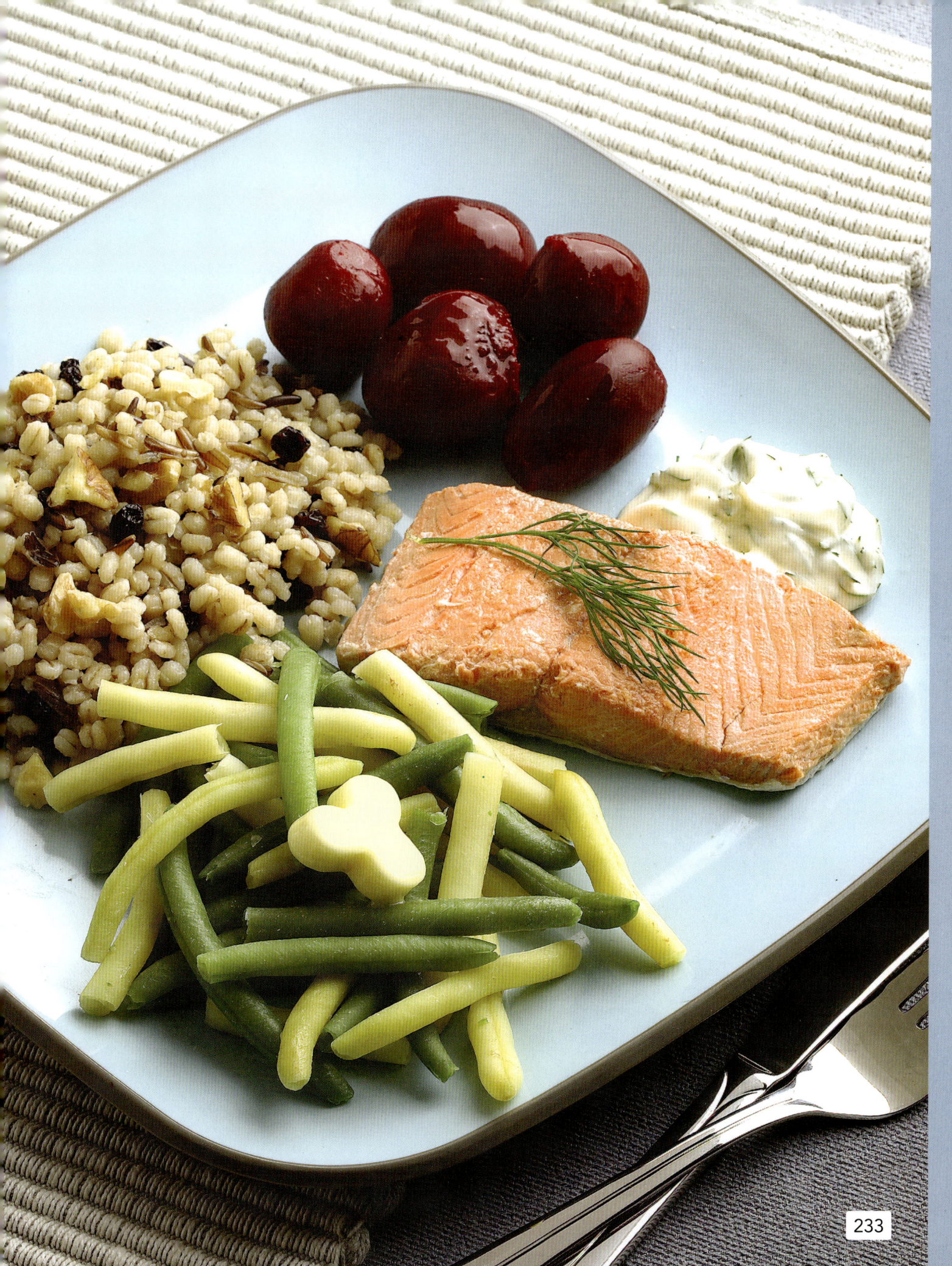

DINNER MEALS

DINNER 35

Sub Sandwich

Sub restaurants usually list the calories of the sandwiches, so you can use this as a guide. You can also look up the carbs on the website before you eat out (see next page).

Beware of the extras: for example, servers can easily squeeze out 3 tablespoons (45 mL) of regular dressing, which adds up to 225 calories. That is half of the entire small meal just in salad dressing. Load up your sub sandwich with their amazing variety of vegetables.

When it comes to selecting your drink, grab the diet version, or choose water, which is always your best option. See page 279 for Sugary Drinks Swaps.

Here is a quick sub sandwich to make at home, served with a small bag of nachos or chips (for the large meal only) and a diet beverage.

HEALTH TIP

Cold cuts contain a lot of salt. For example, 1 oz (30 g) of ham has about 300 mg of sodium. In comparison, 1 oz (30 g) of roast chicken has only 25 mg of sodium.

◯ LOW-CARB SWAP

Swap Sub Sandwich: one 6-inch (15 cm) sub
42 g net carbs

→ For Open-Face Sub with extra cheese: one 6-inch (15 cm) sub; replace the top bun with 2 extra slices of cheese
28 g net carbs

Homemade Sub Sandwich

6-inch (15 cm) whole wheat sub bun

3 oz (90 g) sliced roast chicken, or meat of your choice

1½ oz (45 g) cheese of your choice, sliced

A variety of vegetables of your choice

A few slices of pickles or olives

Black pepper

1 tbsp (15 mL) light mayonnaise or 2 tbsp (30 mL) fat-free mayonnaise

1 tbsp (15 mL) honey mustard

1. Cut the bun in half lengthwise. If desired, toast under the broiler.
2. Add the sandwich ingredients to the bun.

PER SANDWICH	
Calories	567
Carbohydrate	48 g
Fiber	6 g
Net carbs	42 g
Protein	45 g
Fat, total	22 g
Fat, saturated	9 g
Cholesterol	109 mg
Sodium	1102 mg

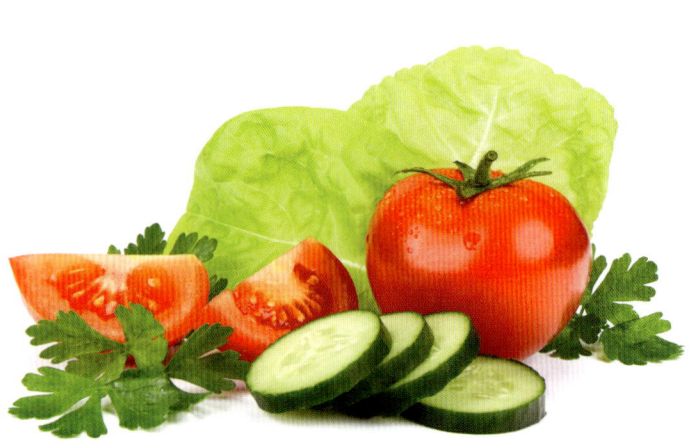

DINNER MEALS

Nutrition, Exercise and Diabetes Apps

If you wear a continuous glucose monitor (CGM), it may have built-in features or connect to an app on your phone that links to nutrition databases or options to take photos of your meal to estimate portions and nutrients. Some of these apps allow you to transfer your food records or CGM blood glucose numbers to your health care provider. Some apps also help you track your blood pressure, medication, activity and weight.

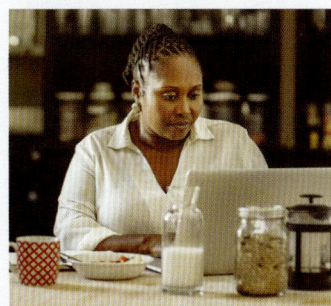

HEALTH TIP

Nutrition Information Online or Apps

1. For accurate information, search for specific foods on government nutrient databases: USDA FoodData Central (American) or Nutrient Value of Some Common Foods (Canadian).

2. A variety of sites and apps, such as FatSecret and Nutritionix, have validated free information displayed in a more friendly format than the government databases. Some apps are free and some offer a premium service for a fee.

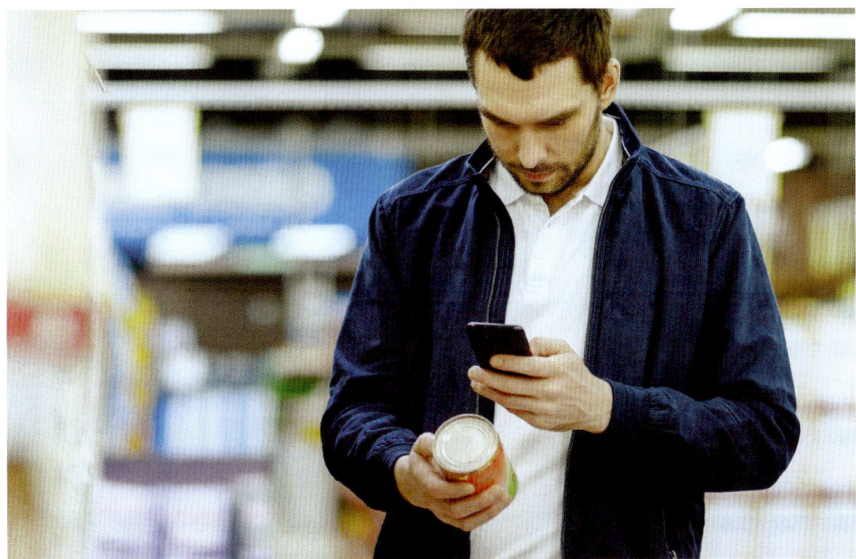

Health apps on their own don't make you healthy. Typically, the more time you spend recording your data into the app, the more benefit you will get.

Once you've established a consistent diet and exercise pattern, you may find you don't need an app anymore. This is good. Now you'll have more time to go for a walk, cook and eat a nutritious meal, and just enjoy time to relax.

YOUR DINNER MENU	Large Meal (730 calories)	Total Carbs	NET CARBS	Small Meal (550 calories)	Total Carbs	NET CARBS
Homemade Sub Sandwich	1 sandwich (6 inch/15 cm)	48	**42**	1 sandwich (6 inch/15 cm)	48	**42**
or Purchased sub sandwich	up to 550 calories			up to 550 calories		
1 bag of nachos or chips or large cookie	1 choice (200–210 calories)	28	**25**	—	—	—
Diet soft drink	Medium (12 oz)	1	**1**	Medium (12 oz)	1	**1**
	TOTAL CARBS	77 g	**68 g**	TOTAL CARBS	49 g	**43 g**
	Total carbs minus fiber = NET CARBS ↑				NET CARBS ↑	
	CARB CHOICES (1 carb choice = 15 g net carbs)		5	CARB CHOICES		3

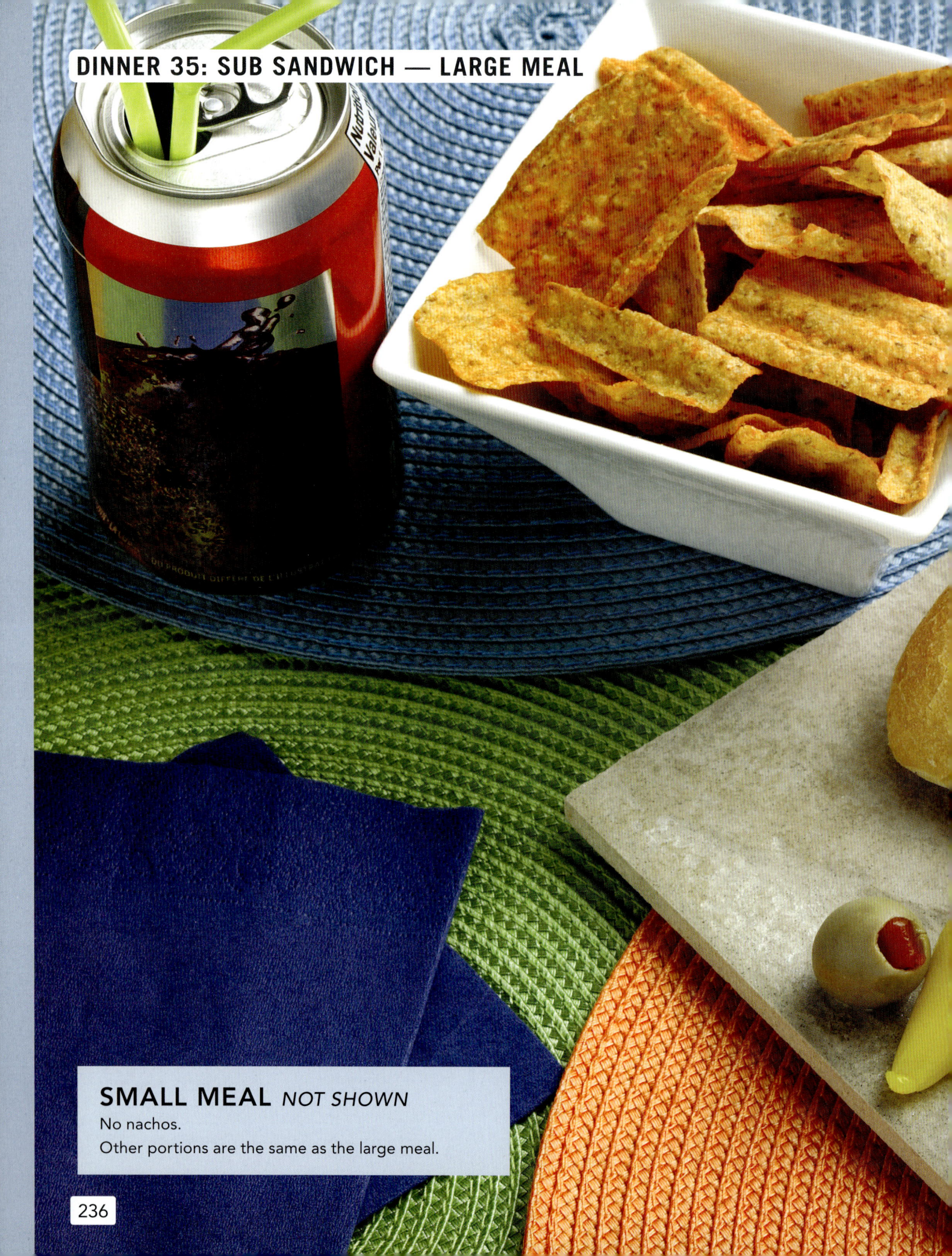

DINNER 35: SUB SANDWICH — LARGE MEAL

SMALL MEAL *NOT SHOWN*
No nachos.
Other portions are the same as the large meal.

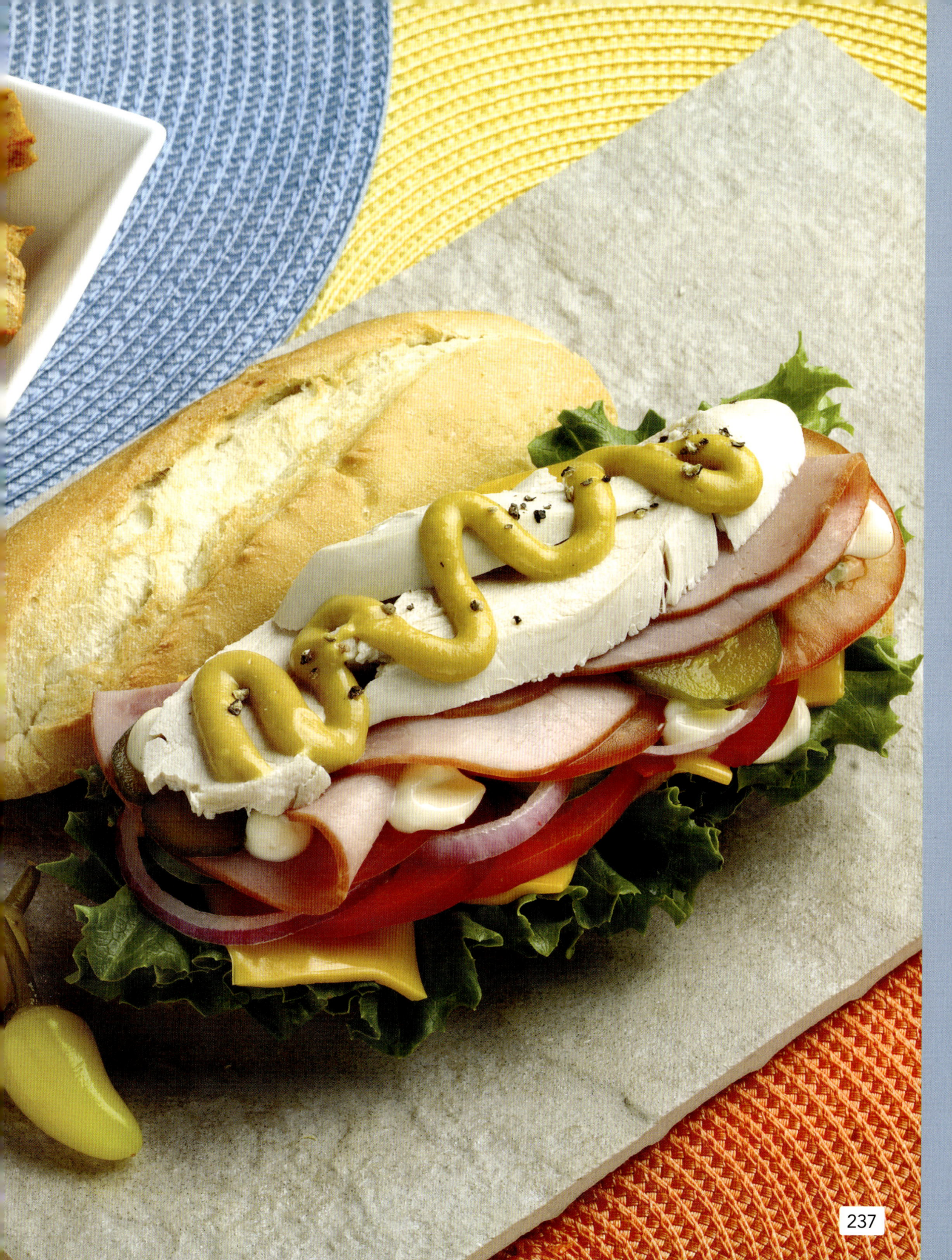

DINNER MEALS

DINNER 36

Beef Parmesan

For Beef Parmesan, you'll need to cook your meat patties first. For your meat patties you could choose frozen beef patties, breaded chicken cutlets, veal cutlets, pork cutlets, pounded minute steak, or the homemade Classic Beef Patties recipe below. While they're hot, cover them with the hot Beef Parmesan Topping.

Serve Beef Parmesan with Mashed Potatoes (see page 126), steamed broccoli and a tasty tossed salad. Finish the meal with frozen yogurt or ice cream for dessert.

Classic Beef Patties

Makes 10 large patties

6 unsalted soda crackers, crumbled

2 lbs (1 kg) lean ground beef

2 large eggs

1 small onion, finely chopped

2 tsp (10 mL) Worcestershire sauce

½ tsp (2 mL) seasoning salt

¼ tsp (1 mL) black pepper

PER PATTY WITH TOPPINGS	
Calories	254
Carbohydrate	7 g
Fiber	0 g
Net carbs	7 g
Protein	23 g
Fat, total	14 g
Fat, saturated	5 g
Cholesterol	92 mg
Sodium	484 mg

1. In a large bowl, mix all ingredients with your hands and shape into 10 patties.
2. Fry, broil or barbecue the patties until there is no pink inside.

Beef Parmesan Topping

TOPPING FOR ONE COOKED MEAT PATTY

3 tbsp (45 mL) pasta sauce

Dash of hot pepper sauce or red pepper flakes

Dash of basil and/or splash of red wine

1½ tbsp (22 mL) Parmesan cheese, shredded

PER PATTY	
Calories	176
Carbohydrate	2 g
Fiber	0 g
Net carbs	2 g
Protein	18 g
Fat, total	10 g
Fat, saturated	3 g
Cholesterol	85 mg
Sodium	150 mg

1. Heat pasta sauce with the added seasonings of your choice.
2. Pour the hot sauce over the hot cooked patty on your plate. Sprinkle the cheese on top.

RECIPE TIP

The wonder of Parmesan cheese in the Beef Parmesan Topping is that with just a small amount, its bold and tangy flavor can change the taste of a meal from good to amazing.

Even though Cheddar and mozzarella cheese are milder tasting, they can be just as satisfying with this meal.

HEALTH TIP

Pasta sauces vary in calories and carbs

Check the Nutrition Facts on the pasta sauce label and look for a mid-range to lower-calorie choice, such as 30 to 60 calories per ½-cup (125 mL) serving.

DINNER MEALS

Add a Cone to Your Frozen Yogurt or Ice Cream

When it is served in a regular ice cream cone, it will only add another 20 calories and 4 grams of carbohydrates.

Bowl Sizes Affect How Much You Eat

When you eat from a smaller bowl, you eat less. Take a look at these three bowls. Each holds a scoop of ice cream. By putting the ice cream in the small bowl, it looks more filling. If you use the large bowl, you just might fill it up with three or four scoops of ice cream, and you would overeat.

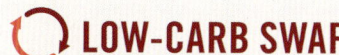

LOW-CARB SWAP

Swap frozen yogurt:
½ cup (125 mL)
16 g net carbs

→ For keto frozen dessert:
½ cup (125 mL)
0–1 g net carbs

See Ice Cream Swaps, page 278.

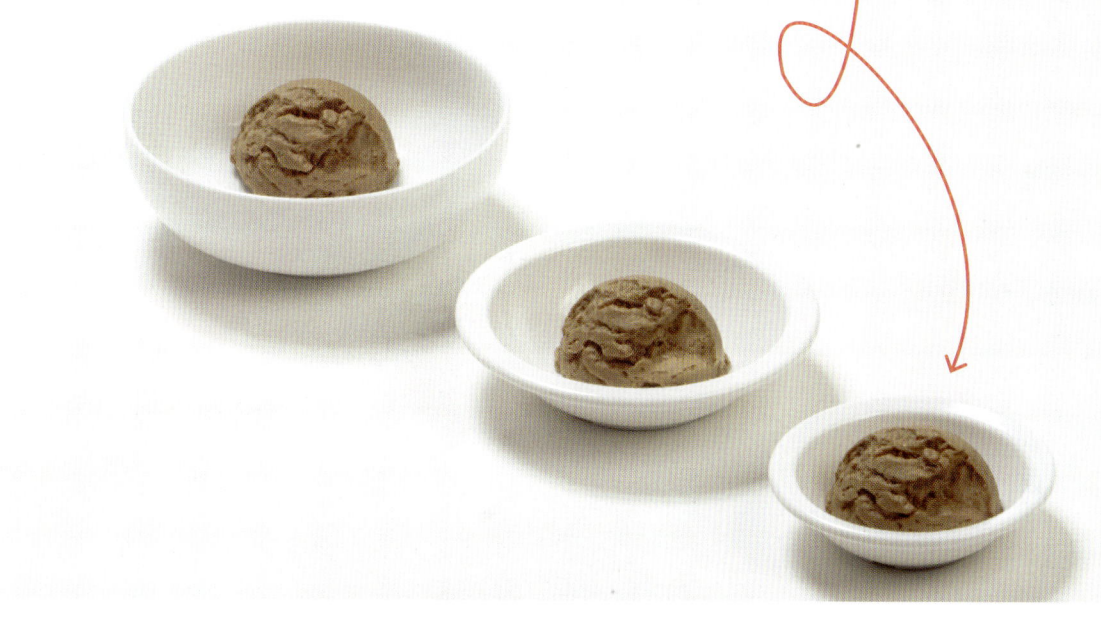

YOUR DINNER MENU	Large Meal (730 calories)	Total Carbs	NET CARBS	Small Meal (550 calories)	Total Carbs	NET CARBS
Beef Parmesan	1½ patties with pasta sauce and cheese	11	11	1½ patties with pasta sauce and cheese	11	11
Mashed Potatoes (see page 126)	1 cup (250 mL)	39	36	¼ cup (60 mL)	10	9
Broccoli	1 to 2 cups (250 to 500 mL)	6	4	1 to 2 cups (250 to 500 mL)	6	4
Tossed salad	Small	2	1	Small	2	1
Fat-free Italian salad dressing	1 tbsp (15 mL)	2	2	1 tbsp (15 mL)	2	2
Frozen yogurt or ice cream (light or regular)	½ cup (125 mL)	16	16	½ cup (125 mL)	16	16
	TOTAL CARBS	76 g	70 g	TOTAL CARBS	47 g	43 g
	Total carbs minus fiber = NET CARBS ↑			NET CARBS ↑		
	CARB CHOICES (1 carb choice = 15 g net carbs)	5		CARB CHOICES	3	

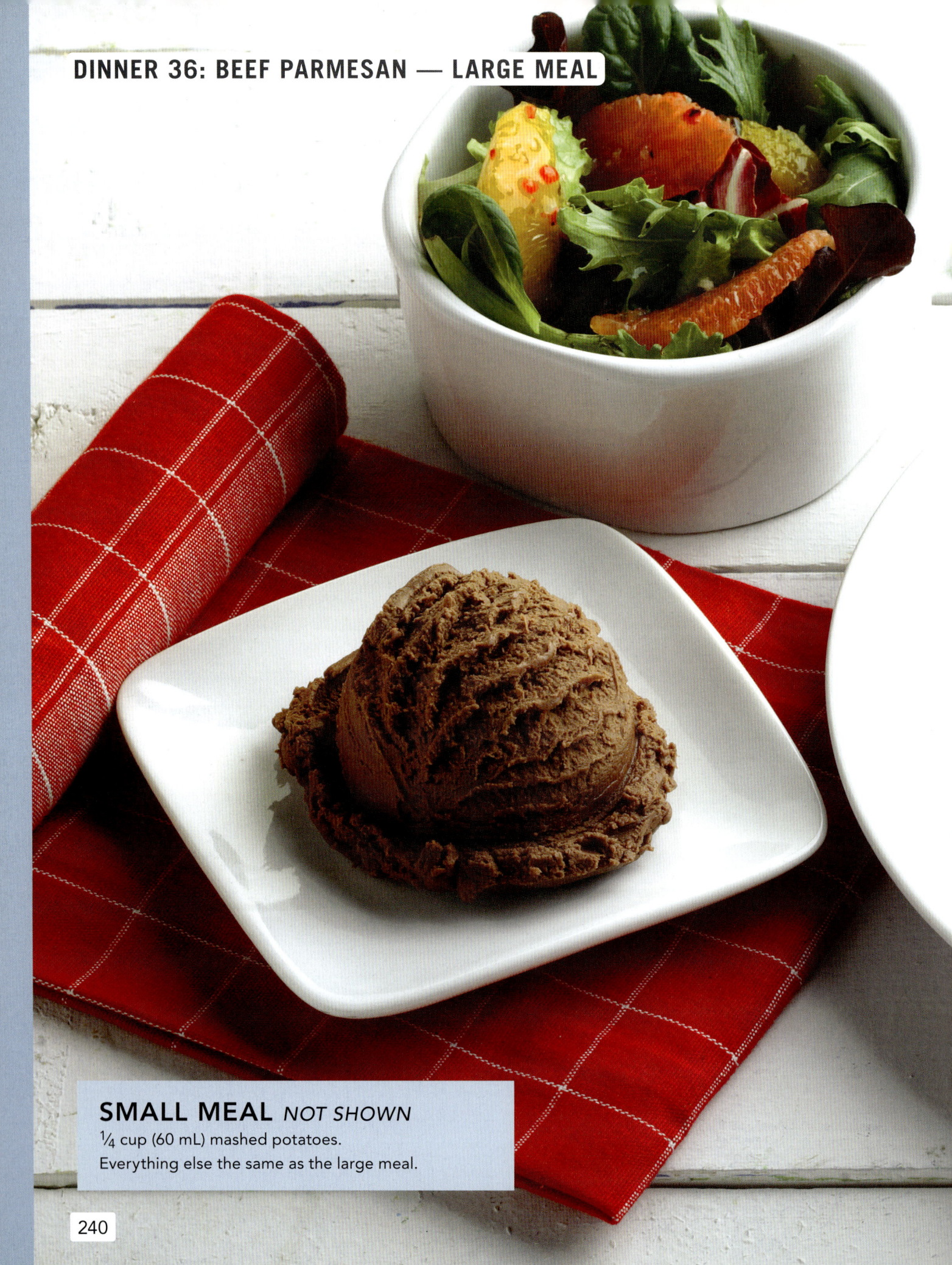

DINNER 36: BEEF PARMESAN — LARGE MEAL

SMALL MEAL *NOT SHOWN*
¼ cup (60 mL) mashed potatoes.
Everything else the same as the large meal.

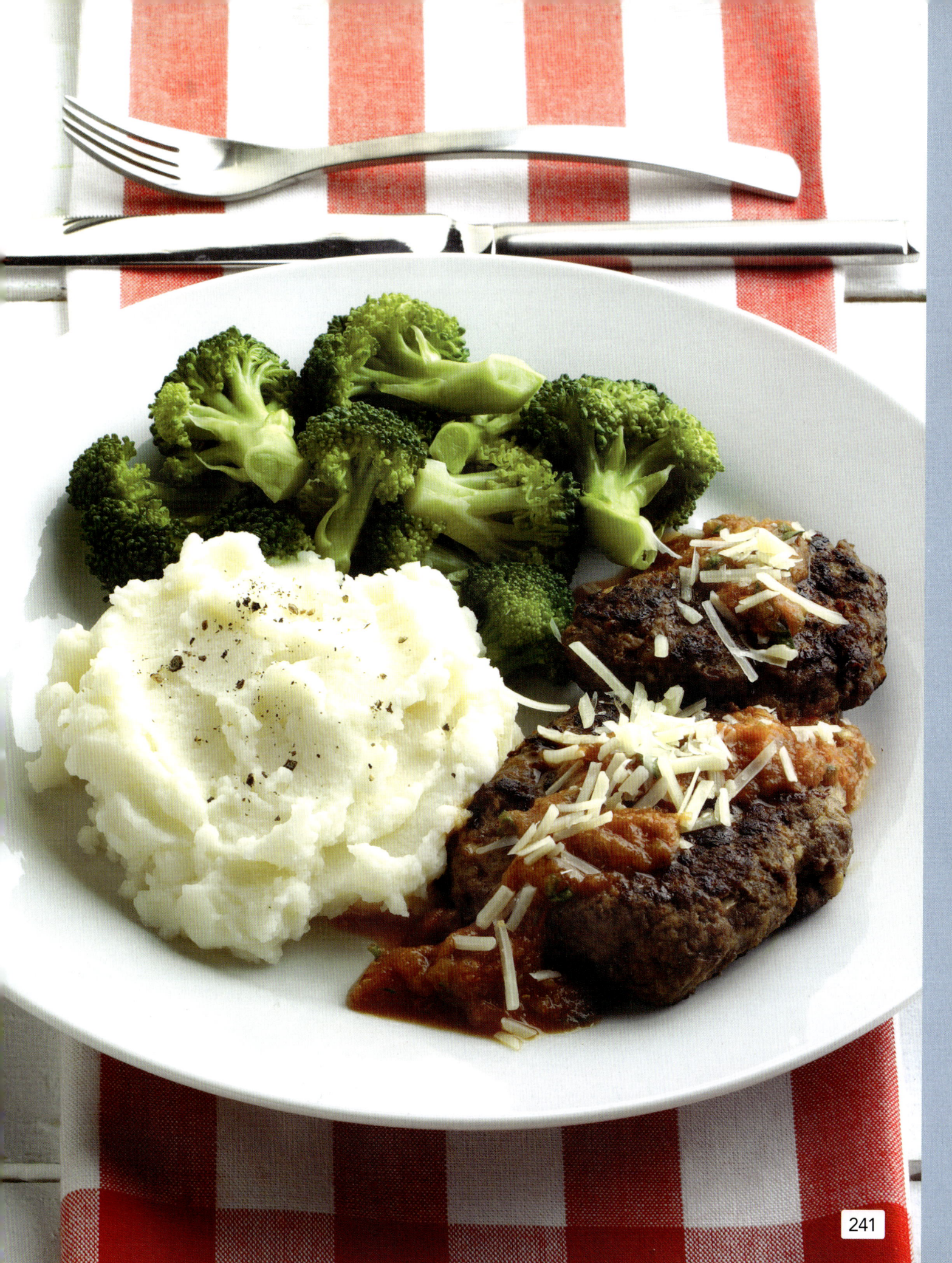

DINNER MEALS

DINNER 37

Santa Fe Salad

This meal is inspired from Mexican American cuisine. It has brilliant color, crunch, sweetness and tanginess, with many flavors and variety in every bite. A slice of Banana Bread is a hearty meal complement. The large meal is served with a handful of tortilla chips.

Santa Fe Salad

Makes 4 servings

12 oz (341 mL) can of corn, drained

19 oz (540 mL) can of black beans, rinsed in cold water and drained

2 to 3 green onions, chopped

1 red pepper, cut into pieces

½ head of lettuce, torn into bite-size pieces

1 tbsp (15 mL) fresh cilantro or parsley, chopped

2–3 tbsp (30–45 mL) light coleslaw dressing

10 oz (300 g) chicken breasts or thighs, boneless and skin removed, cut into chunks or strips

2 tbsp (30 mL) hickory smoke barbecue sauce

½ cup (125 mL) cheese, shredded

PER SERVING	
Calories	336
Carbohydrate	40 g
Fiber	11 g
Net carbs	29 g
Protein	29 g
Fat, total	7 g
Fat, saturated	3 g
Cholesterol	60 mg
Sodium	747 mg

1. In a large bowl, gently toss corn, black beans, green onions, red pepper, lettuce and cilantro. Mix in the coleslaw dressing. Measure out your serving of salad.
2. In a nonstick pan over medium heat, cook chicken pieces with about 2 tbsp (30 mL) of water. When the chicken is no longer pink inside, add the barbecue sauce. Reduce heat and cook for a couple of minutes.
3. Measure out your portion of chicken and cheese and place on top of your serving of salad.

⟲ LOW-CARB SWAP

LARGE MEAL

Swap tortilla chips:
8 chips
9 g net carbs

→ For Cheese Crisps:
2 Cheese Crisps
0 g net carbs
(similar calories)

See Cheese Crisps recipe on page 265.

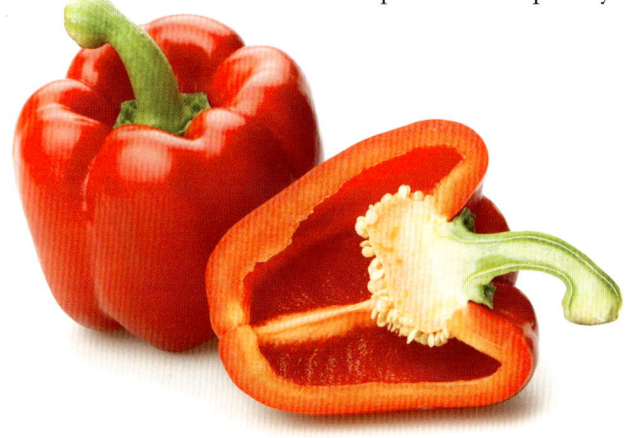

DINNER MEALS

One slice of Banana Bread has 200 calories and can be eaten as a large snack. See the Snacks section (pages 266–267) for other ideas.

Banana Bread

Makes 12 slices

Preheat oven to 350°F (180°C)

1¼ cups (310 mL) flour

1 cup (250 mL) ground flaxseed

1 tbsp (15 mL) baking powder

½ tsp (2 mL) salt

½ tsp (2 mL) nutmeg

2 tbsp (30 mL) margarine or butter

⅓ cup (75 mL) sugar

1 large egg

¼ cup (60 mL) skim milk

3 small bananas

½ cup (125 mL) raisins, packed

¼ cup (60 mL) chopped walnuts or pecans

PER SLICE	
Calories	207
Carbohydrate	30 g
Fiber	4 g
Net carbs	26 g
Protein	6 g
Fat, total	8 g
Fat, saturated	1 g
Cholesterol	16 mg
Sodium	178 mg

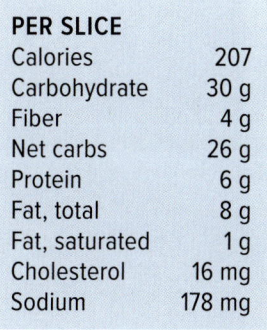
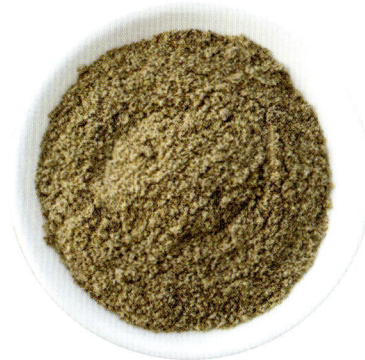

1. Mix flour, ground flaxseed, baking powder, salt and nutmeg in a medium bowl.
2. In a large bowl, cream margarine and sugar with a wooden spoon. Beat in the egg and milk until smooth.
3. Mash the bananas with a fork and add to the egg and milk mixture.
4. Combine the liquid and dry ingredients, mix well, and then add the nuts and raisins.
5. Scrape into a greased 9- by 5-inch (2 L) loaf pan and bake for 50 minutes to 1 hour, until a knife inserted in the center comes out clean. Let cool in the pan, then remove and cut into 12 slices.

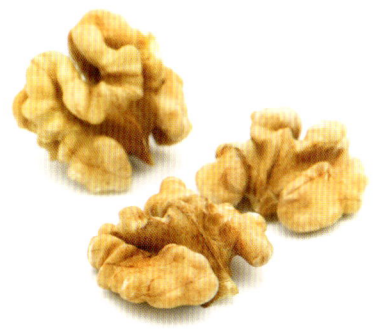

YOUR DINNER MENU	Large Meal (730 calories)	Total Carbs	NET CARBS	Small Meal (550 calories)	Total Carbs	NET CARBS
Santa Fe Salad	1 serving	40	**29**	1 serving	40	**29**
Tortilla chips	8 chips	11	**9**	—	—	—
Banana Bread	1 slice	30	**26**	1 slice	30	**26**
Margarine or butter	1½ tsp (7 mL)	0	**0**	½ tsp (2 mL)	0	**0**
	TOTAL CARBS	81 g	**64 g**	**TOTAL CARBS**	70 g	**55 g**
	Total carbs minus fiber = NET CARBS ↑			NET CARBS ↑		
	CARB CHOICES (1 carb choice = 15 g net carbs)		**4**	CARB CHOICES		**4**

DINNER 37: SANTA FE SALAD — LARGE MEAL

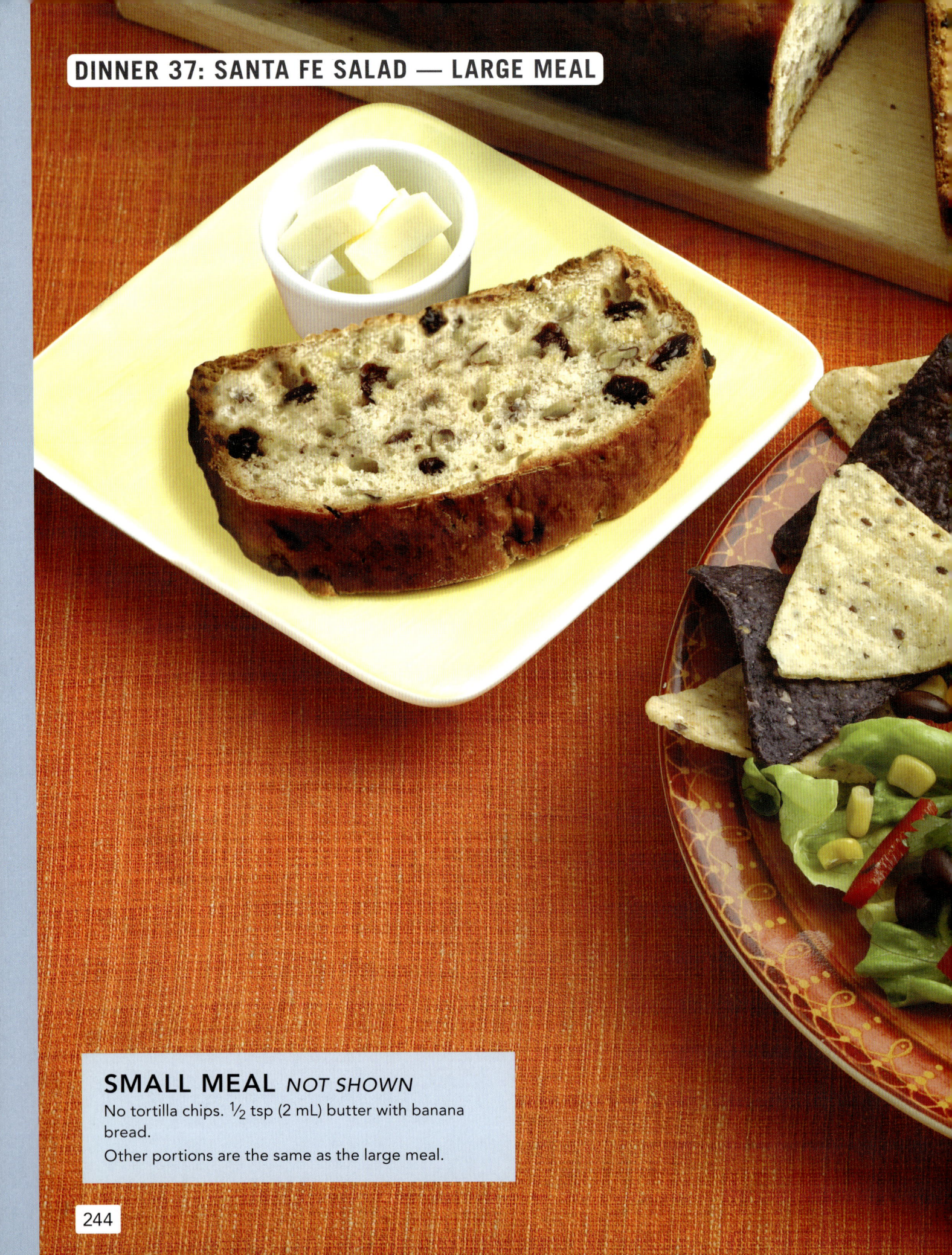

SMALL MEAL *NOT SHOWN*
No tortilla chips. ½ tsp (2 mL) butter with banana bread.
Other portions are the same as the large meal.

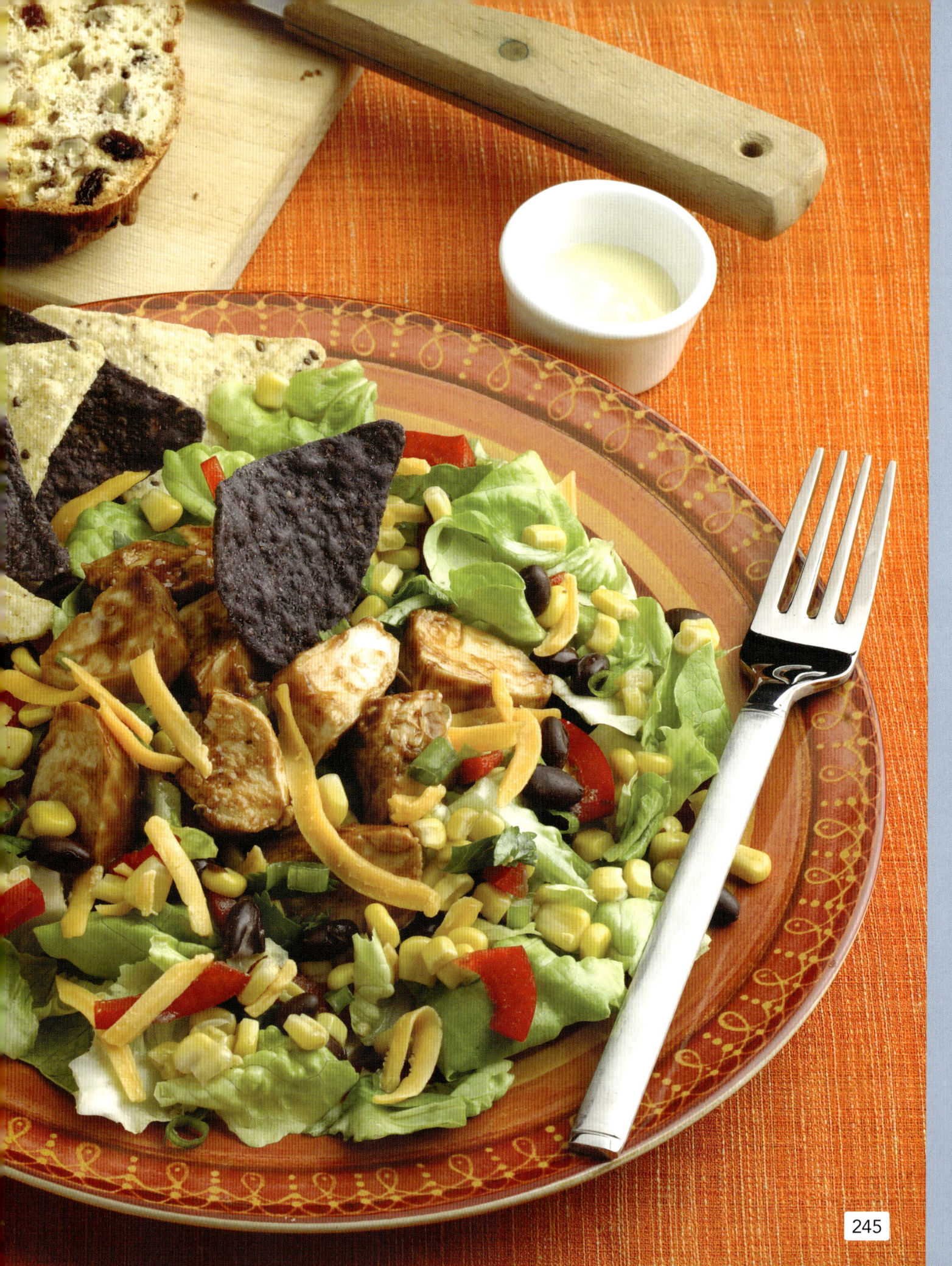

DINNER MEALS

DINNER 38

Pork Chop Casserole

This no-fail casserole, proven to be delicious, only takes an hour to bake in the oven. Once the casserole has baked for 40 minutes, put the rice on to cook. Then, in the last 15 minutes of baking the pork chops, get the tomato in the oven. The plan for this meal is to have pork chops, rice and tomato ready to serve at the same time.

Pork Chop Casserole

Makes 3 servings

Preheat oven to 350°F (180°C)

5 pork chops (thin loin cut), total raw weight with bone about 1¾ lbs (875 g)
1 small onion, thinly sliced
3 stalks celery, sliced
10 oz (284 mL) can of mushroom soup, or other cream soup

PER ONE PORK CHOP WITH SAUCE	
Calories	192
Carbohydrate	6 g
Fiber	1 g
Net carbs	5 g
Protein	21 g
Fat, total	8 g
Fat, saturated	3 g
Cholesterol	62 mg
Sodium	439 mg

1. Trim visible fat from the pork chops. Place in a casserole dish. Evenly add onion and celery on top of the pork chops. Spread the cream soup on top.
2. Bake in a covered casserole dish for 1 hour, or until the pork chops are fork-tender.

HEALTH TIP
Some cream soups are available as low-fat or low-sodium.

Grilled Tomato

Makes 2 servings

Preheat oven to 350°F (180°C)

1 medium tomato
1 tsp (5 mL) dry bread crumbs
1 tsp (5 mL) ground flaxseed
1 tbsp (15 mL) Parmesan cheese, grated
½ tsp (2 mL) dried oregano
1 tsp (5 mL) butter or margarine

PER SERVING	
Calories	51
Carbohydrate	4 g
Fiber	1 g
Net carbs	3 g
Protein	2 g
Fat, total	3 g
Fat, saturated	2 g
Cholesterol	7 mg
Sodium	72 mg

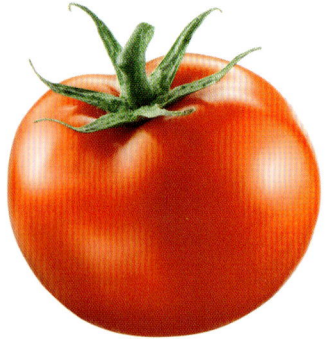

1. Cut the tomato in half crosswise. Place cut side up in a casserole or small baking pan.
2. In a small bowl, combine bread crumbs, ground flaxseed, Parmesan cheese, oregano and butter. Spoon over the open tomato halves and, with the back of the spoon, press down gently.
3. Bake for 15 minutes or until topping is golden brown.

DINNER MEALS

Sugar Snap Peas

This meal is served with raw, crunchy sugar snap peas on the side. They are low-calorie and low-carb, with just 20 calories and 3 g net carbs in 15 snap peas. Sugar snap peas can be added anytime to a stir-fry, or sliced and added to a salad or casserole. They are also great as a snack!

Mandarins and Cottage Cheese is an easy two-ingredient dessert. It is a light yet creamy finish to the meal.

Mandarins and Cottage Cheese

Makes 4 servings

1 cup (250 mL) canned mandarin orange segments in light syrup, drained
¾ cup (175 mL) 2% cottage cheese

1. Gently combine orange pieces and cottage cheese, reserving a few mandarin segments to decorate the top of each serving.
2. Divide among four dessert-size dishes and decorate with the reserved orange segments.

When you sip on a cup of antioxidant-rich green tea with your meal, this helps slow down the speed that you eat. This gives time to feel full. In addition, green and black tea have tannins that help reduce the glycemic index of the meal.

PER SERVING	
Calories	66
Carbohydrate	10 g
Fiber	1 g
Net carbs	9 g
Protein	5 g
Fat, total	1 g
Fat, saturated	1 g
Cholesterol	6 mg
Sodium	157 mg

LOW-CARB SWAP

MANDARINS AND COTTAGE CHEESE RECIPE

Swap recipe made with ¾ cup (175 mL) canned mandarins:
Per serving
9 g net carbs

→ For recipe made with 1 cup (250 mL) fresh mandarin sections:
Per serving
5 g net carbs

See the Complete Diabetes Guide for more information on teas and glycemic index.

YOUR DINNER MENU	Large Meal (730 calories)	Total Carbs	NET CARBS	Small Meal (550 calories)	Total Carbs	NET CARBS
Pork chops with sauce	1 serving	9	8	1 serving	9	8
Rice, long-grain	1 cup (250 mL)	45	44	½ cup (125 mL)	23	22
Grilled Tomato	1 half	3	2	1 half	3	2
Sugar snap peas	15	4	3	15	4	3
Mandarins and Cottage Cheese	1 serving	10	9	1 serving	10	9
Green tea	1 cup (250 mL)	0	0	1 cup (250 mL)	0	0
	TOTAL CARBS	71 g	66 g	TOTAL CARBS	49 g	44 g
	Total carbs minus fiber = NET CARBS ↑			NET CARBS ↑		
	CARB CHOICES (1 carb choice = 15 g net carbs)		4	CARB CHOICES		3

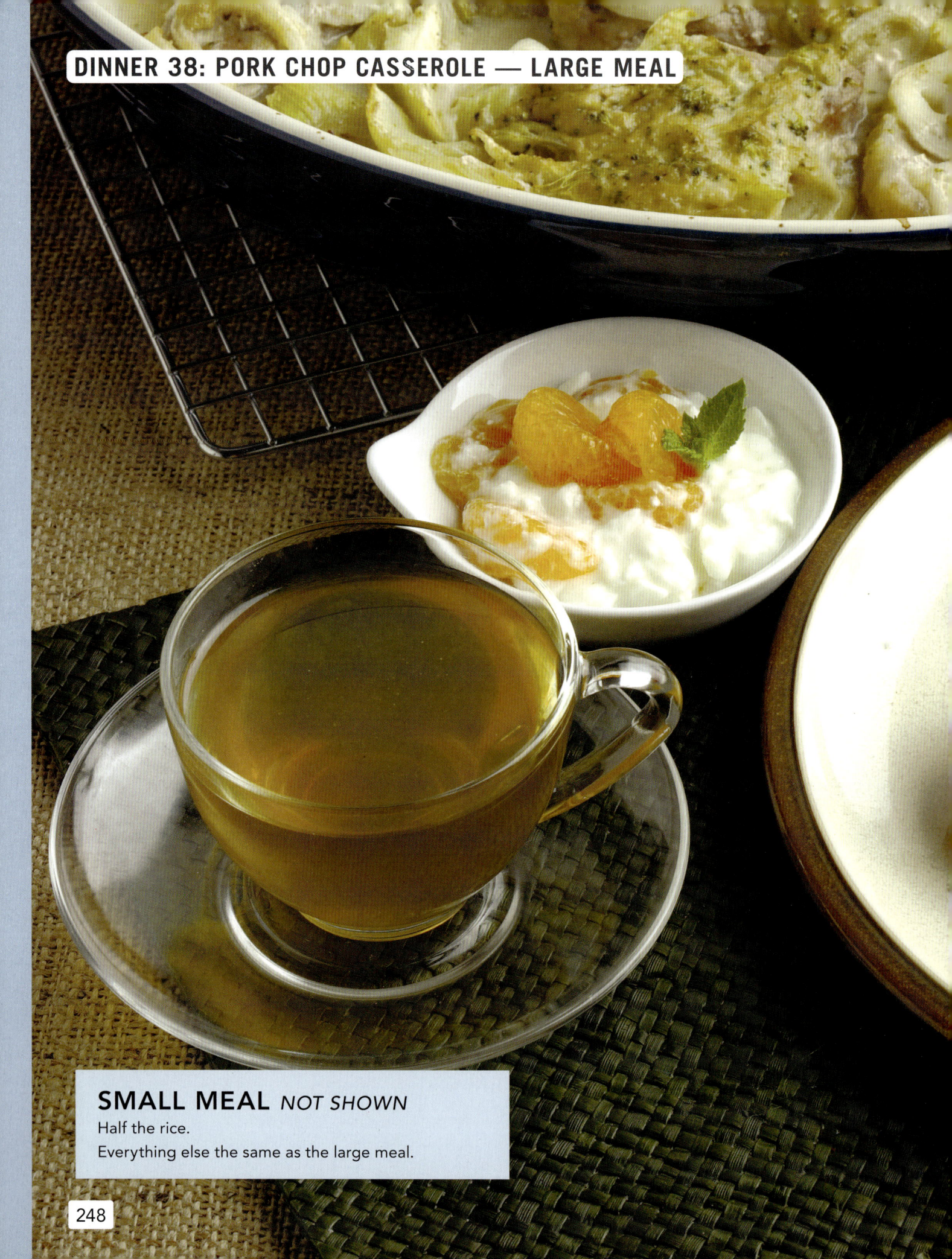

DINNER 38: PORK CHOP CASSEROLE — LARGE MEAL

SMALL MEAL *NOT SHOWN*
Half the rice.
Everything else the same as the large meal.

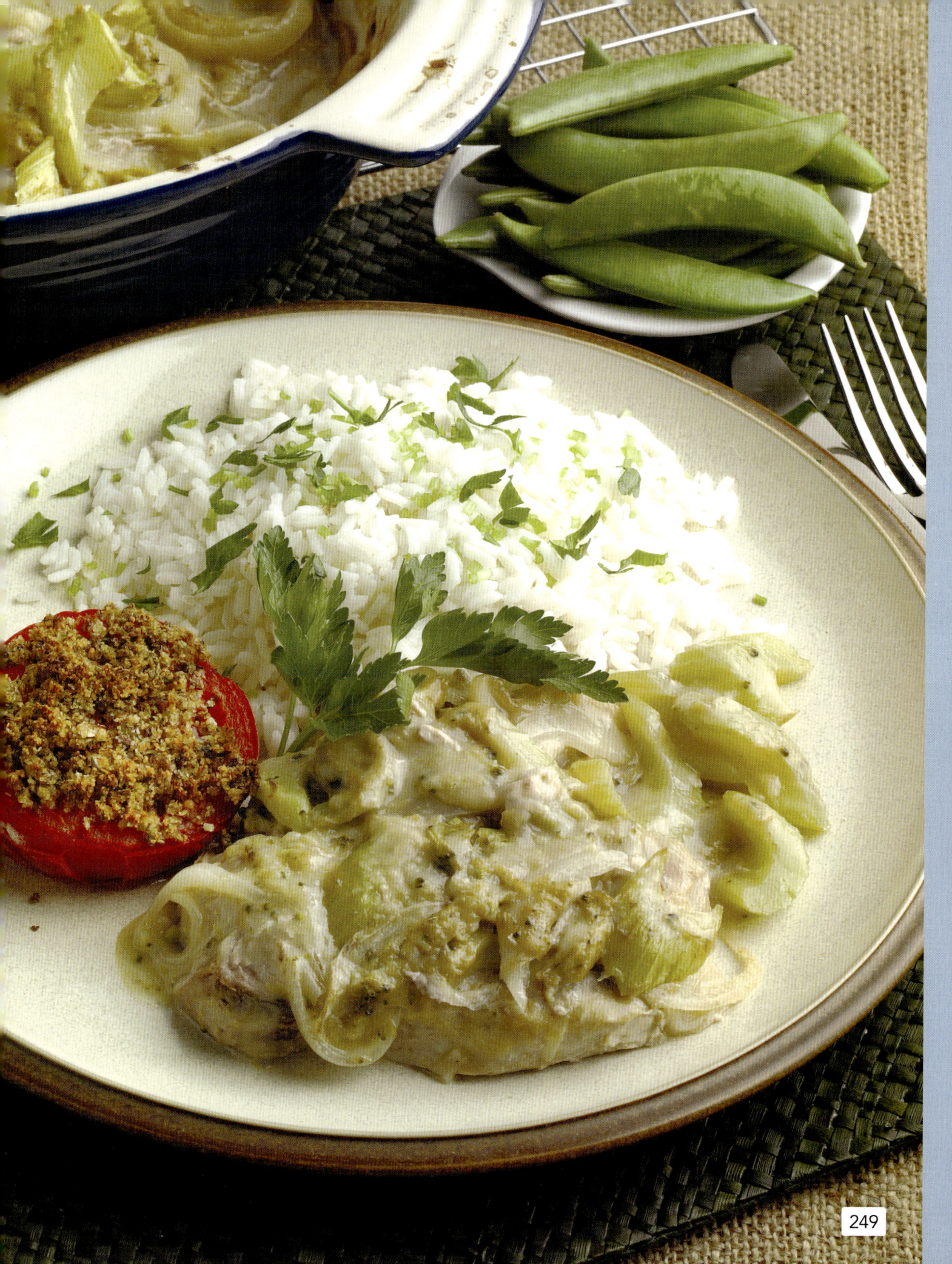

DINNER MEALS

DINNER 39

Shrimp Linguine

Linguine, a flat pasta noodle, is served with a shrimp sauce that takes about 30 minutes to prepare and cook. Halfway through cooking the sauce, remember to boil the pasta. Use 60 g (2 oz) dry linguine for every 1 cup (250 mL) cooked pasta.

Shrimp Linguine Sauce

Makes 4 cups (1 L) (4 servings)

- 1 tbsp (15 mL) olive or vegetable oil
- ⅓ cup (75 mL) water
- 1 small onion, chopped
- 3 large cloves garlic, minced
- 1 cup (250 mL) sliced fresh mushrooms (or one 10 oz/284 mL can, drained)
- 1½ tbsp (22 mL) flour
- 1 packet (4.5 g) reduced-sodium chicken bouillon powder
- ⅛ tsp (0.5 mL) black pepper
- 1 tsp (5 mL) dried dill
- 1¾ cups (425 mL) skim milk
- ½ red or green pepper, cut into 1-inch (2.5 cm) thick strips, or ½ cup (125 mL) other vegetables of your choice
- 10 oz (300 g) cooked frozen shrimp, thawed, shells and tails removed
- ¾ cup (175 mL) cheese of your choice, shredded

PER 1 CUP (250 ML)	
Calories	245
Carbohydrate	11 g
Fiber	1 g
Net carbs	10 g
Protein	27 g
Fat, total	10 g
Fat, saturated	3 g
Cholesterol	133 mg
Sodium	474 mg

1. In a large pan over medium heat, add olive oil, water, onion and garlic and cook until soft.
2. Meanwhile, in a small pan, sauté mushrooms in a bit of water over medium heat until soft. Drain off water and set mushrooms aside.
3. In a small bowl, mix flour, bouillon powder, pepper and dill. Add this mixture to the fried onions and stir until flour is absorbed.
4. Then gradually whisk in milk, stirring constantly for about 5 minutes, until the sauce slightly thickens. Do not let the sauce boil.
5. Mix in vegetables and shrimp and continue stirring until vegetables are tender, about another 5 minutes. Constant stirring prevents the milk from sticking to the bottom of the pot.
6. Lastly, stir in mushrooms and shredded cheese. The sauce will thicken once the cheese melts.
7. Serve over the cooked linguine.

LOW-CARB SWAP

LARGE MEAL

Swap regular linguine:
1¼ cups (310 mL)
48 g net carbs

→ For spelt linguine:
1¼ cups (310 mL)
33 g net carbs

SMALL MEAL

Swap regular linguine:
¾ cup (175 mL)
29 net carbs

→ For spelt linguine:
¾ cup (175 mL)
20 g net carbs

See Pasta Swaps, page 275.

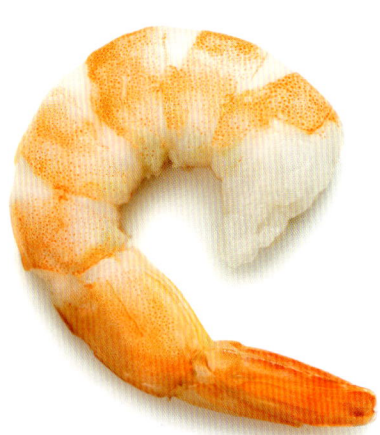

DINNER MEALS

Caesar salad is usually made with dark green romaine lettuce. Dark salad greens are rich in folic acid, a nutrient that is essential for heart health.

Caesar Salad

For 1 serving:

2 cups (500 mL) dark salad greens, torn into bite-size pieces

2 tbsp (30 mL) Parmesan cheese, shredded

¼ cup (60 mL) croutons

Squeeze of fresh lemon juice

PER SERVING	
Calories	88
Carbohydrate	9 g
Fiber	2 g
Net carbs	7 g
Protein	7 g
Fat, total	3 g
Fat, saturated	2 g
Cholesterol	7 mg
Sodium	230 mg

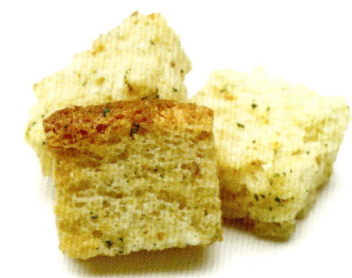

1. Combine greens, cheese, croutons and lemon juice.
2. Top with 1 tbsp (15 mL) Caesar salad dressing.

This cool and delightful beverage is served over ice cubes or crushed ice.

Italian Iced Soda Float

Makes one 12 oz (375 mL) serving

½ cup (125 mL) ice cubes or crushed ice

¾ cup (175 mL) soda water

1 packet (1 tsp/5 mL) cherry- or berry-flavored Crystal Light or Diet Kool-Aid

¼ cup (60 mL) 2% milk

PER SERVING	
Calories	38
Carbohydrate	4 g
Fiber	0 g
Net carbs	4 g
Protein	3 g
Fat, total	1 g
Fat, saturated	1 g
Cholesterol	5 mg
Sodium	84 mg

1. Pour ice into a tall glass.
2. Slowly pour the soda water over the ice, then add the Crystal Light or Diet Kool-Aid and the milk. Stir and enjoy.

YOUR DINNER MENU	Large Meal (730 calories)	Total Carbs	NET CARBS	Small Meal (550 calories)	Total Carbs	NET CARBS
Shrimp Linguine Sauce	1 cup (250 mL)	11	**10**	1 cup (250 mL)	11	**10**
Cooked pasta (linguine)	1¼ cups (310 mL)	50	**48**	¾ cup (175 mL)	30	**28**
Caesar Salad	1 serving	9	**7**	1 serving	9	**7**
Caesar salad dressing, classic	1 tbsp (15 mL)	1	**1**	1 tbsp (15 mL)	1	**1**
Italian Iced Soda Float	12 oz (375 mL)	4	**4**	12 oz (375 mL)	4	**4**
	TOTAL CARBS	**75 g**	**70 g**	**TOTAL CARBS**	**55 g**	**50 g**
	Total carbs minus fiber = NET CARBS ↑			NET CARBS ↑		
	CARB CHOICES (1 carb choice = 15 g net carbs)		5	CARB CHOICES		3

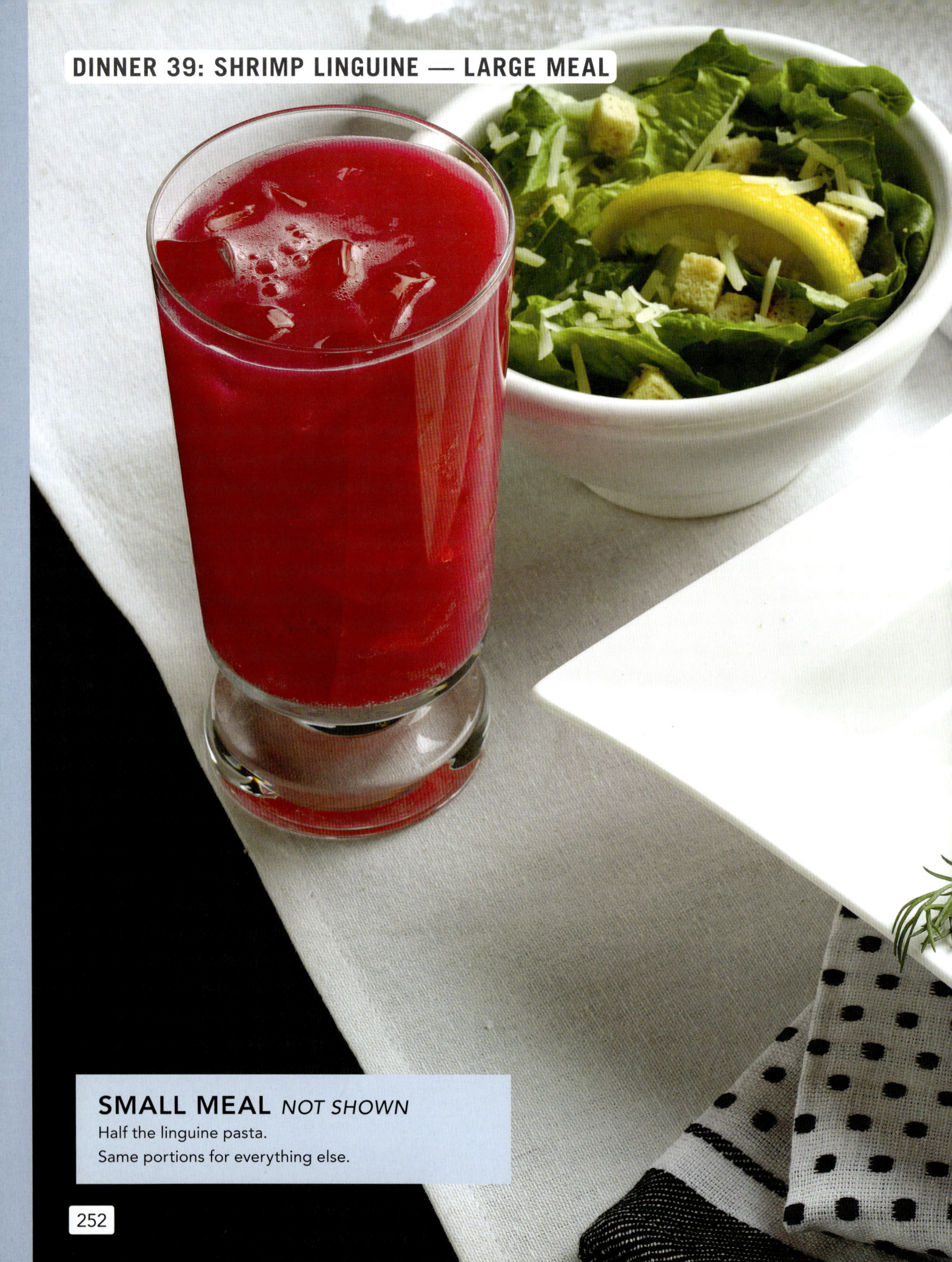

DINNER 39: SHRIMP LINGUINE — LARGE MEAL

SMALL MEAL *NOT SHOWN*
Half the linguine pasta.
Same portions for everything else.

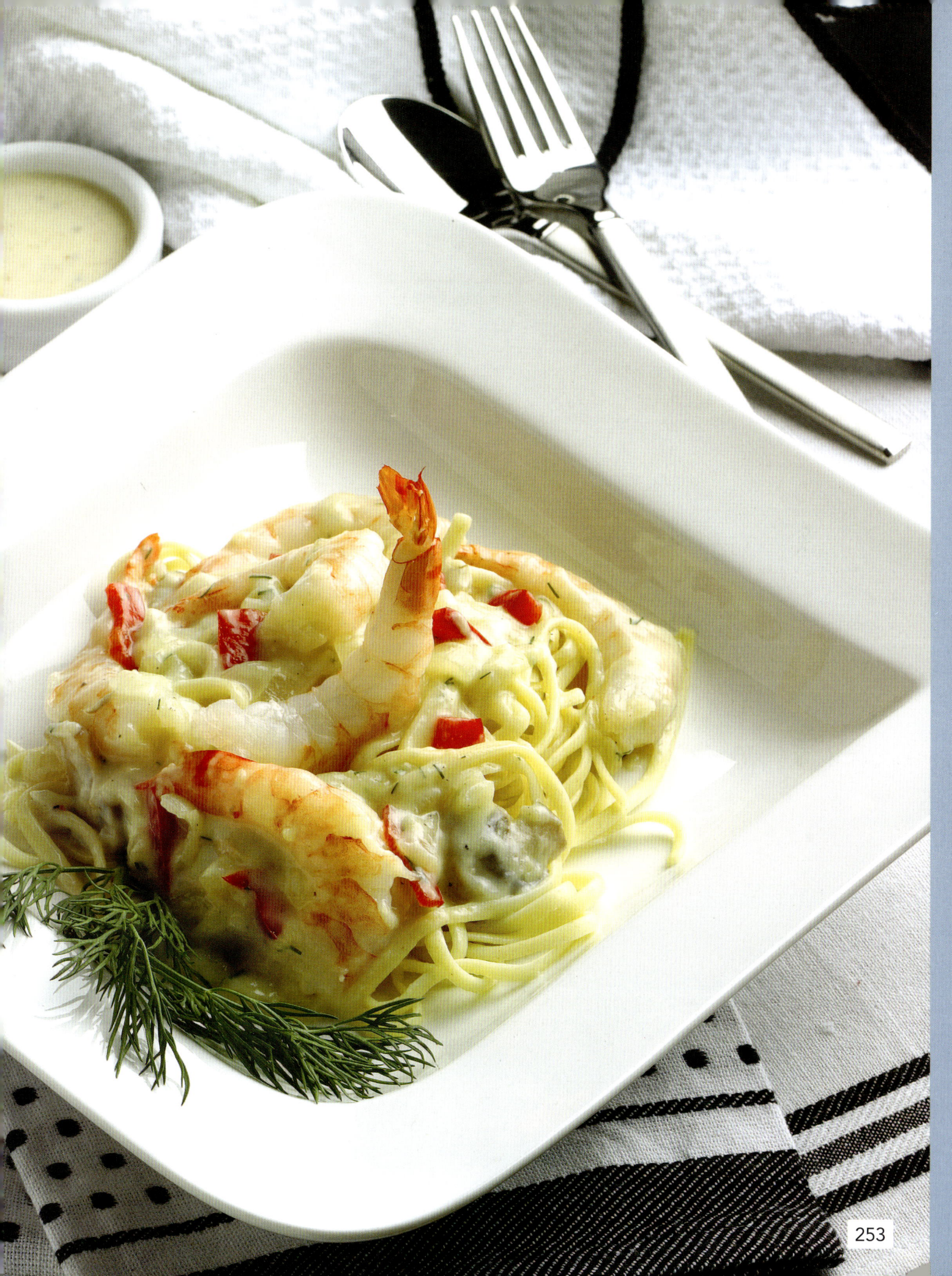

DINNER MEALS

DINNER 40

HEALTH TIP

Raw chicken carries harmful bacteria called Salmonella. Cooking chicken until there is no pink kills the bacteria.

It is essential that you wash your hands, cutting board, sink and countertop – wherever the raw chicken touched. Use hot, soapy water, rinse well and air dry.

◯ LOW-CARB SWAP

IN CHICKEN CORDON BLEU RECIPE

Swap recipe made with ¼ cup (60 mL) bread crumbs:
Per serving
5 g net carbs

→ For recipe made with ⅓ cup (75 mL) almond flour:
Per serving
1 g net carbs

Chicken Cordon Bleu

Cordon Bleu is French for "Blue Ribbon," a famous cooking school in France. Chicken Cordon Bleu has been adapted from the classic French Veal Cordon Bleu.

This dinner includes mashed sweet potatoes, zucchini and parsnips (steamed or baked) and a small salad. For dessert, treat yourself to the exquisite Cream Cheese Pomegranate Burst.

Chicken Cordon Bleu

Makes 4 servings

¼ cup (60 mL) fine dry bread crumbs

Shake of salt and black pepper

1 large egg

4 slices of ham (1 oz/28 g for each chicken breast)

4 slices of part-skim mozzarella cheese (1 oz/28 g for each chicken breast)

4 5 oz (140 g) raw weight boneless, skinless chicken breasts (20 oz/560 g total)

1 to 2 tbsp (15 to 30 mL) butter or margarine

PER SERVING	
Calories	377
Carbohydrate	5 g
Fiber	0 g
Net carbs	5 g
Protein	55 g
Fat, total	15 g
Fat, saturated	7 g
Cholesterol	193 mg
Sodium	637 mg

1. In a bowl, mix bread crumbs with salt and pepper.
2. In another bowl, beat egg with a fork.
3. Slice each chicken breast in half lengthwise, but not all the way through. Gently flatten with a meat pounder or use the edge of a plate; this creates a thinner piece of meat for uniform cooking.
4. Inside each piece of chicken, tuck one slice of ham and one slice of cheese.
5. Dip each filled chicken breast in the egg and coat all over.
6. Then roll each piece in the bread crumbs and place on a plate.
7. In a nonstick pan, melt the butter on medium heat. Fry the chicken for 5 to 8 minutes on one side, then flip and fry on the other side for 4 to 6 minutes. It's cooked when there is no pink in the chicken meat.

Cream Cheese Pomegranate Burst

Makes 4 servings

- 1 packet (1 tsp/5 mL) cherry- or berry-flavored Crystal Light or Diet Kool-Aid
- ¾ cup (175 mL) boiling water
- ¾ cup (175 mL) cold water
- 1 cup (250 mL) pomegranate seeds (about 1 medium)
- ½ of 8 oz package (4 oz/125 g) light or regular cream cheese
- ¼ tsp (1 mL) cinnamon

PER SERVING	
Calories	106
Carbohydrate	9 g
Fiber	2 g
Net carbs	7 g
Protein	4 g
Fat, total	6 g
Fat, saturated	3 g
Cholesterol	20 mg
Sodium	279 mg

HEALTH TIP

Fruit helps fight cancer and keeps your skin healthy. Pomegranate seeds are bursting with extraordinary flavor and are full of vitamin C and antioxidants. They are wonderful in desserts and added to fruit salads and green salads.

1. Put gelatin in a medium glass or metal bowl.
2. Add boiling water and stir immediately, until gelatin is dissolved.
3. Add cold water and stir.
4. Pour ⅓ cup (75 mL) of gelatin mixture into each of four small dessert dishes. You'll have about ¼ cup (60 mL) left over in your bowl.
5. Sprinkle about 2 tbsp (30 mL) pomegranate seeds into each dessert dish. Refrigerate for 1 hour, or until set.
6. To the remaining gelatin mixture in the bowl, add cream cheese and cinnamon and beat with an electric beater until smooth; leave on the counter.
7. Once the gelatin is set in the dessert dishes, divide the cream cheese mixture among the dessert dishes. Use the back of a small spoon to spread evenly.
8. Return to the fridge for 15 minutes for final setting.

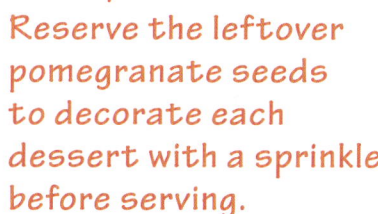

Reserve the leftover pomegranate seeds to decorate each dessert with a sprinkle before serving.

YOUR DINNER MENU	Large Meal (730 calories)	Total Carbs	NET CARBS	Small Meal (550 calories)	Total Carbs	NET CARBS
Chicken Cordon Bleu	5 oz (140 g) serving	5	5	5 oz (140 g) serving	5	5
Mashed sweet potato	⅔ cup (150 mL)	39	34	½ cup (125 mL)	29	26
Zucchini and parsnips	1 cup (250 mL)	11	8	—	—	—
Tossed salad	Small	2	1	Small	2	1
Fat-free Italian salad dressing	1 tbsp (15 mL)	2	2	1 tbsp (15 mL)	2	2
Cream Cheese Pomegranate Burst	1 serving	9	7	1 serving	9	7
	TOTAL CARBS	**68 g**	**57 g**	**TOTAL CARBS**	**47 g**	**41 g**
	Total carbs minus fiber = NET CARBS ↑			NET CARBS ↑		
	CARB CHOICES (1 carb choice = 15 g net carbs)		4	CARB CHOICES		3

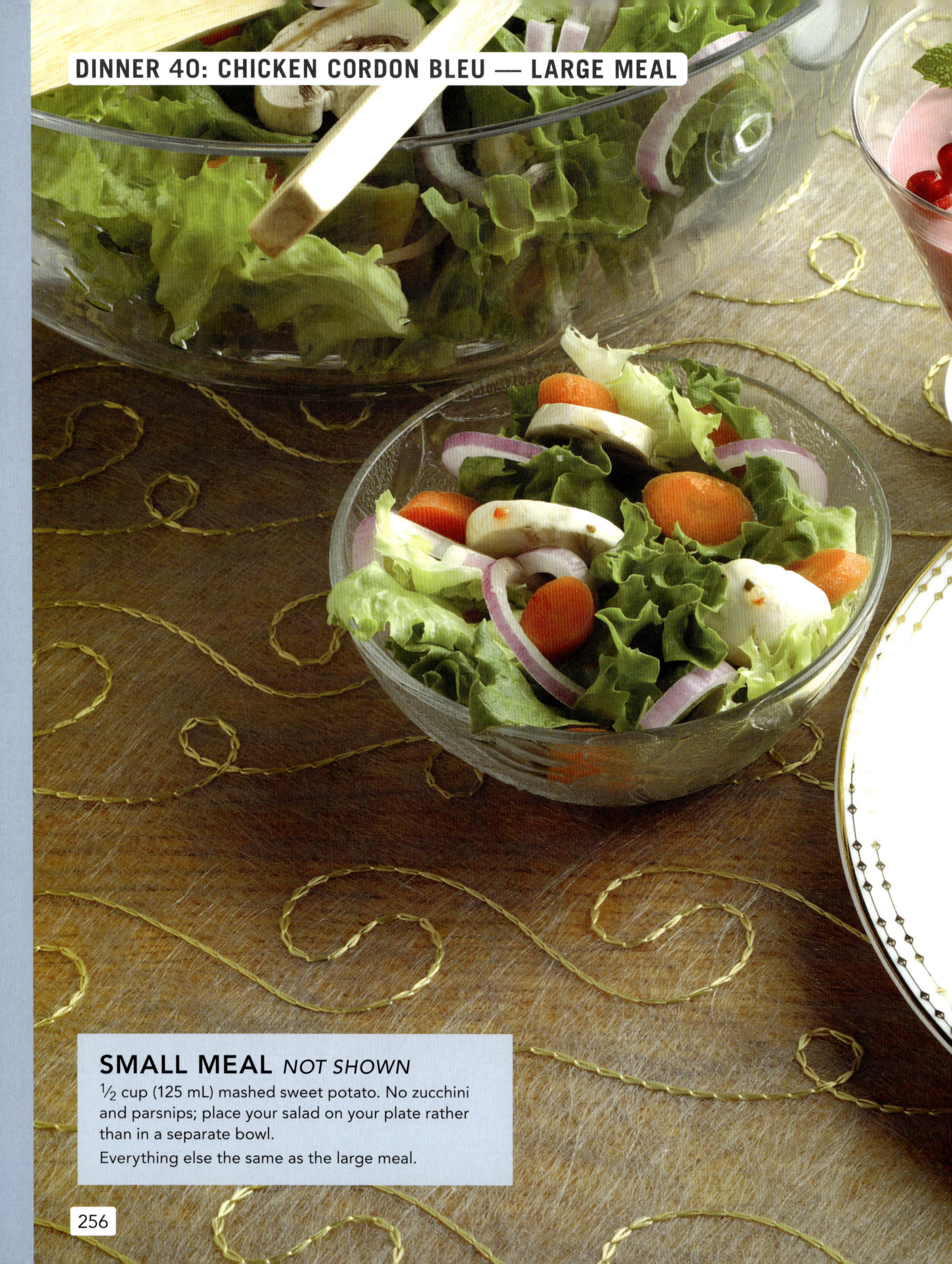

DINNER 40: CHICKEN CORDON BLEU — LARGE MEAL

SMALL MEAL *NOT SHOWN*
½ cup (125 mL) mashed sweet potato. No zucchini and parsnips; place your salad on your plate rather than in a separate bowl.
Everything else the same as the large meal.

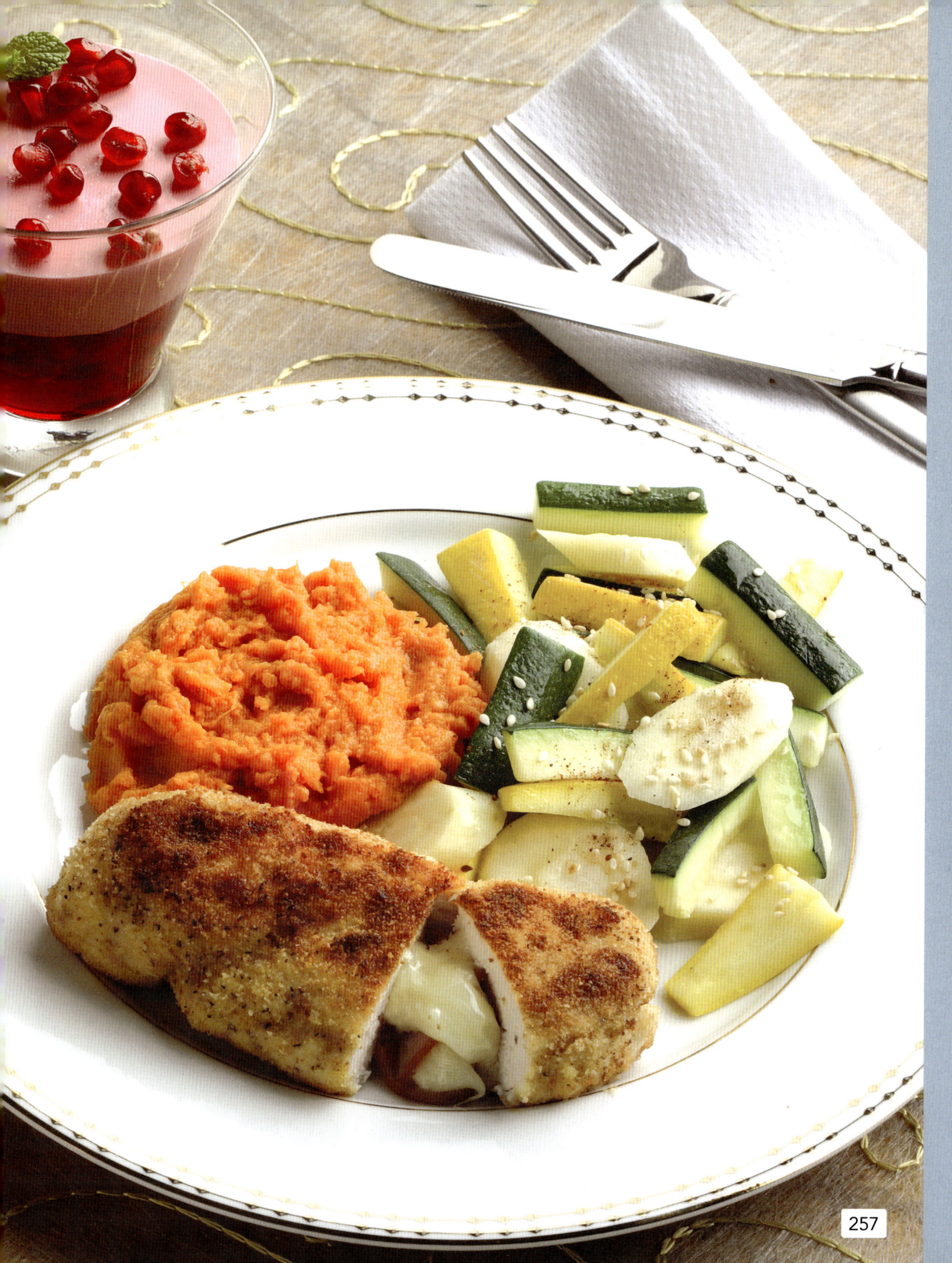

257

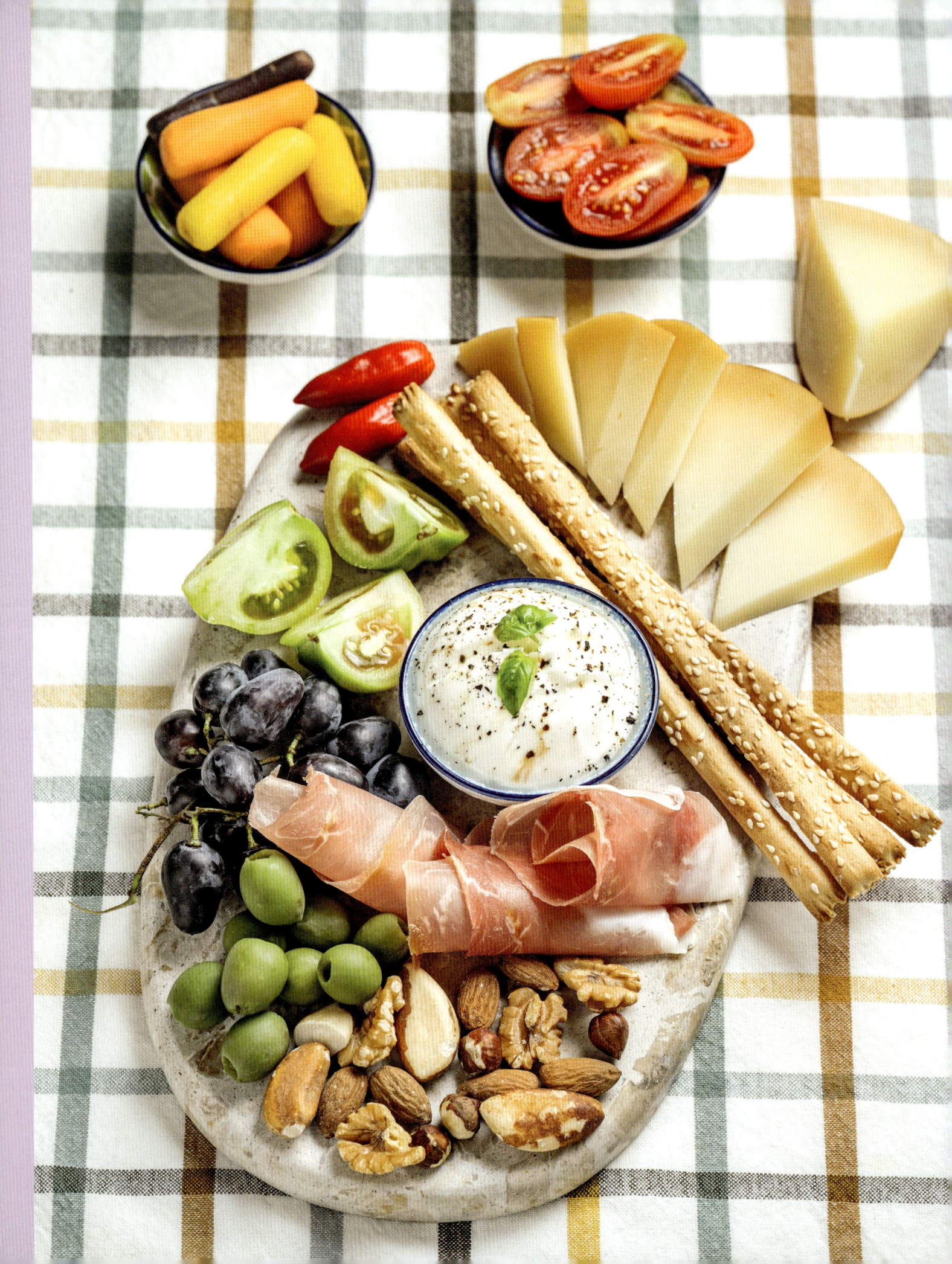

Snacks

> **Freebie Snacks – 20 calories or less**
> (0–5 g net carbs)
>
> **Small Snacks – 50 calories**
> (0–15 g net carbs)
>
> **Medium Snacks – 100 calories**
> (0–20 g net carbs)
>
> **Large Snacks – 200 calories**
> (0–30 g net carbs)

Chaffles (Cheese Waffles)

Makes 4 Chaffles

2 large eggs
2 tbsp (30 mL) almond flour
½ tsp (2 mL) baking powder
1 tsp (5 mL) zero-calorie sweetener
1 cup (250 mL) mozzarella cheese, shredded

1 CHAFFLE	
Calories	148
Total carbs	2 g
Net carbs	1 g

1. Whisk ingredients together in a bowl until smooth, then mix in the shredded mozzarella cheese.
2. Cook in a well-greased waffle iron until golden. These can also be cooked like pancakes in a frying pan.

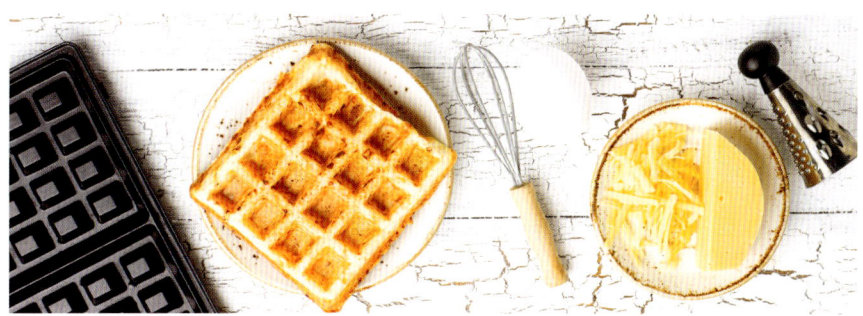

Mug Bread

Makes 2 slices

¼ cup (60 mL) almond flour
½ tsp (2 mL) baking powder
2 tsp (10 mL) vegetable oil
1 large egg

1 SLICE MUG BREAD	
Calories	165
Total carbs	3 g
Net carbs	1 g

1. Place all ingredients in a microwaveable coffee mug that is 3 inches (7.5 cm) wide and that doesn't narrow at the bottom. Stir with a fork until blended.
2. Place the mug in the microwave for 1 minute, or until egg is cooked.
3. Turn the mug upside down and tap it until the bread falls out. Slice it to make a top and bottom slice.

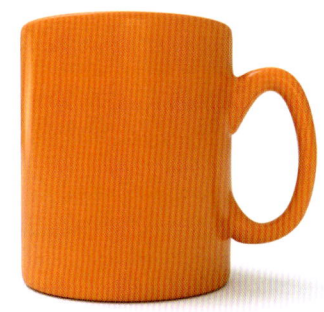

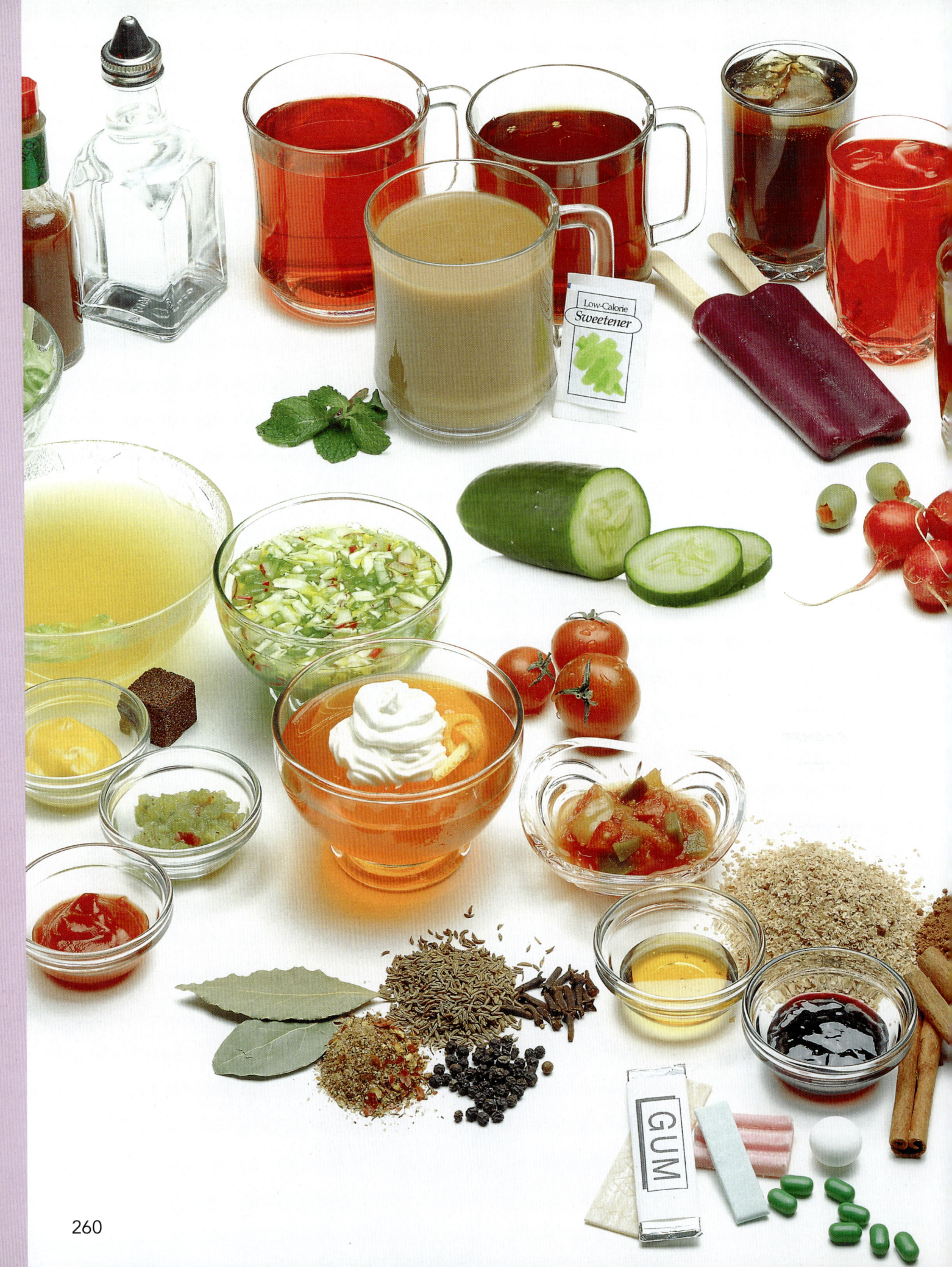

Freebie Snacks

20 calories or less in each snack

0–5 grams of net carbs

Salty snacks with more than 300 mg of salt are marked with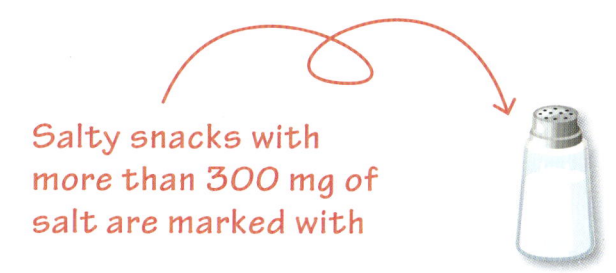

0/0 means: 1st number = total carbs in grams/ 2nd number = net carbs in grams

0–5 g net carbs

FUN SNACKS

- diet soft drinks (diet sodas) and packaged diet drink mixes **0/0**
- ½ cup light gelatin **0/0**
- 3 quartered, marinated artichoke hearts **1/0**
- 1 piece sugar-free gum **1/1**
- herbal tea, coffee or tea, plain **1/1**
- 4 mini-mints (Tic Tac-type) **2/2**
- 1 tbsp no-sugar-added pancake syrup (ED Smith-type) **3/2**
- 1 small hard candy (3 g), sugar-free **3/3**
- 1 sugar-free popsicle **3/3**
- 1 mint or small hard candy **4/4**

GOOD-FOR-YOU SNACKS

- water is always your best choice! **0/0**
- 3 radishes **0/0**
- 2 or 3 small green olives **0/0**
- 1 cup of salad greens **1/0**
- ¾ cup almond beverage, unsweetened **1/0**
- 1 medium stalk celery **2/1**
- ½ tomato **2/1**
- ½ cup Light Jellied Vegetable Salad (page 143) **2/1**
- ½ medium cucumber **3/2**
- 6 spears fresh steamed asparagus **4/2**

SALTY SNACKS YOU MIGHT CRAVE (CHOOSE ONLY OCCASIONALLY)

- 1 dill pickle **1/0**
- 10 hot banana pepper rings **1/0**
- ¼ cup sauerkraut **3/1**
- 1 cup reduced-salt bouillon or broth (4.5 g sachet or cube) **2/2**
- 5 strips roasted red pepper (jarred) **6/4**

ADDITIONS TO YOUR MEALS OR SNACKS

- 1 tsp hot pepper sauce **0/0**
- 1 tsp flavorings, such as cocoa, spices and herbs, lemon or lime **1/0**
- 1 tbsp bran or ½ tbsp ground flaxseed **1–2/0**
- 1 tsp zero-calorie sweetener **4/0**
- 1 tsp mustard, ketchup or relish **1/1**
- 1 tbsp vinegar **1/1**
- 1 tbsp salsa **1/1**
- 1 tbsp frozen whipped topping **1/1**
- 1 tbsp fat-free Italian dressing **1/1**
- 2 tsp diet jam **5/5**

METRIC CONVERSIONS IN SNACKS:
1 cup = 250 mL	1 tbsp = 15 mL
¾ cup = 175 mL	1 tsp = 5 mL
½ cup = 125 mL	½ tsp = 2 mL
¼ cup = 60 mL	¼ tsp = 1 mL

SNACKS

Small Snacks

50 calories in each snack
0–15 grams of net carbs

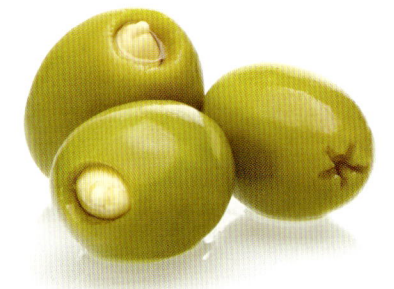

0/0 means: 1st number = total carbs in grams/ 2nd number = net carbs in grams

0–5 g net carbs

- 2 slices (30 g) prosciutto **0/0**
- 3 large green olives each stuffed with an almond **2/0**
- 1 cup Hot Golden Turmeric Milk (page 263) **2/1**
- 1 stalk of celery with 1 tbsp cheese spread (Cheez Whiz-type) **3/2**
- 6 spears fresh steamed asparagus with 1 tsp butter **4/2**
- 1 cup Sugar-Free Jelly with Berries (page 191) **5/3**
- 10 g (1-inch square, ½-inch thick) halva (tahini-based) **4/4**
- ½ cup Greek yogurt, 0%, flavored, zero sugar, with stevia **4/4**
- 1 cup canned tomatoes **8/4**
- ½ cup Greek yogurt, 0%, flavored, with sucralose **6/5**
- 2 Breton-type crackers **6/5**
- ½ cup fruit yogurt, 0%, sweetened with a low-calorie sweetener **6/5**
- Half cucumber sliced with 2 tbsp hummus **7/5**
- **Tomato salad:** 1 large chopped tomato with 1 tbsp fat-free Italian dressing **7/5**
- 1 fiber crispbread (Wasa brand) + thin spread of peanut butter **8/5**
- 4 seed crackers (13 g) **11/5**

ALCOHOLIC SNACKS

- 3 oz dry table wine (6 g alcohol) **3/3**
- 12 oz no-alcohol, low-carb beer (page 282) **5/5**

6–10 g net carbs

- 1 cup Reduced-Salt Instant Cup-of-Soup (page 74) **6/6**
- ½ cup skim or 1% milk **6/6**
- ¾ cup Coleslaw (page 72) **8/6**
- 1 medium carrot **8/6**
- 1 cup zucchini noodles (page 103) topped with ¼ cup spaghetti sauce **9/6**
- ¾ cup Stewed Rhubarb (page 111) **11/6**
- 1 whole-grain rice cake **7/7**
- 1 plain cookie, such as digestive biscuit **8/7**
- 2 melba toasts **8/7**
- 2 bread sticks **8/7**
- 1 cup light hot cocoa (no sugar added) **8/7**
- 4 whole wheat soda crackers **8/7**
- ¼ cup Goldfish Baked Cheddar Snack Crackers **8/8**

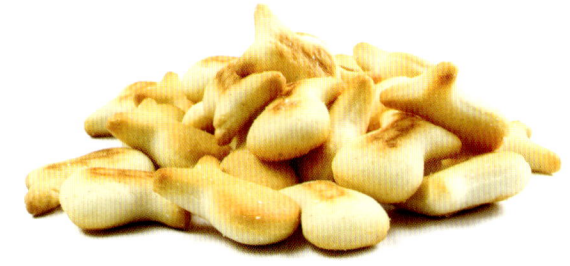

SNACKS

- 1 cup tomato or vegetable juice **9/8**
- 2 poppadoms **10/8**
- 1 cup strawberries **12/8**
- 1 cup Fruit Milkshake (page 107) **15/8**
- 1 medium plum **10/9**
- 1 medium kiwi **12/9**
- ¾ cup bowl of mixed berries **13/9**
- 1 cup puffed wheat cereal with ½ cup almond beverage **11/10**
- 2 prunes or figs **11/10**
- 1 Fig Newton cookie **11/10**
- ½ medium apple **11/10**
- ½ large grapefruit **12/10**
- 2 mandarin oranges **12/10**

11–15 g net carbs

- 2 graham wafer halves **11/11**
- ¾ cup grapes **12/11**
- 2 standard-sized marshmallows **12/12**
- 3 hard candy mints **12/12**
- 12 oz no-alcohol beer **12/12** (see Beer Swaps chart, page 282)
- 1 small orange **14/12**
- ¾ cup Butterscotch Pudding (page 99); try frozen on a popsicle stick **14/12**

Hot Golden Turmeric Milk

Makes 1 cup (250 mL)

Carbs **2/1**

1 cup (250 mL) almond beverage

½ tsp (2 mL) butter

¼ tsp (1 mL) each: turmeric powder, ginger powder and vanilla

Dash of salt and pepper

1-inch (2.5 cm) piece of cinnamon stick

1 tsp (5 mL) zero-calorie sweetener

1. Combine all ingredients in a mug and stir or whisk well. Add piece of cinnamon stick.
2. Microwave for 1 minute or until simmering.

Note: Turmeric milk, if spilled, will stain.

1 CUP	
Calories	50
Total carbs	2 g
Net carbs	1 g

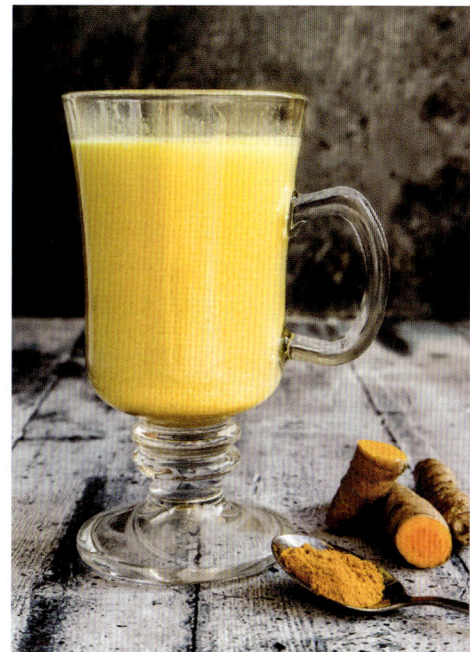

SNACKS

Medium Snacks

100 calories in each snack

0–20 grams of net carbs

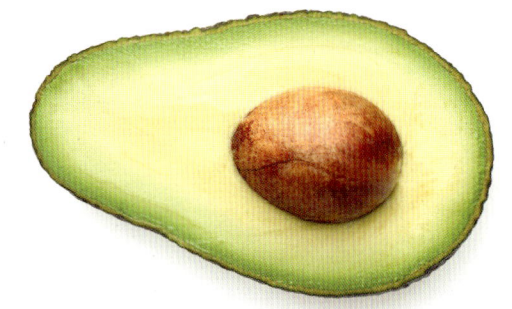

0/0 means: 1st number = total carbs in grams/ 2nd number = net carbs in grams

0–5 g net carbs

- 3 Cheese Crisps (page 265) **0/0**
- 1 oz aged gouda cheese **0/0**
- 1 oz Cheddar or mozzarella cheese **1/1**
- 2 tbsp sunflower seeds **3/1**
- ½ small avocado, plain or chunks, with balsamic vinegar **6/1**
- 8 jumbo shrimp and 2 tbsp shrimp cocktail sauce **3/2**
- 15 almonds **4/2**
- 25 pistachios **5/3**
- ¾ cup canned tomatoes and 3 tbsp shredded cheese (melted on top) **6/3**
- 20 g dark chocolate (80% cocoa) **7/4**
- ⅓ cup steamed edamame beans with 1 tsp sesame seed oil **9/4**
- ½ cup 1% or 2% cottage cheese with ½ medium chopped tomato **6/5**
- Mini high-protein bar (20 g) **8/5**
- 1½ cups roasted low-calorie vegetables, made with ½ tbsp olive oil **8/5**

ALCOHOLIC SNACKS

- 1½ oz alcohol (rye, gin, rum, whiskey), 35–40% alcohol (14 g alcohol), straight or with diet soft drink or water **14/0**
- Light or ultra light beer, 2–4% alcohol (page 282) **3/3**

6–10 g net carbs

- ¾ cup Greek yogurt, 0%, plain **6/6**
- ½ cup Greek yogurt, 0%, less sugar, flavored **6/6**
- 1 cup Tofu Fruit Smoothie (page 52) **9/6**
- 4 whole wheat or plain soda crackers and ½ oz cheese **8/7**
- ⅓ cup pumpkin seeds **11/7**
- ¾ cup Icelandic yogurt, 0%, plain **8/8**
- 1 Low-Carb Homemade Waffle (page 50) with 1 tsp peanut butter **8/8**
- 4 whole wheat or plain soda crackers with 1 tbsp light cream cheese or canned salmon **9/8**
- 1 serving Chocolate Mousse (page 123) **11/10**
- 6 baked tortilla chips or other baked chips with 2 tbsp hummus or salsa sauce **12/10**

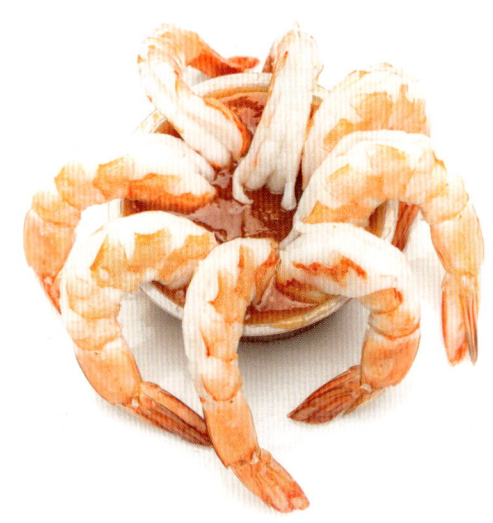

SNACKS

11–20 g net carbs

- ½ cup Icelandic yogurt, 0%, flavored, with stevia **11**/**11**
- ½ medium apple with ½ tbsp peanut butter **13**/**11**
- 24 beet chips (see page 282 for other chip examples for 200 calories) **16**/**11**
- 2 gingersnap cookies with ½ oz cheese **12**/**12**
- 1 cup low-fat milk (or buttermilk) **12**/**12**
- 1 Rice Cake Dessert (page 175) **13**/**12**
- ½ pizza bun **13**/**12**
- ½ cup Greek yogurt, 0%, plain, with ½ cup blueberries **14**/**12**
- 1 piece toast with thin spread of peanut butter **15**/**12**
- Mini 100 g (⅓ cup) container of yogurt, 1.5%, regular, creamy fruit flavored **13**/**13**
- ½ English muffin with thin spread of peanut butter **14**/**13**
- 1 slice raisin bread with 1 tsp margarine **14**/**13**
- 2 to 3 cups raw vegetables with 2 tbsp Vegetable Dip (page 174) **19**/**13**
- 3 cups air-popped popcorn **19**/**15**
- 3 arrowroots or other plain cookies **17**/**16**
- ½ cup frozen yogurt, Dutch chocolate (page 278) **17**/**16**
- ⅔ cup Cheerios-type oat cereal and ½ cup low-fat milk **17**/**16**
- 1 small banana with 1 tsp nut butter **17**/**16**
- 2 Dad's Oatmeal Cookies **18**/**16**
- ⅓ of a 3 oz package of oriental noodles (made with salt-free spice blend) **20**/**19**
- 5 dried apricots **22**/**19**
- ½ small cantaloupe **22**/**20**

Cheese Crisps

Makes 12

3 Cheese Crisps = Carbs **5**/**1**

Preheat oven to 375°F (190°C)

3 CRISPS	
Calories	109
Total carbs	0 g
Net carbs	0 g

FOR EACH CHEESE CRISP:

1 heaping tbsp (15 mL) shredded cheese such as Cheddar, mozzarella or Parmesan

Optional topping: Sprinkle of sesame seeds, dried rosemary, or if you like it hot: chili pepper flakes or a thin slice of jalapeno pepper

1. Cover baking sheet with parchment paper. Drop the spoonfuls of shredded cheese into mounds on top of the parchment paper. Allow room for it to spread as it cooks.
2. Add topping if desired.
3. Bake for 5 minutes, or until edges slightly brown.
4. Let cool for 5 minutes.
5. Store extras in a sealed container on the counter, or for more than a day, in the fridge.

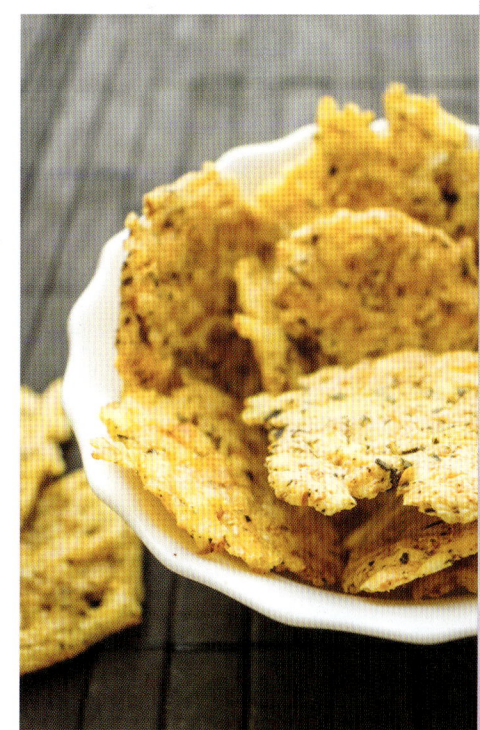

SNACKS

Large Snacks

200 calories in each snack

0–30 grams of net carbs

2/1 means: 1st number = total carbs in grams/ 2nd number = net carbs in grams

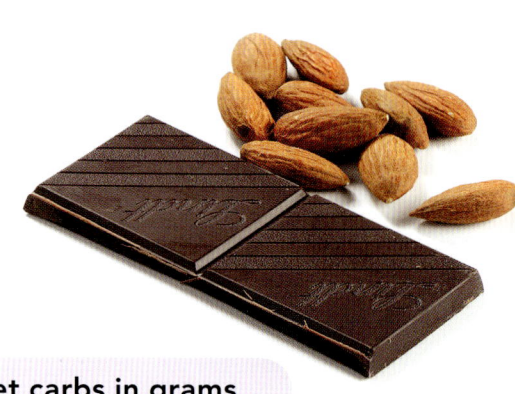

0–5 g net carbs

- **Veggie Scramble:** 1 tsp butter or oil, 1 cup chopped low-carb veggies (page 134), 1 large egg and 3 tbsp shredded cheese **2/1**
- ½ cup keto frozen dessert (page 278) **10/1** (make a float by adding your ice cream to a cold glassful of zero-calorie diet cola)
- 1 slice buttered keto bread topped with 1 oz cheese **8/2**
- Frying pan grilled cheese sandwich made with 2 slices keto bread, 1 oz cheese and 2 tsp margarine/butter **8/2**
- Enlightened Keto ice cream bar **11/2**
- 29 almonds **8/3**
- 1 small avocado (try with a sprinkle of Worcestershire sauce or lemon) **12/3**
- Stuffed Portobello Mushroom (page 267) **5/4**
- 16 peanuts in the shell **6/4**
- **Mixed nuts:** 3 walnuts, 6 almonds and 6 hazelnuts **7/5**
- 40 g high-protein/high-fat snack bar (page 280) **12/5**

6–10 g net carbs

- ¾ oz 80% dark chocolate with 10 almonds (as shown above) **10/6**
- 50 pistachios **10/6**
- 3 oz cooked chicken pieces, 1 medium carrot (sticks); dip into 2 tbsp Vegetable Dip (page 174) **10/8**

- 1.5 oz (40 g) 80% dark chocolate **14/8**
- **Low-Carb Dessert Omelet:** combine 2 large eggs with ½ tbsp zero-calorie sweetener, 1 tbsp milk and a sprinkle of cinnamon and fry; serve with 3 tbsp 40%-less-sugar syrup **14/8**
- 1 cup keto cereal (page 277) with ½ cup almond beverage **18/8**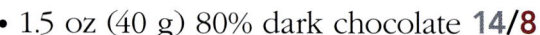
- 4 Breton-style crackers with 2 large sardines **10/9**
- **Protein Shake:** 42 g scoop protein powder (with 10 g carbs) and 1 cup almond beverage **11/9**
- 22 cashews **11/10**

11–20 g net carbs

- 1 cup nut or coconut beverage or buttermilk plus 1 high-protein bar **19/12**
- 1 slice pumpernickel bread with 1 tsp margarine and 1½ oz pickled herring or salmon/tuna salad **16/14**
- 1 serving Greek Salad (page 215) **17/15**
- 18 potato chips **18/16**
- 1 boiled or poached egg and 1 slice toast with 1 tsp margarine **20/17**
- 1 piece of Low-Carb Bannock (page 119) **20/18**
- 1 shredded wheat biscuit with 1 cup nut or coconut beverage plus 2 tbsp chopped nuts **23/18**
- 25 Cheezies **20/20**
- 1 medium apple with 1 oz cheese **22/20**

SNACKS

- 1 Bran Muffin (page 44) and ½ oz cheese **24**/**20**
- Half of a 10 oz can cream of tomato soup made with ½ can nut or coconut beverage plus 2 tbsp cheese, shredded **22**/**20**

- 1 Baked Apple (page 151) plus ½ oz cheese **25**/**23**
- 1 cup cooked cream of wheat with 1 cup almond beverage, 1 tsp butter melted in, and a sprinkle of cinnamon **28**/**24**
- 2 Dad's Oatmeal Chocolate Chip Cookies **26**/**25**
- 1 small cone with ¾ cup regular ice cream **26**/**26**
- **Ham sandwich:** 1 oz meat on 2 slices of whole-grain bread with mustard and lettuce **30**/**26**
- 1 slice Banana Bread (page 243) **30**/**26**
- ½ small (3-inch) bagel with 2 tbsp light cream cheese **27**/**27**
- ¾ cup Rice Pudding (page 115) **31**/**30**

21–30 g net carbs

- Small cake donut **23**/**22**
- 5 pieces of California sushi roll **24**/**22**
- 16 baked tortilla chips and 2 tbsp hummus or salsa **26**/**22**
- 1⅓ oz chocolate bar (3 sticks of a KitKat) **24**/**23**
- 1 slice Crustless Pumpkin Pie (page 163) with 2 to 4 tbsp whipped cream or topping **25**/**23**

Stuffed Portobello Mushrooms

Makes 2 mushrooms (2 servings)

1 Stuffed Mushroom = Carbs **5**/**4**

Preheat oven to 400°F (200°C)

2 large portobello mushrooms – 5 inches (12.5 cm) in diameter; choose mushrooms with a complete unbroken rim (like a bowl)

2 tsp (10 mL) butter, melted

¼ cup (60 mL) spaghetti or marinara sauce

¼ tsp (1 mL) garlic powder

½ tsp (2 mL) oregano

2 tbsp (30 mL) Parmesan cheese, shredded

4 thin slices (14 g/½ oz) pepperoni

½ cup (125 mL) mozzarella cheese, shredded

2–3 baby tomatoes, halved

Fresh herbs, chopped, such as basil

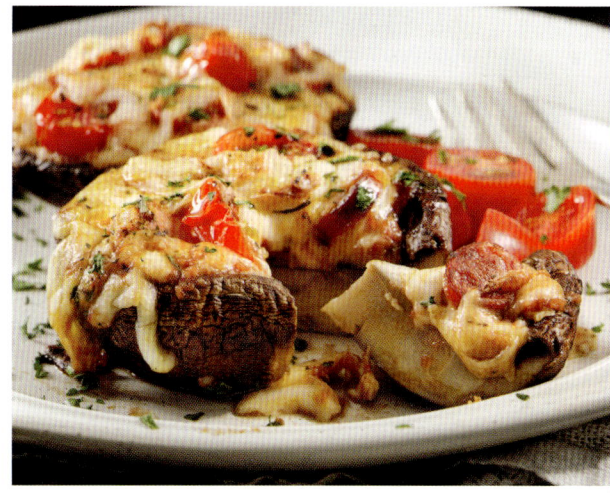

1 STUFFED MUSHROOM	
Calories	198
Total carbs	5 g
Net carbs	4 g

1. Use a small spoon to scrape out the stem and mushroom gills.
2. Brush the melted butter inside the mushroom.
3. Mix together spaghetti sauce, garlic powder, oregano and Parmesan cheese, and add to inside of mushrooms.
4. Layer on top: pepperoni, mozzarella cheese, halved baby tomatoes and herbs.
5. Put parchment paper on your pan and place mushrooms on paper. Bake in oven for 25 minutes, or until cheese bubbles.

READ FOOD LABELS FOR CARBS

Example of a Food Label

NUTRITION FACTS

Serving Size
Nutrition Facts are based on serving size, which can vary between similar products.

Calories
Calories are a total of fat, carbohydrate and protein.

If a yogurt has lower carbohydrate, it will have more calories from fat or protein.

Sodium
This yogurt has 3% sodium. As a general guide, 5% or less sodium per serving is considered low.

INGREDIENTS LIST

CREAMY STRAWBERRY YOGURT

NUTRITION FACTS

Per ¾ cup (175 g)	
Calories	130
Fat	2.5 g
Saturated	1.5 g
Trans	0.1 g
Carbohydrate	29 g
Fiber	0 g
Sugars	17 g
Protein	7 g
Cholesterol	10 mg
Sodium	70 mg 3%

INGREDIENTS:
SKIM MILK, MODIFIED MILK INGREDIENTS, CANE SUGAR, WATER, CREAM, MODIFIED CORN STARCH, STRAWBERRIES, WHEY PROTEIN, ACTIVE BACTERIAL CULTURE, PECTIN, NATURAL FLAVOR, VITAMIN D3.

Ingredients
Ingredients are listed in order from the most to the least.

Sugars
For sweetening, this yogurt has cane sugar added. This increases carbohydrate.

Milk Fat (% MF)
This yogurt has 1.5% milk fat. 0% MF is the lowest; some yogurts are especially high at 14% MF.

Diet or Less Sugar Flavored Yogurts

Instead of sugar, these will have other low-calorie products added for sweetening. For example, you may see aspartame, monk fruit, stevia, sucralose or sorbitol listed.

Read Food Labels for Carbs

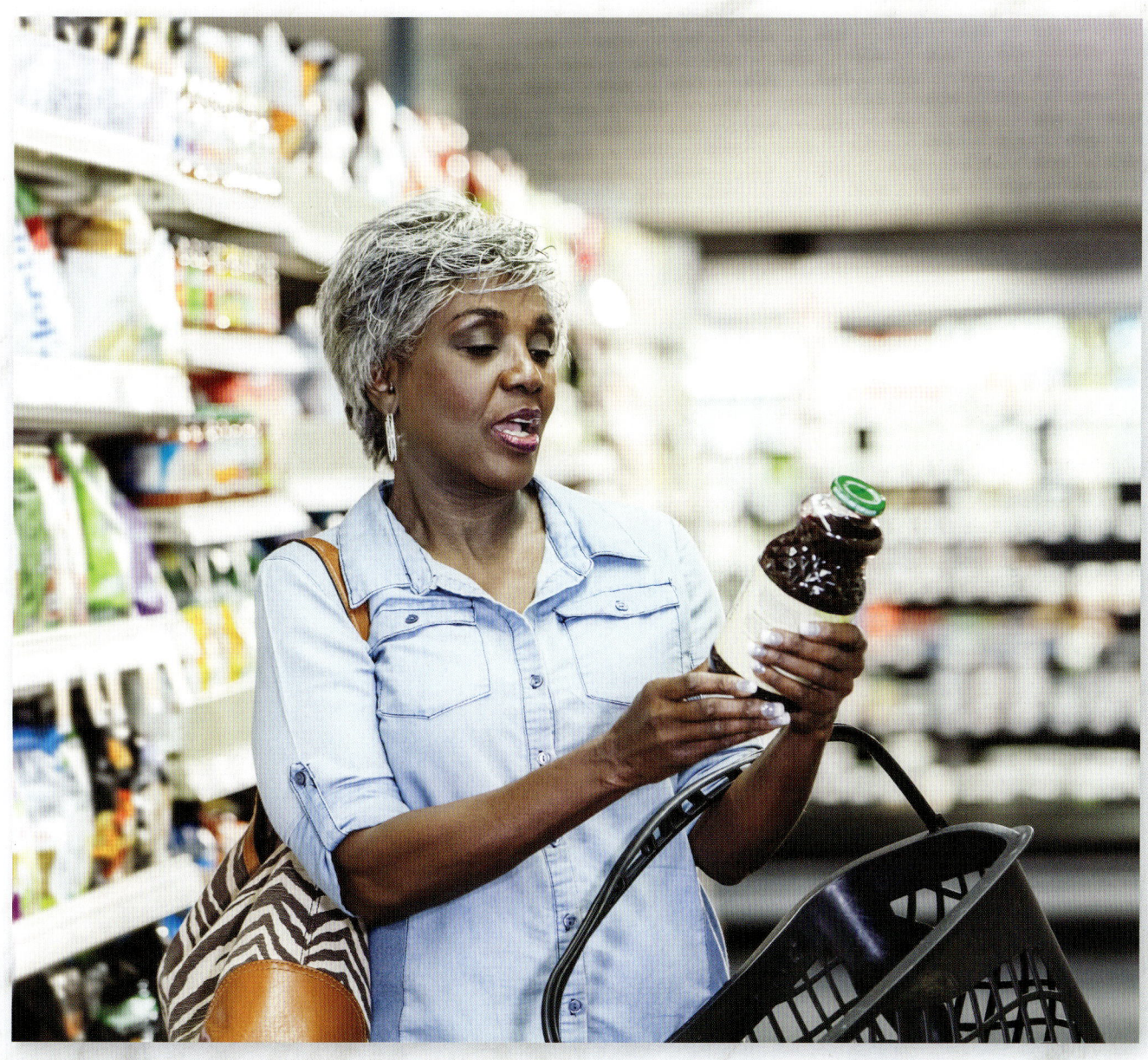

My goodness, this juice has a lot of natural sugar.

READ FOOD LABELS FOR CARBS

How to Calculate Net Carbs from the Nutrition Facts on a Food Label

First, look at the Carbohydrate.
On the food label, Carbohydrate is equal to "Total Carbs" listed in each food menu in this book. It includes:

- Fiber
- Sugar:
  - **natural sugar** from fruits, vegetables or milk
  - **added sugar** from cane sugar, fructose, sucrose and corn syrup
- Sugar alcohols such as sorbitol
- Starches, such as grains and cereals

Good news! You don't need to count Sugars/Added Sugars because these are already counted in the Carbohydrate.

Next, look at the Fiber.
Fiber in its whole (unprocessed) form is not digested, so fiber does not raise blood sugar. To calculate net carbs, subtract the **Fiber** from the **Carbohydrate** number.

Then, look for the Sugar Alcohols.
Most sugar alcohols are half absorbed by the body. To calculate net carbs, you will subtract **half of the Sugar Alcohols** from the Carbohydrate number.

Most sugar alcohols are half absorbed.

The INGREDIENTS list these sugar alcohols:

- isomalt
- lactitol
- maltitol
- mannitol
- sorbitol
- xylitol

There is one exception.
Erythritol is a common sugar alcohol in low-carb products. It is not absorbed at all. Therefore, you **subtract all of the erythritol** from the **Carbohydrate** number.

Erythritol is an exception: it is not absorbed at all = zero net carbs.

Sometimes erythritol is listed on the Nutrition Facts label under Carbohydrate. Other times, the only way you know erythritol is in the food product is by looking at the ingredients list. If erythritol is listed first, second, third or fourth, then you know it's a main ingredient. Go ahead and subtract it from the Carbohydrate when you are working out net carbs.

Erythritol therefore has zero carbs and zero calories just like aspartame, monk fruit, stevia and sucralose.

Let's Calculate Net Carbs

Net Carbs appear on some American food labels but are not regulated. Net Carbs are not listed on Canadian food labels. Use the the information below and on page 272 to more accurately determine the net carbs.

Net carbs = Carbohydrate minus Fiber and minus Sugar Alcohols (most or all, depending on the type of sugar alcohols)

EXAMPLE 1: Sugar-free peppermint chocolate patties made with maltitol and isomalt

The INGREDIENTS show maltitol and isomalt in the top four. Both of these sugar alcohols are half-carb sweeteners.

"Sugar-free" on the label does not mean carb-free.

NUTRITION FACTS

Per 3 pieces (37 g)
Calories	120
Fat	8 g
Saturated	4.5 g
Trans	0 g
Carbohydrate	24 g
Fiber	2 g
Sugar	0 g
Sugar Alcohols	20 g
Protein	8 g
Cholesterol	0 mg
Sodium	5 mg 0%

INGREDIENTS: MALTITOL, CHOCOLATE, ISOMALT, MALTITOL SYRUP, COCOA BUTTER, MILK FAT, OIL OF PEPPERMINT, FLAVORS.

For a serving size of 3 pieces

Carbohydrates	24 g
Fiber	2 g
Sugar Alcohols	20 g

Net carbs

Carbohydrates (24 g) *minus* Fiber (2 g) *minus* half Sugar Alcohols (10 g)
Equals 12 g net carbs

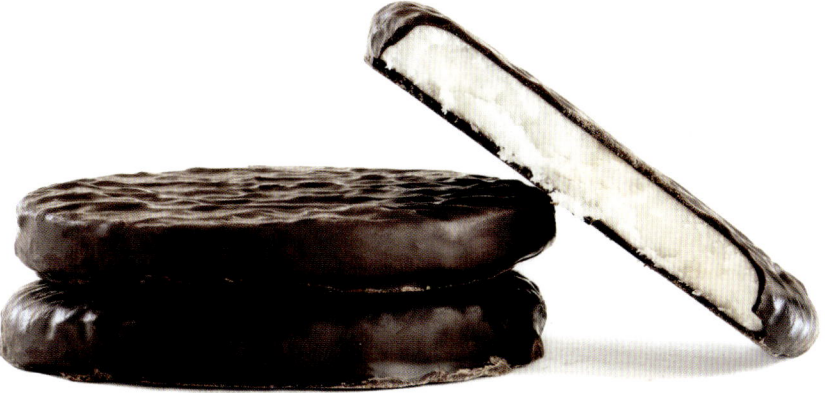

To compare the carbs in these chocolates to other chocolates and candies, see the Candy Swaps chart on page 281.

READ FOOD LABELS FOR CARBS

EXAMPLE 2: Keto chocolate frozen dessert (ice cream) made with erythritol

The INGREDIENTS show erythritol as the fourth ingredient. This sugar alcohol is a zero-calorie sweetener.

NUTRITION FACTS

Per ½ cup (125 mL)	
Calories	**200**
Fat	**17 g**
Saturated	11 g
Trans	0 g
Carbohydrate	**10 g**
Fiber	2 g
Sugar	0 g
Sugar Alcohols	8 g
Protein	**3 g**
Cholesterol	**110 mg**
Sodium	**25 mg 1%**

INGREDIENTS:
CREAM, WATER, EGG YOLKS, ERYTHRITOL, XYLITOL, SOLUBLE CORN FIBER, COCOA, VEGETABLE GLYCERIN, MILK PROTEIN CONCENTRATE, VANILLA, MONK FRUIT JUICE CONCENTRATE, SKIM MILK, CELULLOSE GUM.

For a serving size of ½ cup

Carbohydrates 10 g
Fiber 2 g
Sugar Alcohols 8 g

Net carbs

Carbohydrates (10 g) *minus* Fiber (2 g) *minus* all Sugar Alcohols (8 g)
Equals 0 g (no net carbs)

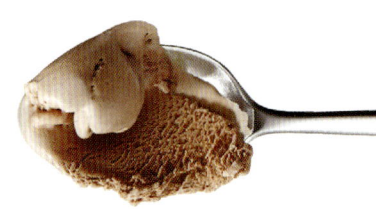

To compare the carbs in this ice cream to other ice creams, see the Ice Cream Swaps chart on page 278.

EXAMPLE 3: No-sugar-added oatmeal cookie made with maltitol

The INGREDIENTS show maltitol in the top three. This sugar alcohol is a half-carb sweetener.

"No Sugar Added" on the label does not mean carb-free.

NUTRITION FACTS

Per 1 cookie (19 g)	
Calories	**85**
Fat	**4 g**
Saturated	1 g
Trans	0 g
Carbohydrate	**14 g**
Fiber	1 g
Sugar	0 g
Sugar Alcohols	6 g
Protein	**1 g**
Cholesterol	**0 mg**
Sodium	**45 mg 2%**

INGREDIENTS:
ENRICHED WHEAT FLOUR, WHOLE GRAIN OATS, MALTITOL, VEGETABLE OIL, MALTITOL SYRUP, WATER, WHOLE GRAIN FLOUR, PALM OIL, SALT, CINNAMON, BAKING SODA, SKIM MILK POWDER, DRIED WHOLE EGG, SOY LECITHIN, NATURAL FLAVOR.

For a serving size of 1 cookie

Carbohydrates 10 g
Fiber 2 g
Sugar Alcohols 6 g

Net carbs

Carbohydrates (10 g) *minus* Fiber (2 g) *minus* half Sugar Alcohols (3 g)
Equals 5 g net carbs

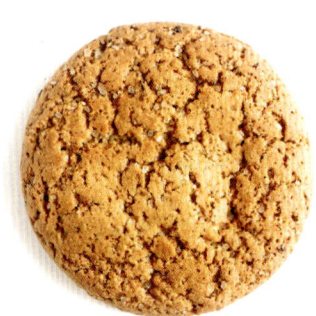

To compare the carbs in this cookie to other cookies, see the Cookie Swaps chart on page 280.

Low-Carb Swap Charts

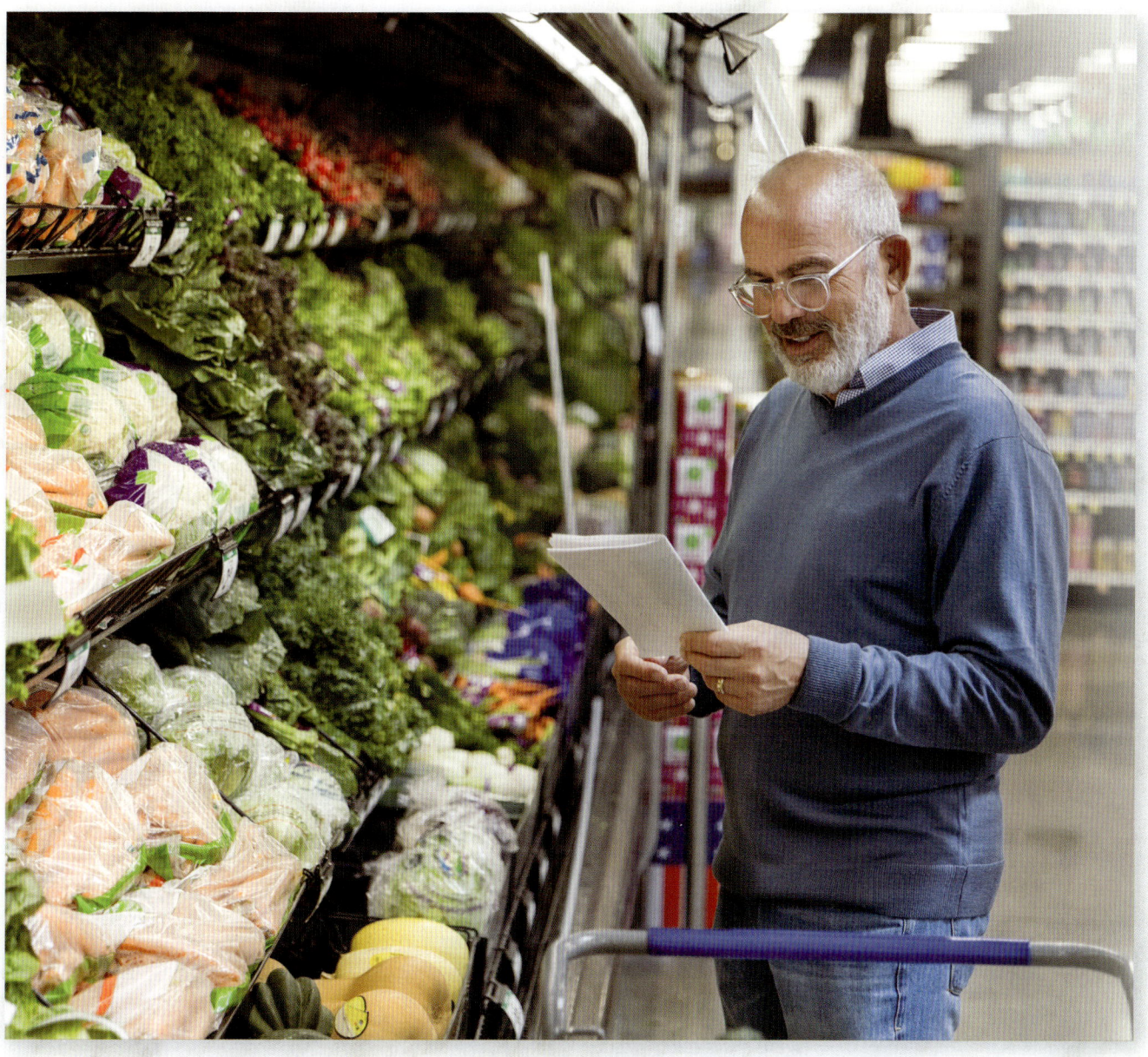

For dinner tonight, I think I'll try the squash instead of potato.

LOW-CARB SWAP CHARTS

Carbs, protein and fat are in grams (g).

Products are listed from lowest to highest carb count.

Bread Swaps

30–40 g slice of bread

Many whole-grain, high-fiber breads are sliced thicker (and could weigh more than 40 g) and so may have more carbs than shown in the chart.

	CALORIES	TOTAL CARBS	FIBER	NET CARBS	PROTEIN	FAT	SODIUM (MG)
STANDARD BREADS							
Whole-grain bread	81	14	2	12	4	1	146
Whole wheat bread	**81**	**14**	**2**	**12**	**4**	**1**	**146**
Rye bread	83	15	2	13	3	1	193
Fiber white bread	77	16	3	13	4	1	154
White bread	98	18	1	17	3	1	180
ALTERNATIVE BREADS OR CRACKERS							
Mug Bread (page 259), 1 slice	163	3	2	1	6	20	99
Homemade Low-Carb Egg Muffin (page 56), half muffin	131	2	1	1	5	12	124
Low-Carb Egg Bread (page 68), 1 piece	65	1	0	1	4	5	82
Low-carb bread (page 46)	90	8	6	2	7	3	115
Breton-type crackers, original, 4 crackers	90	12	1	11	2	4	150
Whole wheat soda crackers (saltines), 7 crackers	84	14	1	13	2	2	252
Soda crackers (regular), 7 crackers	91	15	1	14	2	2	196
FLATBREADS							
Chapati, thin, 6-inch (15 cm)	91	15	3	12	3	2	99
Flour tortilla, half of an 8-inch (20 cm)	85	15	1	14	2	2	125
Naan bread, one third of a 90 g piece	87	15	1	14	3	2	140
Roti shell, dhalpuri, one third of a 13-inch (33 cm)	94	16	1	15	3	2	73
Pita shell, half of a 6-inch (15 cm)	83	17	1	16	3	1	161

Pasta Swaps

25 g dry pasta = ½ cup/125 mL cooked

The cooked volume from 25 g pasta varies slightly between pastas.

	CALORIES	TOTAL CARBS	FIBER	NET CARBS	PROTEIN	NOTES
Konjac spaghetti (shirataki with oat fiber) is an Asian vegetable that is very low in carbs 100 g = ½ cup (125 mL) precooked	15	4	3	1	0	Bland, costly and packaged in heavy plastic. Ready to eat, cold or heated. See page 226. Don't eat konjac pasta daily due to its gelatinous soluble fiber.
Zucchini noodles; also called zoodles	10	2	0	2	0	Very low in carbs and calories. Buy pre-made frozen zoodles or make at home. See page 103.
Edamame (soybean) spaghetti	81	9	6	3	11	Very high in protein and fiber; thin, moist, tasty strands
Spaghetti squash	21	5	1	4	0	
Butternut squash noodles	42	11	3	8	1	
Spelt spaghetti	84	16	3	13	3	Dark brown pasta
Whole-grain spaghetti	**88**	**19**	**2**	**17**	**3**	**Coarser than regular**
Regular spaghetti (durum wheat)	90	20	1	19	3	

Potato Swaps

½ medium potato or equivalent

	CALORIES	TOTAL CARBS	FIBER	NET CARBS	PROTEIN
BAKED – measured as ½ cup (125 mL) raw cubed or ½ medium potato (2–3-inches/ 5–7.5 cm) in size = medium)					
Baked turnip (white inside)	21	5	2	3	1
Baked rutabaga (yellow inside)	35	6	2	4	1
Baked butternut squash	41	11	4	7	1
Baked potato	**80**	**18**	**2**	**16**	**2**
Baked sweet potato (yams)	90	21	4	17	2
MASHED – measured as ½ cup (125 mL), made with milk and butter (pages 126–127)					
Mashed cauliflower	32	5	1	4	2
Mashed Potatoes with Cauliflower (page 127)	43	8	1	6	1
Mashed potato	113	20	2	18	2

LOW-CARB SWAP CHARTS

Rice Swaps

⅓ cup/75 mL, cooked

In this rice chart, the glycemic index (GI) of different types of rice is also compared. Low GI foods raise your blood sugar more slowly than high GI foods.

	CALORIES	TOTAL CARBS	FIBER	NET CARBS	PROTEIN	NOTES
RICE						
Brown rice, short or long grain	73	15	1	14	2	Low GI
Parboiled (converted) rice	67	16	0	15	2	Low GI and lowest net carbs. The rice is precooked, which hardens the rice kernel and changes the starch; it is digested more slowly.
Basmati long-grain rice (white or brown) Or red rice or black rice	68	15	0	15	1	Low GI. These have a compound called amylose which slows carbohydrate digestion.
Long-grain rice	**68**	**15**	**0**	**15**	**1**	**Medium GI**
Jasmine rice (long-grain); short grain; sticky rice	79	17	0	17	1	High GI. Use smaller portions and monitor the effect on your blood sugar.
Day-old rice (cooked, then left to sit in the fridge for a day) develops more "resistant starch." This starch is slower to digest, so it has a lower GI than freshly cooked rice.						
RICE ALTERNATIVES						
Rice-shaped konjac	10	0	5	0	0	100 g = ⅓ cup
Riced cauliflower	8	2	1	1	1	See page 106
Couscous: regular or whole wheat	59	12	1	11	2	See page 139
Quinoa	74	13	2	11	3	
Wild rice	55	12	1	11	2	

LOW-CARB SWAP CHARTS

Cereal Swaps
1 cup/250 mL serving

	CALORIES	TOTAL CARBS	FIBER	NET CARBS	PROTEIN	FAT	SODIUM	NOTES
HOT COOKED CEREAL								
Oatmeal (minute oats)	**133**	**24**	**4**	**20**	**5**	**2**	**1**	**The GI goes down with large-flake oats and steel-cut oats**
Cream of Wheat	132	26	2	24	4	1	43	High in added iron
Quinoa	222	40	5	35	9	4	13	
COLD DRY CEREAL								
Keto cereal, marked low-carb or zero carb	150–200	18	10	8	7	3	280	Keto cereals have added protein, fiber, fat and low-calorie sweeteners.
Shredded Wheat (1 biscuit)	80	19	3	16	3	1	0	
Cheerios, original	**100**	**20**	**3**	**17**	**4**	**2**	**170**	
Multi Grain Cheerios	113	24	2	22	2	1	113	Multi Grain Cheerios have more sugar added than original.
Bran flakes, generic brand	110	25	4	21	3	1	220	
Rice Krispies	110	25	0	25	2	1	153	
Honey Nut Cheerios	140	30	3	27	3	2	211	
Shreddies	200	46	6	40	5	1	210	Whole grain, but high in carbs
Granola	596	66	12	56	18	30	32	High in calories, so just have a sprinkle

LOW-CARB SWAP CHARTS

Yogurt Swaps

¾ cup/175 mL portion

Because yogurt does not contain fiber, total and net carbs are the same.

	CALORIES	FAT	TOTAL CARBS/ NET CARBS	PROTEIN
REGULAR YOGURT				
Balkan yogurt, 6%, plain	140	10	7	6
Yogurt, 0%, strawberry, no added sugar (with stevia)	68	0	9	7
Yogurt, 0%, plain	**70**	**0**	**11**	**6**
Yogurt, 1.5%, creamy strawberry (shown on page 268)	130	3	29	7
GREEK-STYLE YOGURT (has extra protein)				
Greek yogurt, 0%, plain, "No Sugar Added"	100	0	6	17
Greek yogurt, 0%, strawberry, Zero Sugar (with stevia)	68	0	6	12
Icelandic yogurt, 0%, plain	120	0	8	20
Icelandic yogurt, 0%, with berries and stevia	140	0	17	17
Greek yogurt, 0%, "Less Sugar," strawberry	136	0	20	14
Greek yogurt, 5%, extra creamy strawberry	200	7	22	13

Ice Cream Swaps

Per ½-cup/125 mL serving of chocolate ice cream

	CALORIES	TOTAL CARBS	FIBER	SUGAR ALCOHOLS	NET CARBS	FAT	NOTES
Keto frozen dessert, chocolate, marked "0 grams of sugar," see page 272	200	10	2	7 erythritol	1	17	Some are high in fat (cream); others are high in protein (eggs or vegetable proteins).
Ice cream, chocolate, regular	**127**	**17**	**1**	**0**	**16**	**5**	
Frozen yogurt, Dutch chocolate	93	17	1	0	16	2	
Ice milk, chocolate	100	18	1	0	17	2	
Ice cream, rich, chocolate hazelnut divine	320	31	2	0	29	20	Made with regular sugar

Sugary Drinks Swaps

Per 1 cup/250 mL serving

One of the most important changes you can make for your diabetes is to cut out:
- soft drinks (sodas)
- fruit juices
- other sweetened beverages

	TOTAL CARBS/ NET CARBS
• Tap water, plain bottled water, mineral water or soda water • Diet and "zero" soft drinks, Sugar Free Kool-Aid, Sugar Free Tang, Crystal Light, Vitamin Water Zero or Gatorade Zero • Tea, herbal tea, perked or instant black coffee	0
• Soft drinks (soda or pop) • Orange juice or apple juice • Slushies or Slurpees • Iced specialty coffees • Energy drinks • Diabetes meal replacement drinks (check brands)	16 to 28
• Fruit juices like cranberry juice cocktail, grape juice or pineapple juice (unsweetened; sugar comes from natural concentrated sugar) • Commercial milkshakes or fruit smoothies • Eggnog • Commercial milkshakes or meal replacement drinks such as Ensure or Boost High Protein, or Breakfast Essentials or Slim Fast Original made with milk	32 to 40
• Vitamin Water Essential • Gatorade energy drink • Triple Thick Shake • Frappuccino malt coffee • Prune juice, unsweetened	44 to 68

Brands have different amounts of sugar (carbs).

Many beverages are super-size. Check the serving size on the label.

4 grams of carbs = 1 teaspoon of sugar.

Is Diet Coke better than regular Coke?

Yes. Diet Coke has no sugar. Regular Coke has 10 tsp (50 mL) of sugar (39 g carbs) in a 355 mL can.

However, drinking diet soft drinks every day can reduce the number of healthy bacteria in your gut.

Try this over several months. Give yourself time to make this change:

First, replace some of the regular pop with diet pop.

Then, replace some of the diet pop with soda water flavored with lemon or lime.

When you're ready, replace most of the pop (whether regular or diet) with tap water.

Snack Bar Swaps

35–40 g

If palm oil or coconut oil is the main ingredient, these are unhealthy saturated types of fat.

	CALORIES	TOTAL CARBS	FIBER	SUGAR ALCOHOLS	NET CARBS	PROTEIN	FAT	NOTES
Hungry Buddha Keto Bar	170	17	13	0	4	10	10	High fiber and fat; stevia
Love Good Fats Chewy Nutty Peanut Butter Chocolatey bar	200	12	7	0	5	10	14	Has 7 g of unhealthy saturated fat, stevia
Good to Go Raspberry Lemon soft baked bar	170	17	7	5 erythritol	8	6	13	Texture like fig bar; almond flour
Kind Almond & Dark Chocolate	200	16	7	0	9	6	15	
Simply Protein, Dark Chocolate Salted Caramel	150	17	7	0	10	12	5	Has soy and chicory root fiber
Granola Bar, Sweet and Salty, Peanut	170	20	2	0	18	4	8	

Cookie Swaps

For 1 oatmeal cookie; weights vary

	WEIGHT (G)	CALORIES	TOTAL CARBS	FIBER	SUGAR ALCOHOLS	NET CARBS	FAT
Oatmeal cookie, Dad's, Original	12	60	9	1	0	8	3
Oatmeal Cookies, homemade (page 131), made with part zero-calorie sweetener	20	76	10	1	1 erythritol	8	
Oatmeal Cookies, homemade (page 131)	20	82	11	1	0	10	4
Oatmeal cookie, no sugar added (page 272)	19	85	14	1	6 maltitol	10	2
Oatmeal raisin spice cookie, large-sized coffee shop variety	52	210	32	1	0	31	8

Candy Swaps

	WEIGHT (G)	CALORIES	TOTAL CARBS	FIBER	SUGAR ALCOHOLS	NET CARBS	FAT
80% dark chocolate	20	115	7	3	0	4	9
4 wrapped hard candies, zero added sugar (Jolly Rancher type)	**16**	**35**	**15**	**0**	**15 isomalt**	**7**	**0**
2 squares no-sugar-added milk chocolate bar (Lindt type)	25	130	13	0	10 maltitol	8	9
1 peanut butter cup	21	110	12	1	0	11	7
3 sugar-free peppermint patties (page 271)	37	120	24	2	21 maltitol and isomalt	12	8
10 milk-chocolate-covered peanuts	22	105	13	1	0	12	6
2 pieces of a Kit Kat bar	21	109	14	0	0	14	6
5 chocolate kisses	23	114	14	0	0	14	6
3 wrapped hard candies (made with regular sugar)	18	70	17	0	0	17	0
9 small squares of a milk chocolate bar	30	160	18	1	0	17	9
2 peppermint patties	34	120	20	0	0	27	3

Salad Dressing Swaps

1 tbsp/15 mL

	CALORIES	FAT	TOTAL CARBS/ NET CARBS
Oil and vinegar (2 parts oil and 1 part vinegar)	**80**	**10**	**0**
Oil and vinegar (1 part oil and 1 part vinegar)	60	7	0
Citrus Vinaigrette (page 80)	42	5	0
Ranch	65	7	1
Italian	35	3	2
Balsamic vinegar	14	0	3
Light Ranch	29	2	3

LOW-CARB SWAP CHARTS

Potato Chips Swaps

Per 200-calorie portions = Large Snack size

	TOTAL CARBS	FIBER	NET CARBS	PROTEIN	FAT	SODIUM
3 cheese strings	3	0	3	18	11	420
½ cup (125 mL) roasted edamame beans	11	8	3	21	8	308
Protein chips, Quest brand (46 g)	7	1	6	26	9	486
4 stalks of celery and 4 tbsp (60 mL) Cheez Whiz or peanut butter	8	1	7	11	14	1108
24 beet chips, varied sizes (34 g)	16	5	11	3	14	116
18 potato chips	**18**	**2**	**16**	**2**	**13**	**198**
8 soda crackers with 1 oz (30 g) cheese	18	1	17	9	11	450
2 cups (500 mL) raw crunchy veggies, ¼ cup (60 mL) dip and 1 cheese string	25	6	19	10	5	480
4 cups (1 L) popped popcorn + 2 tsp (10 mL) oil	25	5	20	4	10	2
18 baked tortilla chips (37 g)	24	4	20	2	11	81
Quinoa vegetable puffs (44 g)	24	3	21	5	10	296
20 Bacon Dippers crackers (42 g)	24	2	22	4	10	500
56 small Garden Veggie wavy chips (42 g); potato is still main ingredient	24	1	23	2	11	340
40 small Veggie Crispy Minis, made with rice (50 g)	38	3	35	3	6	350
25 rice crackers (50 g)	40	2	38	4	2	35

Beer Swaps

341–355 mL = 12 ounces

Always check the carbohydrate. There is no fiber in beer, so total and net carbs are equal.

	ALCOHOL CONTENT	CALORIES	TOTAL CARBS/ NET CARBS	NOTES
Standard beer	**4–6%**	**140–185**	**10–12 g**	
LOW-CARB BEERS WITH NO ALCOHOL				
Non-alcoholic beer (Look for specialty names like IPA brands)	0.3%–0.5%	10–40	2–5 g	No alcohol and is low-carb.
LOW-CARB BEERS WITH ALCOHOL				
Light or ultralight beer (e.g., Michelob Ultra; Sleemans Clear 2)	2%–4%	80–110	3–4 g	Light does not mean less alcohol.
NO-ALCOHOL BEERS WITH CARBS				
Non-alcoholic beer (e.g., Corona Sunbrew or Budweiser ZERO)	0%	50–60	12–13 g	De-alcoholized beer. These are not low-carb beers.

Index

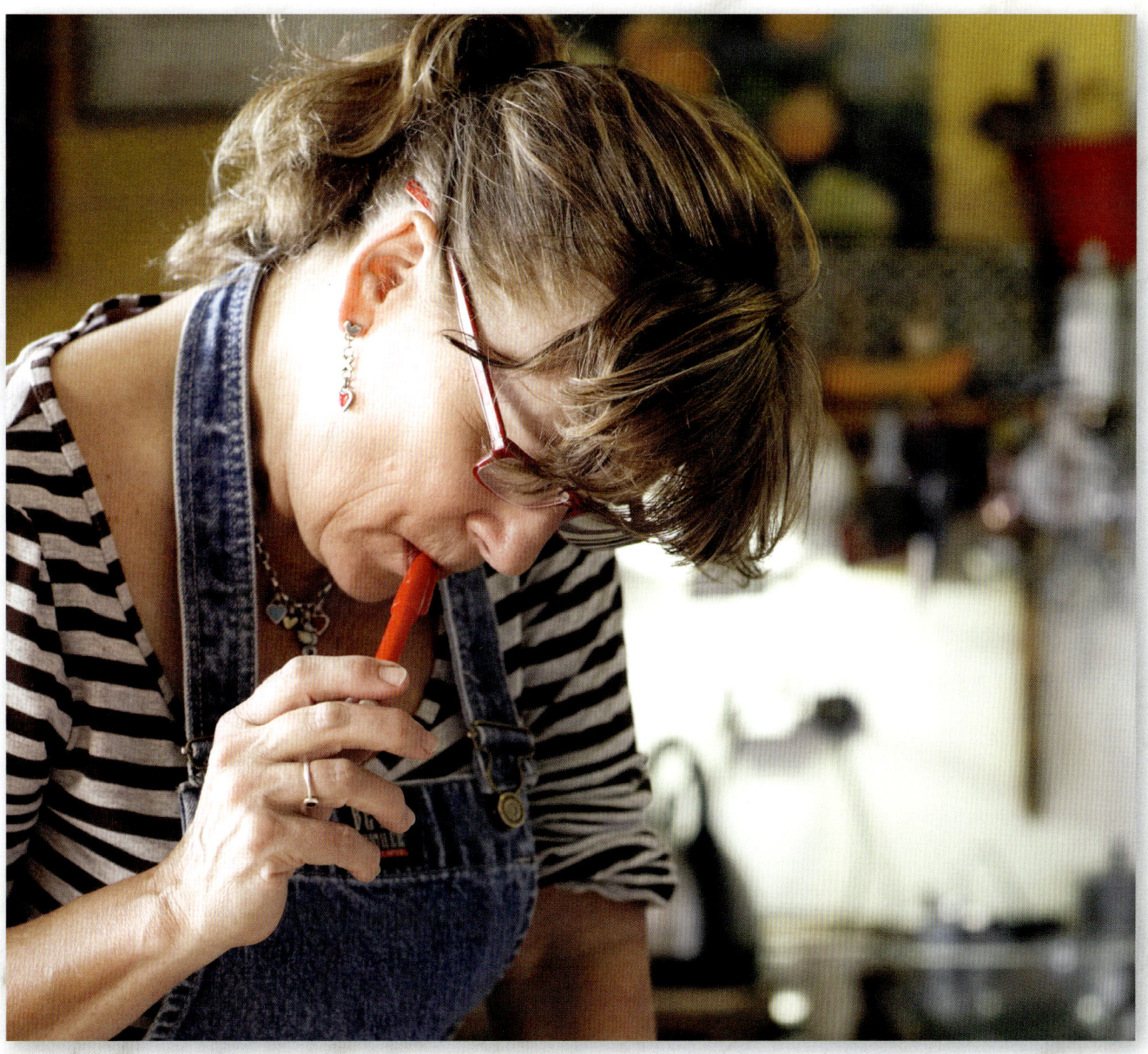

I love the index because it lists all the recipes, low-carb swaps and charts. I can quickly find the page I want to go to.

INDEX

LOW-CARB SWAPS, LOW-CARB SWAP RECIPES AND LOW-CARB SWAPS CHARTS

LOW-CARB SWAPS

angel food cake ➡ Rice Cake Dessert, 175
bagel ➡ Mug Bread, 70; bun, 186
baguette slices ➡ zucchini slices, 90
banana ➡ onion, 76
beer ➡ low-carb beer, 94
bread ➡ avocado, 36
bread ➡ bell pepper, 66
bread ➡ cheese, 82, 138
bread ➡ egg bread, 68
bread ➡ low-carb/keto bread, 46, 72, 210
bread crumb crust ➡ crustless, 60
bread crumbs ➡ almond flour, 254
bun ➡ cheese, 202, 234
bun ➡ cottage cheese, 74
bun ➡ egg or chicken, 80
cake ➡ with zero-calorie sweetener, 62
cereal, Bran Flakes ➡ Chia Pudding, 34
chocolate pudding ➡ dark chocolate, 84, 123
cookies ➡ cheese, 78
cookies ➡ light gelatin, 231
cookies ➡ with zero-calorie sweetener, 131
corn ➡ crab cake, 92
corn ➡ low-carb veggies, 118, 191
English muffin ➡ homemade egg muffin, 56
frozen yogurt ➡ keto frozen dessert, 239
high protein bar ➡ dark chocolate, 52
ice cream ➡ Greek yogurt, 111
ice cream ➡ keto frozen dessert, 111, 147
jam ➡ light cream cheese, 40
mandarins, canned ➡ mandarins, fresh, 247
milk ➡ almond beverage, 86, 107
pancake ➡ adapted recipe, 38
pasta ➡ spelt pasta, 250
pasta ➡ whole wheat pasta, 103, 166
pasta ➡ zucchini noodles, 103
pear dessert ➡ pear and nuts, 223
perogy ➡ cheese, 154
pineapple dessert ➡ pineapple and nuts, 195
pita ➡ egg bread, 78; low-carb pita, 78
pizza crust ➡ cauliflower crust, 198
potato salad ➡ with rutabaga, 159
potatoes ➡ rutabaga/turnip, 98
potatoes, mashed ➡ cauliflower, mashed, 127, 162
pudding with milk ➡ with soy beverage, 171
rice ➡ cauliflower, riced, 106, 150, 183, 218
rice ➡ couscous, 54, 214
rice ➡ frozen mixed veggies, 207
rice ➡ quinoa, 186, 214
rice noodles ➡ edamame spaghetti, 226
rice noodles ➡ konjac noodles, 226
rice pudding ➡ with zero-calorie sweetener, 115
roti shell ➡ tortilla shell, 178
spaghetti ➡ zucchini noodles, 103
squash, acorn ➡ spaghetti squash, 142
sweet potato ➡ butternut squash, 134
tacos ➡ taco salad, 174
tortilla chips ➡ Cheese Crisps, 242
waffle ➡ Chaffle, 50
yogurt, Greek ➡ cheese, 44
yogurt, Greek ➡ sour cream/mascarpone, 58

LOW-CARB SWAP RECIPES

Chia Pudding, 34
Homemade Low-Carb Egg Muffin, 56
Low-Carb Cauliflower Pizza Crust, 198
Low-Carb Egg Bread, 68
Mashed Potatoes with Cauliflower, 127
Rice Cake Dessert, 175
Roasted Rutabaga, 98
Vegetable Noodles, 103

LOW-CARB SWAPS CHARTS

Beer Swaps, 282
Bread Swaps, 274
Candy Swaps, 281
Cereal Swaps, 277
Cookie Swaps, 280
Flour Swaps, 27
Ice Cream Swaps, 278
Milk Swaps, 28
Pasta Swaps, 275
Potato Chips Swaps, 282
Potato Swaps, 275
Rice Swaps, 276
Salad Dressing Swaps, 281
Snack Bar Swaps, 280
Sugar Swaps, 29
Sugary Drink Swaps, 279
Yogurt Swaps, 278

Red shows the recipes
Burgundy shows the Low-Carb Swaps charts

A

A1C (average blood sugar), 18
alcohol. *See also* beer, sugar alcohols, wine
  alcoholic snacks, 262, 264
  and diabetes, 24
  and low blood sugar, 24
almond beverage, 26
  as snack, 261, 263, 266, 267
  Cinnamon Coffee, 54
  Hot Golden Turmeric Milk, 263
  Milk Swaps chart, 28
  smoothies, 52
almond flour, 26
  Flour Swaps chart, 27

apples, as snack, 263, 265, 266, 267
  Baked Apples, 151
  Cinnamon Apple Slices, 215
apps, for diabetes, 235
Arugula Pear Salad, 199
Arugula Salad, 48
aspartame, 268, 270
  Sugar Swaps chart, 29
Atkins diet, transitioning off, 18
avocado, as snack, 264, 266
  Avocado Salad, 90
  Tuna Sandwich option, 86

B

bacon
  Liver & Onions, 182
  Pancakes & Bacon, 38
  Roasted Cabbage with Bacon, 194
bagels. *See also* breads
  Chicken Soup & Bagel, 70
  Sun Burgers, 186
Baked Apples, 151
baking, low-carb, 25–29
bananas, as snack, 265
  Banana Bread, 243
  Fried Peanut Butter & Banana Sandwich, 76
Bannock, Low-Carb, 119
barley, benefits, 231
  Walnut Barley Medley, 231
BEANS MAIN COURSES
  Bean and Meat Filling, 174
  Beans & Toast, 68
  Beans & Wieners, 122
  Chili Con Carne, 150
  Low-Salt Home-Baked Beans, 122
  Mexican Rice & Beans, 54
  Nachos in a Pan, 94
  Santa Fe Salad, 242

INDEX

Stir-Fry (tip), 206
Sun Burgers, 186
BEEF MAIN COURSES
   Beef Dip Sandwich, 66
   Beef Parmesan, 238
   Beef Stew, 138
   cheeseburger, 158, 202
   Cheesy Hamburger Casserole, 194
   Chili Con Carne, 150
   Classic Beef Patties, 238
   Grandma's Swiss Steak, 222
   Hamburger Soup, 118
   Liver & Onions, 182
   Moroccan Beef Stew, 139
   Roast Beef, 110
   Spaghetti Meat Sauce, 102
   steak, 126
   Tacos, 174
beer. *See also* alcohol
   alcoholic snacks, 262–264
   and diabetes, 24
   Beer Swaps chart, 282
beets
   Easy Beet Soup, 155
   Oven-Roasted Beets, 110
berries. *See also* DESSERTS, SALADS
   as snack, 263, 265
beverages. *See also* alcohol, soft drinks
   Chai Latte, 219
   Cinnamon Coffee, 54
   cocoa, as snack, 262
   Fruit Milkshake, 107
   Ginger Tea, 207
   Hot Golden Turmeric Milk, 263
   Italian Iced Soda Float, 251
   smoothies, 52
   Sugary Drinks Swaps chart, 279
   Wine Spritzer, 162
blood pressure, 14, 211
blood sugar (glucose)
   and meal planning 14–19
   what affects blood sugar, 21–24
Bran Muffins, 44
breads. *See also* sandwiches
   Banana Bread, 243
   Bread Swaps chart, 274
   Low-Carb Bannock, 119
   Low-Carb Egg Bread, 68
   Mug Bread, 259
breakfasts, 30, 33–63
   and weight loss, 16
Bruschetta, 90
buns, 10. *See also* breads
burgers
   fast-food, 202
   Hamburger with Potato Salad, 158
   Sun Burgers, 186
   veggie/plant-based, 203
Butterscotch Pudding, 99

C

CGM. *See* continuous glucose monitoring
cabbage
   Coleslaw, 72
   Roasted Cabbage with Bacon, 194

Caesar Salad, 251
cake
   angel food cake, 175
   Irish Currant Cake, 62
calcium, for nutrition, 15, 88
calorie calculator, 9
calories, 9, 19, 30
   very-low-calorie diets, 18
candy
   as snack, 261, 263, 267
   food label, 271
   Candy Swaps chart, 281
carbs/carbohydrates
   calculating net carbs, 270–272
   carb choices, 10, 16, 30
   carb counting, 11, 17, 19, 20
   effects on blood sugar, 22–24
   net and total carbs, 11, 30
   very-low-carb diets, 18, 23
Caribbean Chicken Roti, 178
cauliflower
   Cilantro Riced Cauliflower, 218
   Low-Carb Cauliflower Pizza Crust, 198
   Mashed Potatoes with Cauliflower, 127
cereal, as snacks, 263, 265, 266, 267
   Cereal Swaps chart, 277
   Chia Pudding, 34
   Cold or Hot Cereal, 34
   Crunchy Nut Granola, 58
Chai Latte, 219
Chef's Salad, 80
CHEESE MAIN COURSES
   Cheese & Crackers, 88
   Cheese Omelet, 130
   Cheese Waffles (Chaffles), 259
   Creamy Mac & Cheese, 166
   Homemade Low-Carb Egg Muffin, 56
   Muffin & Cheese, 44
   Toasted Cheese & Tomato Sandwich, 72
Cheese Crisps, 264, 265
Chia Pudding, 34
CHICKEN MAIN COURSES
   Baked Chicken & Potato, 98
   Caribbean Chicken Roti, 178
   Chicken Cordon Bleu, 254
   Chicken Soup & Bagel, 70
   Homemade Sub Sandwich, 234
   Santa Fe Salad, 242
   Tandoori Chicken and Sauce, 218
   Thai Chicken, 226
children and youth with diabetes, 15, 19
Chili con Carne, 150
chips, as snack, 15, 264–267
   Potato Chips Swaps chart, 282
Chocolate, as snack, 264, 266
   Candy Swaps chart, 281
Chocolate Mousse, 123
cholesterol, 36, 46, 52, 90, 182, 231
Cilantro Riced Cauliflower, 218
Cinnamon Apple Slices, 215
Cinnamon Coffee, 54
Citrus Vinaigrette, 80
Classic Beef Patties, 238

coffee
   Cinnamon Coffee, 54
   Sugary Drinks Swaps chart, 279
Cold Plate lunch, 74, dinner, 114
Coleslaw, 72
Complete Diabetes Guide, 16, 20, 22, back cover
continuous glucose monitoring, 17, 19, 235
cookies
   as dessert, 78, 231, 235
   as snack, 262, 263, 265, 267
   Cookie Swaps chart, 280
   Oatmeal Cookies, 131, 272
Cornbread or Corn Muffins, 146
cottage cheese
   Mandarins and Cottage Cheese, 247
couscous, 139
   Rice Swaps chart, 276
Crab Cakes, Maryland, 92
crackers, 210
   Cheese & Crackers, 88
cream cheese
   Cream Cheese Pomegranate Burst, 255
   Rice Cake Dessert, 175
Creamy Mac & Cheese, 166
Crunchy Nut Granola, 58
Crustless Pumpkin Pie, 163
Currant Cake, Irish, 62

D

Denver Sandwich & Soup, 210
DESSERTS. *See also* cookies, fruit, ice cream, yogurt
   angel food cake, 175
   Baked Apples, 151
   baking, 25–29
   Banana Bread, 243
   Bran Muffins, 44
   Butterscotch Pudding, 99
   Chia Pudding, 34
   chocolate and almonds, 266
   Chocolate Mousse, 123
   chocolate pudding, 84
   Cinnamon Apple Slices, 215
   Cream Cheese Pomegranate Burst, 255
   Crustless Pumpkin Pie, 163
   Dream Delight, 187
   Irish Currant Cake, 62
   Lemon Pear-fection, 223
   light gelatin, 102
   Low-Carb Dessert Omelet, 266
   Mandarins and Cottage Cheese, 247
   Pineapple Surprise, 195
   Rice Cake Dessert, 175
   Rice Pudding, 115
   Sour Cream and Fruit, 227
   Stewed Rhubarb, 111
   Sugar-Free Jelly with Berries, 191
   Tapioca Pudding, 171
   Whipped Gelatin, 135
diabetes
   exchanges, 10, 16
   gestational, 15

285

INDEX

diabetes *(continued)*
   health care team, 14–24, 235
   prevention/prediabetes, 14
   remission diets, 18
   type 1, 19
   type 2, 15–18
Diabetes Essentials, 20, 22, back cover
Diabetes Healthy Plate, 7
Dill Topping, 230
dinners, 30, 97–257
Dr. Shomali Says, 14–20
Dream Delight, 187

E

Easy Beet Soup, 155
eating out
   Fast-Food Breakfast, 56
   Fast-Food Dinner, 202
   Sub Sandwich, 234
edamame beans, 134, 206
   as snack, 264
   Potato Chips Swaps chart, 282
EGGS MAIN COURSES
   Cheese Omelet, 130
   Denver Sandwich, 210
   Egg & Toast, 36
   French toast, 38
   Homemade Low-Carb Egg Muffin, 56
   Low-Carb Egg Bread, 68
   Prairie Quiche, 60
   Spinach & Eggs, 42
   Tuna Scramble, 48
   Veggie Scramble, 266
erythritol. *See* sugar alcohols
exercise, 15, 18, 24, 211, 235

F

fast food. *See* eating out
fats
   and blood sugar, 11, 23
   healthy, 86, 88, 106
fiber
   calculate net carbs, 11, 270–272
   effect on blood sugar, 23
   sources, 36, 88, 150, 191, 231
Fiesta Breakfast, 54
FISH AND SEAFOOD MAIN COURSES
   Chicken Soup & Bagel, 70
   Cold Plate Dinner, 114
   Fish & Chips, 142
   Fish with Rice, 106
   Maryland Crab Cakes, 92
   Poached Salmon with Dill, 230
   Salmon Potato Dish, 190
   Shrimp Linguine, 250
   Tuna Sandwich, 86
   Tuna Scramble, 48
Five Spice Blend, 98
flaxseed, 26, 27
Flour Swaps chart, 27
food groups for health, 88
food labels, 268–272
French fries, 142, 203
French Onion Soup, 82

Fresh Salsa, 42
fruit, 88. *See also* DESSERTS
   exchanges, 10, 34, 46
   fresh berry combo, 183
   Fruit Milkshake, 107
   juice, 36, 60
   Spinach Fruit Smoothie, 52
   Tofu Fruit Smoothie, 52

G

gelatin. *See* DESSERTS
   Light Jellied Vegetable Salad, 143
German Bean Salad, 170
gestational diabetes, 15
Ginger Tea, 207
grains, 88. *See also* barley, cereals, couscous, oats, rice
Grandma's Swiss Steak, 222
Granola, Crunchy Nut, 58
grapefruit and medications, 46
Greek Salad, 215
gut bacteria, 23

H

ham, as snack, 267
   Ham & Sweet Potato, 134
Hamburger Casserole, Cheesy, 194
Hamburger Soup, 118
Hamburger with Potato Salad, 158
Homemade Low-Carb Egg Muffin, 56
Homemade Sub Sandwich, 234
Homemade Thin-Crust Pizza, 198
Hot Golden Turmeric Milk, 263

I

ice cream, 111, 127, 147, 239
   Ice Cream Swaps chart, 278
   keto frozen dessert label, 272
infants/toddlers, 17
infections, 22
insulin, 12, 17–19, 22, 24
   insulin-to-carb ratio, 19
   insulin dosing, 19
Irish Currant Cake, 62
isomalt. *See* sugar alcohols
Italian Iced Soda Float, 251

J

Jalapeno Corn Cornbread, 146
jam, no added sugar, 40
juice, fruit, 36, 60
   Sugary Drinks Swaps chart, 279

K

kebabs
   Chicken Souvlaki, 214
   Shish Kebabs, 214
keto chocolate frozen dessert, 272
keto diet, transitioning off, 18
konjac pasta or konjac rice
   Pasta Swaps chart, 275
   Rice Swaps chart, 276

L

lamb, Shish Kebabs, 214
Lemon Pear-fection, 223
life-size photographs, 8, 20
lifestyle changes, 14
Light Iced Tea, 159
Light Jellied Vegetable Salad, 143
Liver & Onions, 182
low blood sugar, 17, 23, 24
Low-Carb Bannock, 119
Low-Carb Cauliflower Pizza Crust, 198
low-carb cooking, 25–29
Low-Carb Dessert Omelet, 266
Low-Carb Egg Bread, 68
Low-Carb Egg Muffin, 56
Low-Carb Homemade Waffle, 50
low-carb shopping, 26
LOW-CARB SWAPS Index. *See* 284
LOW-CARB SWAPS CHARTS Index. *See* 284
LOW-CARB SWAP RECIPES Index. *See* 284
low-carb vegetables, 134
Low-Salt Home-Baked Beans, 122
lunches, 30, 65–95

M

Mac & Cheese, Creamy, 166
maltitol/mannitol. *See* sugar alcohols
Mandarins and Cottage Cheese, 247
marinades, 206, 214, 218
Maryland Crab Cakes, 92
Mashed Potatoes, 126
Mashed Potatoes with Cauliflower, 127
meal size, small and large, 9, 16
meal timing, 23
meals, 7–9, 30. *See also* snacks
meat substitutes, 78, 186, 203, 206
medications, 12, 16, 17, 22–24, 46
metformin, 22
Mexican Rice & Beans, 54
milk, 88. *See also* almond beverage, soy beverage
   Milk Swaps chart, 28
monk fruit, sweetener, 268, 270, 272
Moroccan Beef Stew, 139
muffins, as snacks, 265, 267
   Bran Muffins, 44
   Corn Muffins, 146
   English muffin, 56
   Homemade Low-Carb Egg Muffin, 56
Mug Bread, 259
mushrooms
   Stuffed Portobello Mushrooms, 267

N

Nachos in a Pan, 94
net carbs. *See* carbs
noodles, as snack, 265. *See also* konjac, pasta, Vegetable Noodles
Pasta Swaps chart, 275
nutrient information, 202, 235. *See also* individual recipes in the book

INDEX

sorbitol. See sugar alcohols
soups, as snacks, 262, 267
   Chicken Rice Soup, 70
   Denver Sandwich & Soup, 210
   Easy Beet Soup, 155
   French Onion Soup, 82
   Hamburger Soup, 118
Sour Cream and Fruit, 227
soy beverage, 26, 28
   Butterscotch Pudding, 99
   Milk Swaps chart, 28
Spaghetti & Meat Sauce, 102
spinach, 134, 191
   Poppy Seed Spinach Salad, 227
   Spinach & Eggs, 42
   Spinach Fruit Smoothie, 52
Spritzer, Wine, 162
squash. See also zucchini
   Microwaved Squash, 142
   Moroccan Beef Stew, 139
   Pasta Swaps chart, 275
   Potato Swaps chart, 275
   Roasted Acorn Squash, 142
starches, 7, 11, 88, 207. See also carbs
Steak, Swiss, Grandma's, 222
Steak & Potato, 126
stevia. See zero-calorie sweeteners
Stewed Rhubarb, 111
Stir-Fry, 206
stress and blood sugar, 23
Stuffed Portobello Mushrooms, 267
Sub Sandwich, Homemade, 234
sucralose. See zero-calorie sweeteners
sugar. See also blood sugar
   label reading, 268, 270–272
   no sugar added, 272
   Sugar Swaps chart, 29
   sugar-free, 271
   Sugary Drinks Swaps chart, 279
sugar alcohols, 11, 270–272, 278, 280
   Sugar Swaps chart, 29
Sugar-Free Jelly with Berries, 191
Sun Burgers, 186

sushi, as snack, 267
SWAPS Index. See 284
sweet potatoes, 255
   Ham & Sweet Potato, 134
   Potato Swaps chart, 275
sweeteners. See sugar; zero-calorie sweeteners
Swiss Steak, Grandma's, 222
syrup. See pancake syrup

T

Tacos, 174
Tandoori Chicken and Sauce, 218
Tapioca Pudding, 171
tea, 247
   Chai Latte, 219
   Ginger Tea, 207
   iced, 88
Thai Chicken, 226
timing of meals, 23
Toast & Peanut Butter, 40
Toasted Cheese & Tomato Sandwich, 72
tofu, 78, 206
   Tofu Fruit Smoothie, 52
Tomato, Grilled, 246
tortilla chips. See chips
total carbs. See carbs
Tropical Green Salad, 179
Tuna Sandwich, 86
Tuna Scramble, 48
Turkey Dinner, Roast, 162
type 1 diabetes, 19
type 2 diabetes, 15–18

V

Vegetable Dip, 174
Vegetable Noodles, 12, 103
   as snack, 262
   Pasta Swaps chart, 275
vegetables, 7, 88
   low-carb/low-calorie, 134

Vegetables, Quick-Fry, 167
veggie burgers. See burgers
Veggie Scramble, 266, as snack
very-low-calorie diets, 18
very-low-carb diets, 18, 23

W

waffles
   Chaffles (Cheese Waffles), 259
   Homemade Low-Carb Waffles, 50
walking. See exercise
Walnut Barley Medley, 231
water, benefits, 23, 48, 166
websites, nutrient, 202, 235
weight gain, 18, 24
weight loss, 9, 14, 16, 20, 24
Whipped Gelatin, 135
wieners, 122
wild rice, 106, 231
wine. See also alcohol
   alcoholic snacks, 262
   and diabetes, 24
   spritzer, 162
   with a meal, 102

Y

yogurt, 10, 23
   as snack, 262, 264, 265
   food label, 268
   homemade diet yogurt, 44
   Yogurt Swaps chart, 278

Z

zero-calorie sweeteners, 26, 151, 159, 268, 270, 272, 278, 280
   Sugar Swaps chart, 29
zucchini, 134, 147
   as snack, 262
   Nachos in a Pan, 94
   Ratatouille, 146
   Vegetable Noodles, 103

LIBRARY AND ARCHIVES CANADA CATALOGUING IN PUBLICATION

Title: Diabetes meals for good health cookbook : low-carb recipes & swaps for every meal / Karen Graham, RD, CDE, Registered Dietitian & Certified Diabetes Educator, Mansur Shomali, MD, CM, endocrinologist & diabetes expert.
Other titles: Diabetes meals for good health
Names: Graham, Karen, author. | Shomali, Mansur, author.
Description: Fourth edition. | Series statement: Health & wellness series | Includes index. | Originally published under the title: Diabetes meals for good health. Toronto : Robert Rose Inc., 2008.
Identifiers: Canadiana 20230187366 | ISBN 9780778807162 (softcover)
Subjects: LCSH: Diabetes—Diet therapy—Recipes. | LCSH: Diabetes—Nutritional aspects. | LCGFT: Cookbooks.
Classification: LCC RC662 .G72 2023 | DDC 641.5/6314—dc23

Additional Image Credits: Front cover: top photo © Andrew Lipsett and on page 16 (bottom) and 31. Photos of Karen Graham by David McIlvride/Jenny McKinney (Makeup Artist) on page 25, 26, 64 and back cover. Photos of Mansur Shomali by Eric Stocklin on page 21 and back cover. Photos on pages: 2, 4, 5, 6, 10, 11, 12, 13, 14, 15, 16, 17, 18, 19, 20, 22, 23, 24, 26, 36, 40, 74, 76, 78, 80, 84, 99, 103, 110, 111, 118, 119, 122, 123, 126, 127, 130, 131, 134, 135, 138, 139, 142, 143, 146, 150, 151, 154, 155, 162, 163, 166, 167, 170, 171, 175, 178, 179, 182, 183, 186, 187, 190, 191, 194, 195, 199, 206, 207, 211, 214, 215, 222, 223, 226, 227, 230, 234, 235, 242, 243, 246, 250, 251, 255, 258, 259, 260 (drop cucumber), 262, 263, 264, 265, 267, 268, 269, 271, 272, 273 and 283 © Getty Images. Texture page 5, 13, 21, 25, 31, 33, 65, 97, 269, 273, 283 © Getty Images. Salt icon (pages 261–267) © Getty Images.

INDEX

nutrition facts on labels, 268–272
nuts
  as snacks, 264, 266
  with meals, 34, 50, 88

O

oats
  Cereal Swaps chart, 277
  Flour Swaps chart, 27
  oatmeal cookie, no-sugar-added, 272
  Oatmeal Cookies, 25, 131
oils, 88, 280
olives, 88
  as snacks, 261, 262
  Greek Salad, 215
  Nachos in a Pan, 94
onions
  French Onion Soup, 82
  Liver & Onions, 182
oranges, 36, 44, 70, 119, 263
  Kale and Orange Salad, 187
  Mandarins and Cottage Cheese, 247
  Tropical Green Salad, 179
Oven-Roasted Beets, 110

P

pancake syrup, 26
  as snack, 261
  Sugar Swaps chart, 29
pancakes, 13, 38
pasta
  Cheesy Hamburger Casserole, 194
  Creamy Mac & Cheese, 166
  Pasta Swaps chart, 275
  Shrimp Linguine, 250
  Spaghetti & Meat Sauce, 102
peaches, 46, 52, 74, 155
peanut butter, 78, 226
  as snack, 262, 264, 265. See also nuts
  Fried Peanut Butter & Banana Sandwich, 76
  Potato Chips Swaps chart, 282
  Snack Bar Swaps chart, 280
  Toast & Peanut Butter, 40
pears, 82
  Arugula Pear Salad, 199
  Lemon Pear-fection, 223
peppers, bell, 115, 177
  Roasted Pepper Strips, 223
perogies, 154
pickles, as snack, 261
Pie, Pumpkin, Crustless, 163
pineapple, 134
  Pineapple Surprise, 195
  Tropical Green Salad, 179
Pita Sandwich, 78
pizza, 198
plant-based beverages, 26. See also almond beverage, soy beverage
  Milk Swaps chart, 28
plant-based burgers. See burgers.
pomegranates
  Arugula Pear Salad, 199
  Cream Cheese Pomegranate Burst, 255

popcorn, as snack, 265
  Potato Chips Swaps chart, 282
poppadoms, 218
PORK MAIN COURSES
  Ham and Sweet Potatoes, 134
  Pork Chop & Applesauce, 170
  Pork Chop Casserole, 246
  Stir-Fry, 206
portions, correct, 8, 14, 17, 20
  bowl sizes, 239
potatoes, 10. See also chips, French fries, sweet potatoes
  Mashed Potatoes, 126
  Mashed Potatoes with Cauliflower, 127
  Potato Salad, 159
  Potato Swaps chart, 275
  Salmon Potato Dish, 190
Prairie Quiche, 60
prediabetes/prevention, 14
pregnancy, 15
probiotics, 23
protein bars, 52
  Snack Bar Swaps chart, 280
Protein-Power Pancakes, 13, 38
Protein Shake, as snack, 266
proteins, 7, 88
  in carb counting, 11, 23
puddings. See DESSERTS
Pumpkin Pie, Crustless, 163

Q

Quesadilla, 84
Quiche, Prairie, 60
Quick-Fry Vegetables, 167

R

Ratatouille, 146
remission diets, transitioning off, 18
restaurant meals. See eating out
Rhubarb, Stewed, 111
rice, 10
  Chicken Rice Soup, 70
  Cilantro Riced Cauliflower, 218
  Fried Rice, 207
  Rice Cake Dessert, 175
  Rice Pudding, 115
  Rice Swaps chart, 276
  Riced Cauliflower, 183
rice flour, 27
Roast Turkey Dinner, 162
Roasted Cabbage with Bacon, 194
Roasted Pepper Strips, 223
Roti, Caribbean Chicken, 178
Rutabaga, Roasted, 98

S

SALADS
  Arugula Pear Salad, 199
  Arugula Salad, 48
  Avocado Salad, 90
  Caesar Salad, 251
  Chef's Salad, 80
  German Bean Salad, 170
  Greek Salad, 215

  Kale and Orange Salad, 187
  Light Jellied Vegetable Salad, 143
  Poppy Seed Spinach Salad, 227
  Potato Salad, 159
  Santa Fe Salad, 242
  Tropical Green Salad, 179
salad dressings, 199, 234, 261
  Salad Dressing Swaps Chart, 281
  Citrus Vinaigrette, 80
salmon. See FISH AND SEAFOOD MAIN COURSES
Salsa, Fresh, 42
salt. See sodium
sandwiches. See also burgers
  as snacks, 266, 267
  Beef Dip Sandwich, 66
  Denver Sandwich, 210
  Fried Peanut Butter & Banana Sandwich, 76
  Homemade Sub Sandwich, 234
  Pita Sandwich, 78
  Quesadilla, 84
  Toasted Cheese & Tomato Sandwich, 72
  Tuna Sandwich, 86
Santa Fe Salad, 242
saturated fat, 14, 146, 268, 280
sauerkraut, 154
  as snack, 261
sausages, 155, 198
  Sausages & Cornbread, 146
seasonings, 222, 261
  Five Spice Blend, 98
  Salt-Free Taco Seasoning Mix, 174
  Steak Seasoning, 126
Shish Kebabs, 214
shrimp, as snack, 264
  Shrimp Linguine, 250
  Shrimp Linguine Sauce, 250
sleep and blood sugar, 23
smoking and blood sugar, 22
smoothies
  Spinach Fruit Smoothie, 52
  Tofu Fruit Smoothie, 52
Snack Bar Swaps chart, 280
snack recipes
  Chaffles (Cheese Waffles), 259
  Cheese Crisps, 265
  Hot Golden Turmeric Milk, 263
  Low-Carb Dessert Omelet, 266
  Mug Bread, 259
  Protein Shake, 266
  Stuffed Portobello Mushrooms, 267
  Veggie Scramble, 266
snacks, 9, 20, 30, 258–267
  freebie, 260–261
  large, 266–267
  medium, 264–265
  small, 262–263
sodas. See soft drinks
sodium, 14, 268
  high-salt foods, 122, 146, 203, 261
  tips to cut back, 66, 74, 82, 118, 122, 126, 150, 154, 158, 174, 190, 210, 234
soft drinks, 15, 203
  as snacks, 261, 266
  Sugary Drinks Swaps chart, 279